CONTEMPORARY DIABETES

ARISTIDIS VEVES, MD, DSc, SERIES EDITOR

For further volumes:
http://www.springer.com/series/7679

Gautam V. Shrikhande • James F. McKinsey
Editors

Diabetes and Peripheral Vascular Disease

Diagnosis and Management

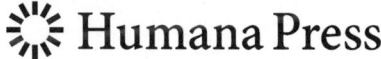

Editors
Gautam V. Shrikhande, MD
Division of Vascular Surgery and
 Endovascular Interventions
Columbia University College of
 Physicians and Surgeons
New York Presbyterian Hospital
New York, NY
USA

James F. McKinsey, MD, FACS
Division of Vascular Surgery and
 Endovascular Interventions
Columbia University College of
 Physicians and Surgeons
New York Presbyterian Hospital
New York, NY
USA

ISBN 978-1-62703-157-8   ISBN 978-1-62703-158-5 (eBook)
DOI 10.1007/978-1-62703-158-5
Springer New York Heidelberg Dordrecht London

Library of Congress Control Number: 2012949162

© Springer Science+Business Media New York 2012
This work is subject to copyright. All rights are reserved by the Publisher, whether the whole or part of the material is concerned, specifically the rights of translation, reprinting, reuse of illustrations, recitation, broadcasting, reproduction on microfilms or in any other physical way, and transmission or information storage and retrieval, electronic adaptation, computer software, or by similar or dissimilar methodology now known or hereafter developed. Exempted from this legal reservation are brief excerpts in connection with reviews or scholarly analysis or material supplied specifically for the purpose of being entered and executed on a computer system, for exclusive use by the purchaser of the work. Duplication of this publication or parts thereof is permitted only under the provisions of the Copyright Law of the Publisher's location, in its current version, and permission for use must always be obtained from Springer. Permissions for use may be obtained through RightsLink at the Copyright Clearance Center. Violations are liable to prosecution under the respective Copyright Law.
The use of general descriptive names, registered names, trademarks, service marks, etc. in this publication does not imply, even in the absence of a specific statement, that such names are exempt from the relevant protective laws and regulations and therefore free for general use.
While the advice and information in this book are believed to be true and accurate at the date of publication, neither the authors nor the editors nor the publisher can accept any legal responsibility for any errors or omissions that may be made. The publisher makes no warranty, express or implied, with respect to the material contained herein.

Printed on acid-free paper

Humana Press is part of Springer Science+Business Media (www.springer.com)

To those who have trained us when we were students, residents, and fellows and to the students, residents, and fellows that we are fortunate to train in our quest to advance the field of vascular and endovascular interventions.

Preface

The incidence and prevalence of peripheral vascular disease continues to rise in our aging population. Diabetic patients are at a higher risk of atherosclerotic disease in all arterial beds of the human body. We have asked leaders in the field of medicine, podiatry, and vascular and endovascular therapy to assimilate the latest literature for an in-depth review of the management of peripheral vascular disease. The objective of this textbook is to provide an overview of the management of diabetes and diabetic foot changes as well as providing a view of cutting-edge and emerging topics in optimization of arterial status. We have addressed pathophysiology, anatomy, diagnosis, and management of diabetic peripheral vascular disease emphasizing a multidisciplinary approach.

The first chapter of the book provides an overview of this complex disease process and discusses the teamwork required for optimal management. The chapters continue with the basic pathophysiology of diabetic atherosclerosis and a contemporary review of the management of diabetes. Next, we discuss the genesis of diabetic foot ulceration and prevention and management strategies. The effects of neuropathy and microvascular changes in the diabetic foot are highlighted. We then specifically address the microbiology of diabetic foot infections. Assessment of arterial status is discussed as improving blood flow becomes paramount in peripheral vascular disease. The role of endovascular interventions and vascular surgery as well as the management of the complications of these procedures are described in the setting of diabetes. As a last resort, the process of amputation is discussed for those patients who have progressed beyond a limb salvage situation. The effects of diabetes on the cerebrovascular system as well as its implications in patients with aortoiliac disease are discussed. The book concludes with a chapter on emerging endovascular technologies including drug eluting balloons and stents. The chapters throughout the book will describe and evaluate the results of recent, applicable clinical trials.

The intended audience for this book includes internists, family practitioners, surgeons, podiatrists, wound care specialists, and vascular specialists. Students, residents, and fellows in surgical and medical specialties should also find this book of significant value and interest, as it may help them shape how they will approach peripheral vascular disease, diabetes, and their subsequent complications.

We are fortunate to have benefited from the expertise of the renowned authors who contributed to this book. We want to thank them for the time and effort that they contributed to this project; they represent the multidisciplinary approach required for management of this difficult problem. It is our hope that this book will be an invaluable reference for all clinicians concerned with diabetes and peripheral vascular disease.

New York, NY, USA Gautam V. Shrikhande, M.D.
New York, NY, USA James F. McKinsey, M.D.

Contents

1 **General Considerations in the Diabetic Patient with Peripheral Vascular Disease** 1
Rishi Kundi, Andrew J. Meltzer, and Danielle Bajakian

2 **The Pathogenesis of Diabetic Atherosclerosis** 13
Jeffrey J. Siracuse and Elliot L. Chaikof

3 **Diabetes Mellitus and Peripheral Vascular Disease** 27
Matthew J. Freeby

4 **Diabetic Neuropathy** 39
Francesco Tecilazich, Thanh L. Dinh, and Aristidis Veves

5 **Microvascular Changes in the Diabetic Foot** 53
Thomas S. Monahan

6 **Diabetic Foot Ulceration and Management** 63
Peter A. Blume, Akhilesh K. Jain, and Bauer Sumpio

7 **Diabetic Foot Infections: Microbiology and Antibiotic Therapy** 93
Brian Scully

8 **Arterial Imaging** 103
Rodney P. Bensley and Marc L. Schermerhorn

9 **The Role of Endovascular Therapy in Peripheral Arterial Disease** 119
Andrew J. Meltzer and James F. McKinsey

10 **Surgical Treatment of Infrainguinal Occlusive Disease in Diabetes** 133
Shant M. Vartanian and Michael S. Conte

11 **Managing Complications of Vascular Surgery and Endovascular Therapy** 149
Salvatore T. Scali and Timothy C. Flynn

12 **Diabetes and Lower Extremity Amputation** 167
Roman Nowygrod and Nii-Kabu Kabutey

13 **Diabetic Considerations in Cerebrovascular Disease** 181
Christine Chung, Sharif Ellozy, Michael L. Marin, and Peter L. Faries

14	**Diabetic Considerations in Aortoiliac Disease**	197
	In-Kyong Kim and Rajeev Dayal	
15	**Abdominal Aortic Aneurysms in Patients with Diabetes**	211
	William F. Johnston and Gilbert R. Upchurch Jr.	
16	**Evolving Technology in the Treatment of Peripheral Vascular Disease**	227
	Francesco A. Aiello and Nicholas J. Morrissey	
Index		237

Contributors

Francesco A. Aiello, M.D. Division of Vascular and Endovascular Surgery, University of Massachusetts Medical School, Worcester, MA, USA

Danielle Bajakian, M.D., F.A.C.S. Critical Limb Ischemia Program, Columbia University Medical Center, New York Presbyterian Hospital, New York, NY, USA

Rodney P. Bensley, M.D. Division of Vascular and Endovascular Surgery, Department of Surgery, Beth Israel Deaconess Medical Center, Boston, MA, USA

Peter A. Blume, D.P.M., F.A.C.F.A.S. Department of Anesthesia, Yale School of Medicine, New Haven, CT, USA

Department of Orthopedics and Rehabilitation, Yale School of Medicine, New Haven, CT, USA

Elliot L. Chaikof, M.D., Ph.D. Department of Surgery, Beth Israel Deaconess Medical Center, Harvard Medical School, Boston, MA, USA

New York-Presbyterian Hospital, Columbia University and Weill Cornell Medical Centers, New York, NY, USA

Christine Chung, M.D. Department of Vascular Surgery, Mount Sinai School of Medicine, New York, NY, USA

Michael S. Conte, M.D. Department of Surgery, University of California San Francisco, San Francisco, CA, USA

Rajeev Dayal, M.D. Department of Surgery, North Shore University Hospital, Great Neck, NY, USA

Thanh L. Dinh, D.P.M. Division of Podiatry, Beth Israel Deaconess Medical Center, Harvard Medical School, Boston, MA, USA

Sharif Ellozy, M.D. Department of Vascular Surgery, Mount Sinai School of Medicine, New York, NY, USA

Peter L. Faries, M.D., F.A.C.S. Department of Vascular Surgery, Mount Sinai School of Medicine, New York, NY, USA

Timothy C. Flynn, M.D., F.A.C.S. Division of Vascular Surgery and Endovascular Therapy, Department of Surgery, University of Florida College of Medicine, Shands Hospital at the University of Florida, Gainesville, FL, USA

Matthew J. Freeby, M.D. Department of Medicine, Columbia University, New York, NY, USA

Akhilesh K. Jain, M.D. Section of Vascular Surgery, Yale University, New Haven, CT, USA

William F. Johnston, M.D. Division of Vascular and Endovascular Surgery, Department of Surgery, University of Virginia, Charlottesville, VA, USA

Nii-Kabu Kabutey, M.D. Department of Surgery, Columbia University Medical Center/Weill Cornell, New York, NY, USA

In-Kyong Kim, M.D. Department of General Surgery, Columbia University, New York Presbyterian Hospital, New York, NY, USA

Rishi Kundi, M.D. Department of Vascular Surgery, Columbia University Medical Center, New York Presbyterian Medical Center, New York, NY, USA

Michael L. Marin, M.D., F.A.C.S. Department of Vascular Surgery, Mount Sinai School of Medicine, New York, NY, USA

James F. McKinsey, M.D., F.A.C.S. Division of Vascular Surgery and Endovascular Interventions, New York Presbyterian Hospital, New York, NY, USA

Andrew J. Meltzer, M.D. Division of Vascular Surgery and Endovascular Interventions, New York Presbyterian Hospital, New York, NY, USA

Thomas S. Monahan, M.D. Division of Vascular Surgery, Department of Surgery, University of Maryland Medical Center, University of Maryland School of Medicine, Baltimore, MD, USA

Nicholas J. Morrissey, M.D. Division of Vascular Surgery and Endovascular Interventions, Columbia University College of Physicians and Surgeons, New York Presbyterian Hospital, New York, NY, USA

Roman Nowygrod, A.B., M.S., M.D. Department of Surgery, Columbia University Medical Center, New York, NY, USA

Salvatore T. Scali, M.D. Division of Vascular Surgery and Endovascular Therapy, Department of Surgery, University of Florida College of Medicine, Shands Hospital at the University of Florida, Gainesville, FL, USA

Marc L. Schermerhorn, M.D. Division of Vascular and Endovascular Surgery, Department of Surgery, Beth Israel Deaconess Medical Center, Boston, MA, USA

Brian Scully, M.B., B.Ch. Department of Medicine & Infectious Disease, New York Presbyterian Hospital, New York, NY, USA

Jeffrey J. Siracuse, M.D. Department of Surgery, Beth Israel Deaconess Medical Center, Harvard Medical School, Boston, MA, USA

New York-Presbyterian Hospital, Columbia University and Weill Cornell Medical Centers, New York, NY, USA

Bauer Sumpio, M.D., Ph.D. Department of Vascular Surgery, Yale School of Medicine, New Haven, CT, USA

Francesco Tecilazich, M.D. Microcirculation Lab, Joslin Beth Israel Deaconess Foot Center, Harvard Medical School, Boston, MA, USA

Gilbert R. Upchurch Jr., M.D. Division of Vascular and Endovascular Surgery, Department of Surgery, University of Virginia, Charlottesville, VA, USA

Shant M. Vartanian, M.D. Department of Surgery, University of California San Francisco, San Francisco, CA, USA

Aristidis Veves, M.D., M.Sc., D.Sc. Microcirculation Lab, Joslin Beth Israel Deaconess Foot Center, Harvard Medical School, Boston, MA, USA

General Considerations in the Diabetic Patient with Peripheral Vascular Disease

Rishi Kundi, Andrew J. Meltzer, and Danielle Bajakian

Keywords

Diabetic • Vasculopathy • Ischemic • Foot • Neuropathic • Ulcer • Amputation

Introduction

The prevalence of peripheral arterial disease (PAD) among American adults is estimated at 4% [1]. Among the elderly, the prevalence exceeds 20%, affecting over four million individuals, and accounting for over $20 billion in annual healthcare costs [1, 2]. Its most advanced form, critical limb ischemia (CLI), is a highly morbid condition with 1-year mortality and major amputation rates estimated at 20% and 35%, respectively.

The frequent coexistence of diabetes mellitus (DM) and PAD is readily apparent to healthcare providers involved in the care of patients with either condition [3]. The co-prevalence of these conditions is not simply an association due to shared risk factors; DM plays a fundamental role in the pathophysiology of PAD.

The relationship between diabetes and vasculopathy is complex, and despite a significant research effort in molecular, animal, and translational models, the details of this relationship have yet to be completely elucidated. At present, the end result of peripheral ischemia is thought to result from the interplay between hemodynamic, neurohumoral, and metabolic factors, culminating in endothelial dysfunction [4]. This, in turn, leads to medial smooth muscle cell dysfunction, platelet hyperactivity, and impaired fibrinolysis coupled with hypercoagulability [5]. Fundamental concerns remain unanswered. An example is the phenomenon that the regression in microvascular disease following strict blood glucose control is not observed in the larger vessels encountered by the vascular specialist [6].

R. Kundi, M.D. (✉)
Department of Vascular Surgery, Columbia University Medical Center, New York Presbyterian Medical Center, 353 East 17th Street Apt. 22B,
New York, NY 10032, USA
e-mail: rik2010@nyp.org

A.J. Meltzer, M.D.
Division of Vascular Surgery and Endovascular Interventions, New York Presbyterian Hospital, Presbyterian Hospital, 526 East 68th Street, P706, New York, NY 10021, USA
e-mail: andrewjmeltzer@gmail.com

D. Bajakian, M.D., F.A.C.S.
Critical Limb Ischemia Program, Columbia University Medical Center, New York Presbyterian Hospital, New York, NY, USA

Despite a considerable research effort, as well as improvements in patient education, attention to risk factor modification, and aggressive medical management, the natural history of DM is progressive and frequently includes renal disease, cardiac disease, retinopathy, and PAD [7]. Even more concerning are current statistics that identify significant geographic and socioeconomic variation in lower extremity amputation in this patient population [8, 9].

These findings highlight the need for an aggressive, multidisciplinary approach to limb salvage in the diabetic population. As an introduction to this multidisciplinary textbook, the objective of this chapter is to describe the epidemiology, pathophysiology, and management of coexistent DM and PAD. The development of a multidisciplinary team is paramount to achieving limb salvage in patients with DM and CLI. Collaboration between vascular specialists, podiatrists, medical physicians, wound care specialists, and allied health professionals has proven beneficial to the management of patients with coexisting DM and PAD; it is our hope that this introductory chapter and those that follow will provide a framework for the development of multidisciplinary efforts, resulting in improved limb salvage rates among diabetic patients and elimination of geographic disparities in care.

Epidemiology of Diabetes and Peripheral Arterial Disease

The prevalence of DM among the US elderly population approaches 20% by self-report; these CDC estimates are thought to underestimate the true prevalence by as much as 33% [10]. The dreaded complication of diabetic foot ulceration may result from acute or chronic cutaneous injury, diabetic neuropathy, or arterial insufficiency; however, it is frequently multifactorial [11]. Despite advances in diabetes management and increased awareness of PAD, the majority of diabetic foot ulcerations are now attributable to PAD alone or in combination with neuropathy (neuroischemic) [12]. The significance of neuroischemic ulceration in diabetics has been well demonstrated; it is the precipitating event for the vast majority of non-traumatic lower extremity amputations performed worldwide [13]. While primary prevention of neuroischemic ulceration may therefore appear to be an effective means of amputation prevention, there is dramatic variation in amputation rates in the US population, with clustering of high amputation rates among diabetic Medicare recipients by hospital referral region [14]. These discrepancies are not unique to the USA; in Sweden amputation rates at specialized centers can be as low as 10%, whereas rates in centers without specialization may be twice as high [13].

The tremendous variation in amputation rates among diabetics with neuroischemic ulceration suggests significant room for improvement, not only with primary prevention of neuroischemic ulceration, but with the response of healthcare providers. Through aggressive revascularization and wound care, the impressive limb salvage rates at specialized centers should be attainable irrespective of geography.

In the US population, lower socioeconomic status is itself associated with diabetes. The Boston Community Health Survey was an NIH-supported community health survey of more than 5,500 residents equally distributed amongst racial/ethnic and socioeconomic categories conducted between 2002 and 2005. The results of the survey demonstrated that lower socioeconomic class was correlated with a higher likelihood of both diagnosed and undiagnosed diabetes [15]. Moreover, ethnic differences in the prevalence of diabetes have been well documented, with nonwhite Americans being at higher risk for the disease [16]. CDC data indicate that the prevalence of diabetes among Hispanics was almost double that among whites [17]. Racial differences in the metabolic syndrome have also been demonstrated, with a resultant unequal distribution of the cardiovascular risk increase attendant to the syndrome [18].

Compounding the discrepant effects of diabetes in the USA is the well-established discrepancy in healthcare delivery that exists, particularly that regarding diabetes. 2004 CDC data indicate that Hispanics with diabetes are significantly less likely to have had their HbA1c or their feet checked for either neuropathy or ulcer within the previous year compared to white diabetics. This reduction in healthcare provision persisted even when adjustments were made for socioeconomic status and availability of care [19]. A similar examination of CDC data from 1994 to 2002 showed a similar decrease in glycemic control monitoring among blacks in Missouri [20]. Veterans' Administration data confirm that minority patients were less likely to achieve sufficient glucose control or receive adequate monitoring than whites [21].

The combination of an increased risk of diabetes and a disparity in provision of diabetic care in those patients at highest risk has resulted in an increased risk of diabetic complications in minority patients, particularly among the vascular diseases. Community-based studies have shown that Hispanics and blacks are at significantly greater risk for neuropathy than whites and less likely to receive professional foot care [22]. African Americans and Hispanic Americans are similarly more likely to suffer from dialysis-dependent, diabetes-related end-stage renal disease and yet are less likely to have been cared for by a nephrologist before the initiation of hemodialysis [23].

Perhaps most alarming is the relatively high rate of lower extremity amputation amongst minority populations. Race was an independent risk factor for amputation among patients in a multi-institutional, 8 year study of patients in Chicago hospitals, with black patients being 1.7 times likely to undergo primary amputation than whites [24]. Among patients in Texas, the age-adjusted incidence of diabetic amputation among blacks was more than twice that of whites with Hispanic patients being between the two. Exacerbating this difference is evidence showing that the mortality of diabetes-related amputation is further increased amongst minorities [25]. There is also a disparity in overall vascular care. Using inpatient Medicare data, Holman et al. examined vascular care delivered in the 2 years prior to amputation. They found that blacks were significantly less likely to have undergone any wound debridement, toe amputation, attempted revascularization, or any limb-related admission at all prior to their major amputation [26].

The population at increased risk for diabetes and its vascular complications is also the population at increased risk for insufficient treatment for diabetes and its vascular manifestations, whether that care concerns glycemic control, kidney disease, foot care, wound care, or vascular disease. From the perspective of the vascular surgeon, the multifactorial nature of diabetic vasculopathy contributes to the problem, since without the care provided by several different specialties, the prevention of vascular disease and the success of any vascular intervention are improbable.

Pathophysiology of Diabetes and Peripheral Arterial Disease

As is detailed in Chap. 2, diabetes affects the vasculature in its entirety. Altered metabolism associated with the hyperglycemic state leads to altered arterial structure and function at the tissue, cellular, and molecular levels. Specifically, DM is a pro-inflammatory condition, as evidenced by elevations in C-reactive protein (CRP), which is associated with both DM and PAD [27, 28]. More than a mere inflammatory marker, CRP binds to endothelial cell receptors and has numerous molecular effects, including inhibition of endothelial nitric oxide synthase (eNOS), stimulates tissue factor production, and increases production of anti-fibrinolytic factors including plasminogen activator inhibitor (PAI)-1 [29].

While a comprehensive discussion of nitric oxide (NO) metabolism and its vascular smooth muscle and endothelial cell effects is beyond the scope of this text, it is important to note that alterations in NO metabolism are prevalent among patients with PAD, and these alterations are thought to play an important role in atherogenesis [30]

In diabetics, alterations in NO metabolism result from hyperglycemia and insulin resistance. The immediate result is the development of a pro-inflammatory state that eventually leads to atheroma formation via well-established molecular and cellular pathways.

Additional effects of diabetes on the peripheral vasculature, as previously mentioned, include vascular smooth muscle cell dysfunction and alterations in platelet function and fibrinolysis that lead to a hypercoagulable state, further potentiating atherogenesis and potentially contributing to the adverse outcomes after revascularization discussed later [31].

Diagnosis of PAD in the Diabetic Patient

Patients with diabetes should undergo a comprehensive history and physical examination with specific attention to symptoms suggestive of PAD, including claudication, rest pain, or known ulceration. It is important to consider that the spectrum of PAD ranges from asymptomatic patients to those with advanced tissue loss and gangrene. The physical examination must include a complete vascular examination and specific evaluation of the feet, with attention not only to evident ulceration but also temperature, dependent rubor, pallor on elevation, hairlessness, and dystrophic nails. If there is evidence of any of these stigmata of peripheral vascular disease, particularly in the setting of non-palpable pedal pulses, assessment of the ankle-brachial index is warranted. The ratio of the systolic blood pressure in the ankle divided by the systolic blood pressure at the arm is easily determined with a blood pressure cuff and handheld Doppler at the bedside. In practice, this is generally performed in the vascular laboratory, although the technique and principle should be known to all practitioners caring for diabetic patients. The ABI is considered normal if >0.91. Mild obstruction manifests as an ABI as 0.7–0.9; moderate obstruction 0.4–0.69, and severe obstruction consistent with CLI generally results in an ABI < 0.4. In patients with noncompressible arteries (such as may be found in the setting of diabetes and renal insufficiency), the ABI may be noncompressible (>1.0).

Screening ABI's are recommended by the American Diabetes Association (ADA) in asymptomatic patients over the age of 50, or younger in the presence of other risk factors for PAD. Diagnostic testing is warranted in symptomatic patients. Referral to the vascular laboratory permits formal measurement of ABI as well as pulse volume recordings (PVRs) that permit localization of the anatomic distribution of disease. Additional studies that may be performed in the vascular laboratory, and are discussed in detail later in this text, include exercise (treadmill) testing, toe pressure measurement, and duplex ultrasound.

Medical Management and Lifestyle Modification

Although medical management of patients with PAD and DM will be discussed in detail in Chap. 3, there are several fundamental points that warrant discussion in this introductory section. Diabetes and smoking are the two most significant risk factors for eventual amputation among patients with PAD. Therefore, smoking cessation must be achieved in the diabetic smoker. It is the single most significant modifiable risk factor for amputation, PAD progression, and adverse cardiovascular events.

As previously discussed, tight glucose control does not appear to inhibit PAD to the extent that it permits avoidance of microvascular complications. Nonetheless, general guidelines advise that Hgb A1C <7.0% is a good target, provided it can be achieved without complications related to hypoglycemic events.

Hypertension is associated with atherosclerosis and the development of symptomatic PAD. The hemodynamic consequences of diabetes are irrevocably tied to hypertension, from which over 70% of type II diabetics suffer [32]. Several studies have demonstrated that inhibition of the renin–angiotensin axis with ACE modifiers can result in a decrease in vascular morbidity, most notably the MICRO-HOPE trial which demonstrated a 17% reduction in the risk of vascular disease requiring revascularization among patients who were treated with ramipril [33]. Not only was this reduction too great to attribute to the blood pressure effects alone, but animal studies employing doses of ACE inhibitors subtherapeutic for hypertension control have demonstrated decreases in vascular remodeling [34]. Treatment recommendations, however, are based primarily on the generalized cardiovascular benefit [35]. Recommendations include blood pressure control with lifestyle modifications and medications to achieve blood pressure <130/80 mmHg in patients with PAD and diabetes.

Similarly, dyslipidemia should be addressed; although studies evaluating specific effects of LDL cholesterol levels on PAD progression in diabetic patients are lacking, guidelines recommend a target LDL cholesterol level <100 mg/dl to avoid adverse cardiovascular events. Antiplatelet therapy is recommended in DM; the role of dual antiplatelet therapy remains controversial. Current guidelines suggest aspirin is sufficient for asymptomatic patients with DM and PAD, although ADA documents suggest that clopidogrel may have greater benefit in diabetics [7, 30, 31, 35].

For symptomatic patients with claudication, therapy may include exercise therapy, medical treatment, and revascularization. Diabetic patients presenting with evidence of chronic CLI necessitate an aggressive approach to revascularization and wound care in order to avoid amputation.

In claudicants, supervised exercise therapy has proven an effective and cost-sensitive alternative to immediate revascularization. While non-supervised exercise therapy is insufficient, the results from the recently published Claudication: Exercise Versus Endoluminal Revascularization (CLEVER) trial suggested that supervised exercise therapy was as effective as endovascular revascularization [36]. With respect to the diabetic population, however, these results should be applied cautiously, as only 23% of patients in CLEVER were diabetic. Given the aforementioned effects of the hyperglycemic state on the vascular endothelium, smooth muscle cells, and angiogenesis, it is reasonable to hypothesize that the mechanism of improvement (i.e., collateral development secondary to neovascularization) may be impaired in diabetic patients, although to our knowledge this has not been specifically addressed.

Proven medical treatment for claudication is limited to cilostazol, an oral phosphodiesterase inhibitor. Although cilostazol was approved after pentoxifylline, it is the only drug that reproducibly improves walking distance in the setting of claudication. It is recommended as medical therapy for patients with DM and intermittent claudication, provided there is no evidence of congestive heart failure, which is a contraindication to its use.

Peripheral Bypass Surgery and Endovascular Therapy

While medical management and supervised exercise therapy are reasonable alternatives to patients with DM and symptomatic PAD manifest as claudication, for those patients with CLI (rest pain or ulceration with evidence of vascular insufficiency), an aggressive approach is warranted.

Current treatment options include surgical bypass and endovascular therapy (ET). Although these approaches will be discussed in detail in Chaps. 9 and 10, some general principles warrant discussion.

Although diabetes is highly prevalent among patients with CLI, the observation that DM is associated with a poor outcome following any revascularization has been reported [37]. The pervasiveness of this opinion, even among vascular specialists, may partially explain the high amputation rates in some geographic regions in the USA.

The association between DM and poor outcomes with revascularization is perhaps secondary to the typical pattern of arterial disease seen in DM, in which infrapopliteal disease with relative sparing of the pedal vessels predominates, and multilevel disease is commonplace [37]. Moreover, the comorbidities often associated with CLI include coronary artery disease, heart failure, and renal insufficiency. In the pre-endovascular era, these associated comorbidities rendered many patients with DM and CLI unsuitable for open revascularization, thus propagating a tendency towards primary amputation.

Although some early reports suggested the futility of distal bypass surgery in these patients, 5-year patency rates for autogenous vein bypass grafts to infrapopliteal targets range from 50 to 70% in retrospective series; limb salvage rates exceed 80% [38]. The preconception that DM is associated with poor outcomes after surgical bypass appears to be misguided, as it is not DM per se, but rather associated comorbidities and the anatomic pattern of disease in these patients that results in poor outcome [39]. With appropriate patient selection, adequate conduit, and attention to the technical details of the procedure, surgical bypass remains the gold standard approach to achieve limb salvage in the patient with DM and CLI [39].

For patients without suitable venous conduit, or in whom medical comorbidities are believed to prohibit surgical bypass, endovascular therapy has assumed an integral role in the management of patients with DM and PAD. Although the durability of peripheral bypass surgery is proven, it is associated with significant perioperative morbidity and mortality [40]. Conversely, endovascular interventions are associated with reduced durability and may require serial interventions to achieve limb salvage [41–43]. However, due to the minimally invasive nature of these procedures, they are associated with reduced perioperative risk.

Given the high prevalence of medical comorbidities among patients with PAD, many vascular specialists advocate aggressive use of endovascular therapy as first-line treatment for PAD. We recently reported a series of 1,220 patients undergoing intervention for claudication (22.5%) or CLI (77.5%) [42]. By multivariate analysis, predictors of primary patency loss included TASC C/D disease (HR: 1.375 [1.164–1.624]; $P<0.001$), chronic total occlusion (1.225 [1.041–1.443]; $P=0.015$); DM (1.243 [1.056–1.463]; $P=0.009$), congestive heart failure (1.204 [1.011–1.434]; $P=0.038$), and current smoking (1.529 [1.223–1.913]; $P=0.001$).

The reduced durability associated with endovascular therapy is well established; however, it is expected that serial interventions to maintain patency may permit durable limb salvage. It is therefore essential to examine those factors associated with reduced secondary patency. In the aforementioned series, these included: TASC C/D disease (1.400 [1.111–1.764]; $P=0.004$), DM (1.279 [1.017–1.608]; $P=0.036$), congestive heart failure (1.463 [1.168–1.833]; $P=0.001$), current smoking (1.789 [1.338–2.392]; $P<0.001$), and CLI (4.007 [3.106–5.169]; $P=0.001$). By multivariate analysis, the only independent risk factors for limb loss were current smoking (2.3 [1.24–4.01]; $P=0.007$), end-stage renal disease (1.9 [1.018–3.587]; $P=0.044$), and diabetes (2.13 [1.21–3.76]; $P=0.008$).

The significance of diabetes as an independent predictor of poor outcome after endovascular therapy in our series is supported by prior reports. Abularrage and colleagues at the Massachusetts General Hospital performed a retrospective analysis of over 1,000 limbs to assess the importance of diabetes on outcome after endovascular intervention. In this series, which compared 533 diabetic to 542 nondiabetic limbs, actuarial primary patency at 5 years was 42%±2.4%, assisted patency was 81%±2.0%, and limb salvage was 89%±1.6%. By univariate analysis, diabetes was associated with inferior 5-year primary patency (37%±3.4% vs. 46%±3.3%; $P=0.009$), reduced limb salvage (84%±2.6% vs. 93%±1.8%, $P<0.0001$), and survival (52%±3.5% vs. 68%±3.1%; $P=0.0001$). There was no difference between diabetic and nondiabetic patients with respect to assisted patency. By multivariate analysis, diabetes was associated with reduced primary patency (1.25 [1.01–1.54]; $P=0.04$), along with single-vessel peroneal runoff (HR, 1.54; 95% CI, 1.16–2.08; $P<0.003$), and dialysis dependence (HR, 1.59; 95% CI, 1.10–2.33; $P<0.02$). Multivariate analysis to identify those factors predicting limb loss included CLI (HR, 9.09; 95% CI, 4.17–20.00; $P<0.0001$) and dialysis dependence (HR, 2.94; 95% CI, 1.39–5.00; $P=0.003$; HR, 4.24; 95% CI, 2.80–6.45; $P<0.0001$) [37].

Guidelines and Outcome Metrics

Understanding the success of various treatment options for PAD and diabetes requires familiarity with the language of outcomes assessment as it pertains to this group of patients. It is imperative that vascular specialists treating PAD are familiar with treatment guidelines, reporting standards, and outcome definitions.

A general overview of the management of patients with DM and PAD has been released by the ADA. This document summarizes the global approach to these patients, and includes recommendations ranging from routine preventive care to medical management and revascularization [29]. With regard to surgical revascularization, formal reporting standards have been endorsed by the Society for Vascular Surgery. This document, also known as the Rutherford Reporting Guidelines, contains an overview of the classification and surgical treatment for PAD [44]. As will be discussed in later chapters, decision-making with respect to appropriateness of endovascular (versus surgical) revascularization may be guided by the Inter-Society Consensus Guidelines for the Management of Peripheral Arterial Disease TASC-II (revised) document [45]. Recently, the Society for Vascular Surgery published Objective Performance Goals for the management of CLI, in an effort to standardize clinical studies involving the application of new technology to the management of patients with chronic CLI [46].

With respect to the outcomes of revascularization, commonly reported outcome metrics include, clinical response, primary patency, assisted primary patency, secondary patency, target lesion (or limb) revascularization, and limb salvage. Additional measures include freedom from bypass surgery, and composite endpoints (such as amputation-free survival). The following definitions of accepted outcome measures represent a summary of pertinent points from these documents.

Technical success after revascularization may be claimed in the setting of (1) antegrade flow through the treated lesion; (2) less than 25–30 % residual stenosis; (3) in-line flow to the pedal arch. Post-intervention vascular laboratory studies should reveal a peak systolic velocity ratio of 2.5 or less at the treatment site and/or an ABI improvement of 0.15 or greater. Ongoing hemodynamic success relies on vascular laboratory evaluation, with a maintained ABI increase greater than 0.15 from the early post-procedural level, biphasic or triphasic waveforms. For clinical success to be claimed, these hemodynamic and technical measures must be attained in the setting of clinical improvement [44]. Clinical success is perhaps the most ambiguous outcome measure, yet at the same time the most important from a patient-centered standpoint. Clinical improvement requires improvement by at least one Rutherford–Becker clinical category, with the exception of patients with tissue loss (Rutherford–Becker 5/6) who must advance two categories, to claudication or rest pain, respectively. In each case, wound healing must occur. Moreover, improvement must be clearly attributable to the intervention, and requires hemodynamic confirmation of success: a minimum change in ABI of 0.1 is recommended [44]. Primary patency implies freedom from thrombosis and restenosis. It is generally reported using life-table analysis or Kaplan–Meier survival function. Generally some degree of restenosis is allowable (30–50 %), which correlates with noninvasive vascular studies indicating a systolic velocity ratio greater than 2–2.5 or ABI decrease greater than 0.15 results in loss of primary patency. Assisted patency, also referred to as primary-assisted patency or assisted primary patency, refers to interventions necessitating a subsequent interventional procedure to maintain patency. Secondary patency refers to restoration of patency after re-occlusion. As duplex ultrasound surveillance is generally recommended after peripheral endovascular interventions, these outcome measures are generally comparable, with secondary patency calculations including those in which patency is maintained in the setting of restenosis detected by ultrasound (assisted patency) as well as re-interventions for occlusion. Assisted patency and secondary patency are reported with Kaplan–Meier function estimation or life-table analysis.

The most relevant outcome measure for patients with CLI is limb salvage. Minor amputations (at the toe or trans-metatarsal level) are not considered limb loss. When evaluating long-term limb salvage data, it is important to note that due to the high prevalence of significant comorbidities among these patients, survival is generally poor and therefore many patients are censored due to death throughout follow-up. This fact, combined with an unclear yet significant success rate with medical therapy and wound care alone, may artificially inflate limb salvage estimates after any revascularization procedure.

It is noteworthy that, in addition to these generally accepted outcome metrics, there has been a recent paradigm shift towards the study of patient-centered outcomes that attempt to measure quality of life, permitting comparisons of the efficacy of interventions from a patient-centered perspective.

Some progressive outcomes investigators have applied various objective quality of life assessment tools to patients with CLI undergoing revascularization. These utilities range from simple postoperative functional status assessments to generalized quality of life metrics (e.g., Short Form-36, EuroQol, Nottingham Health Profile) to disease-specific (e.g., VascuQol and Walking Impairment Questionnaire) tools that account for social functioning, emotional well-being, pain, symptomatology, and overall quality of life [47–49]. It is anticipated that, given current trends in healthcare, increasing importance will be placed on these instruments in an effort to individualize clinical decision-making and outcomes reporting.

Wound Care, Debridement, Minor Amputation, and Pedal Sepsis

While neuropathic ulceration is frequently found on the plantar surface, ischemic ulceration tends to occur around the edges of the foot, in the toe or heel, at the most distal sites of perfusion. Frequently ulceration follows minor trauma, such as may occur from the use of inappropriate footwear. This phenomenon emphasizes the importance of routine preventive foot care for the diabetic patient.

Once the diabetic patient has developed ischemic or neuroischemic ulceration, timely involvement of all members of the multidisciplinary team is essential. The prior sections in this introduction, and following chapters, highlight the importance of aggressive medical management, evaluation for ischemia, and revascularization by either open or endovascular therapy, as appropriate.

This involves the work of medical physicians, endocrinologists, vascular specialists specializing in limb salvage, podiatrists, and wound care specialists.

In addition to aggressive medical management, PAD evaluation, and treatment, it is imperative to address the visible manifestation of PAD and diabetes: the pedal ulcer or wound itself. Techniques include surgical debridement, the application of bioactive dressings, and minor amputation. Although a fundamental goal of the multidisciplinary approach to limb salvage is avoiding amputation, there is still a role for primary major amputation, particularly among patients presenting with pedal sepsis in whom less aggressive options pose a threat to life.

When debridement is warranted, frequent sharp debridement is the preferred method of treatment when necrotic tissue is present. Localized fluctuance, suggesting underlying purulence, must be drained. The presence of air in the soft tissues on radiography, or crepitance on examination, should alert providers to significant underlying infection and prompt plans for immediate surgical management in addition to administration of intravenous antibiotics. These findings suggest wet gangrene; such a diabetic foot infection must be regarded as a surgical emergency.

Incision and drainage must be sufficiently wide as to allow for egress of purulence and facilitate subsequent dressing changes. One must balance this need with the desire to spare tissue; as a result the use of "counter incisions" remains somewhat controversial. In cases of localized sepsis, toe amputation may be necessary for drainage and removal of necrosis. Review of results with minor amputation (at the toe or forefoot level) suggests that these techniques, followed by revascularization efforts and local wound care, may permit control of infection and long-term limb salvage, although wound healing may be slow [49].

Major Amputation

While the ultimate goal of care in the management of PAD and diabetes is avoidance of amputation, in some cases major amputation is inevitable (discussed further in Chap. 12). In the setting of sepsis and extensive gangrene, for example, emergent guillotine amputation may be necessary as a lifesaving measure. Although there remains a role for primary amputation (i.e., amputation without efforts at revascularization), this probably applies to a smaller subgroup of patients than previously recognized. While extensive tissue loss, non-ambulatory status, the presence of significant contractures, and the absence of target vessels are indications to consider primary amputation, the role of systemic comorbidities in clinical decision-making remains ill defined. Using propensity score matched National Surgical Quality Improvement Program data, Barshes and colleagues at the Brigham and Women's Hospital recently reported that, in the most systemically ill patients with CLI, amputation was no less morbid than surgical revascularization [50]. This study does not even take into consideration the possibility of endovascular revascularization, which is associated with reduced perioperative morbidity and mortality. Given these findings, considered in the context of the endovascular era, it would appear that comorbidities should not preclude efforts at revascularization.

A Multidisciplinary Approach to Limb Salvage

This introduction provides an overview of general considerations in the management of coexistent DM and PAD. These topics, from risk factor modification to revascularization and amputation will be individually emphasized in subsequent chapters. Clearly, there has been great improvement in limb salvage rates worldwide in the past several decades. This phenomenon cannot be attributed to the efforts of any group of specialists in isolation. Rather, there is considerable evidence to suggest that a multidisciplinary approach is mandated to achieve successful limb salvage.

Logerfo and colleagues at the Beth Israel Deaconess Medical Center (formerly the New England Deaconess Hospital) and Joslin Diabetes Center were pioneers in the implementation of a team approach to limb salvage in patients in PAD and DM [51, 52]. Numerous reports from this group and other pioneers, utilizing a team-centered approach, identified reduced amputation rates, shorter hospitalizations, and total cost reduction [52, 53].

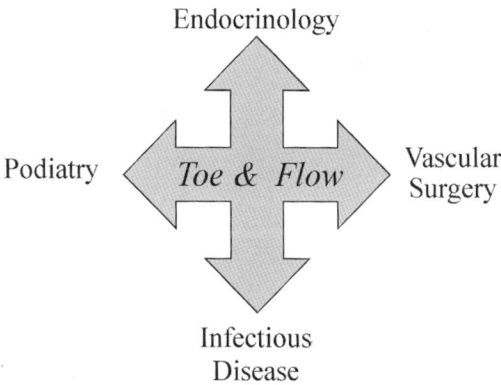

Fig. 1.1 The "toe and flow" model of the multidisciplinary team is designed to coordinate care of the diabetic wound, the diabetic foot, and perfusion through cooperation between a podiatrist and a vascular surgeon. The addition of other specialists enables more comprehensive and more detailed attention to all aspects of the disease process [based on data from Rogers LC, Andros G, Caporusso J, et al. Toe and flow: essential components and structure of the amputation prevention team. J Am Podiatr Med Assoc. 2010;100(5):342–8]

At a minimum, the team approach to diabetes must consist of a vascular surgeon or vascular specialist dedicated to treating CLI and podiatrist [48, 54, 55]. In reality, the multidisciplinary team should include these specialists, in addition to an orthopedist, wound care specialist, diabetologist, infectious disease specialist, prosthetist, and associated internists, cardiologists and allied health professionals.

The podiatrist is frequently the point of contact for the diabetic patient with a potentially limb-threatening condition. As a vital member of the so-called "toe and flow" construct (Fig. 1.1), the podiatrist's duties frequently include initial management of diabetic foot infections, initiation of the neurovascular evaluation, and wound management. The vascular surgeon must have a commitment to aggressive management of PAD, and in the present era should be well versed in both surgical and endovascular techniques as applied to PAD. In addition, vascular surgeons are frequently involved in wound care, and perform minor or major amputations, as necessary.

The commitment of an infectious disease specialist is essential. While medical management and antibiotic therapy should never supplant aggressive surgical debridement in the setting of complex diabetic foot infection, selection of appropriate antibiotics for an adequate duration is of great importance in the treatment of acute infections as well as osteomyelitis. Given the ever-changing microbial environment, evolving antibiotic resistance patterns, immunocompromised state associated with diabetes, and prevalence of multiresistant organisms in nursing facilities and hospitals, the infectious disease specialist plays a critical role on the team.

The endocrinologist or diabetologist has a crucial role. While management of diabetes is frequently straightforward, in many patients—particularly in the setting of infection—blood glucose levels may prove markedly difficult to normalize. In addition to management of DM in the inpatient setting, the diabetologist will frequently play a critical role in the outpatient management of these patients, assuming a leadership role in the risk factor modification and general medical care.

Depending on institutional particularities, general surgeons and orthopedists may have a role in the multidisciplinary team, particularly as adjunctive specialists in wound care management.

The conception of diabetic vascular disease, from molecular pathophysiology to clinical outcomes, is one of multiplicity. From one cause come many disease pathways, culminating in the phenomenon of clinical diabetic peripheral vascular disease. For that clinical disease to be adequately treated, then, all contributing disease pathways must be addressed and treated. The social and economic context of diabetes has presented an obstacle to the sufficient treatment of all of the elements of diabetic peripheral vascular disease, leaving those most at risk of vascular complications with the least comprehensive care. For these reasons, our institution among others has adopted a multidisciplinary approach to the prevention, assessment (Fig. 1.2), and treatment

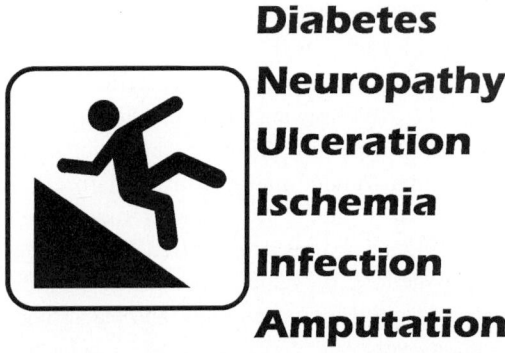

Fig. 1.2 The stairway to amputation. The evolution of the infected diabetic foot involves neuropathy and ischemia acting to progress from the ulcer to infection treatable only by infection. This sequence can be arrested by treatment of both neuropathy and ischemia as well as the consequent traumatic ulceration or infection [based on data from Rogers LC, Andros G, Caporusso J, et al. Toe and flow: essential components and structure of the amputation prevention team. J Am Podiatr Med Assoc. 2010;100(5):342–8]

of diabetic PAD. The result of this method has, around the world, proven to be both efficacious and economically sound. The understanding of diabetic vascular disease as fundamentally multifactorial and deserving of correspondingly multidisciplinary care is the single most important consideration of peripheral vascular disease in diabetic patients.

References

1. Pande RL, Perlstein TS, Beckman JA, Creager MA. Secondary prevention and mortality in peripheral artery disease: National Health and Nutrition Examination Study, 1999 to 2004. Circulation. 2011;124(1):17–23.
2. McDermott MM. Peripheral arterial disease: epidemiology and drug therapy. Am J Geriatr Cardiol. 2002;11(4):258–66.
3. Kannel WB, McGee DL. Diabetes and cardiovascular disease. The Framingham study. JAMA. 1979;241(19):2035–8.
4. Cooper ME, Bonnet F, Oldfield M, Jandeleit-Dahm K. Mechanisms of diabetic vasculopathy: an overview. Am J Hypertens. 2001;14(5 Pt 1):475–86.
5. Rahman S, Rahman T, Ismail AA, Rashid AR. Diabetes-associated macrovasculopathy: pathophysiology and pathogenesis. Diabetes Obes Metab. 2007;9(6):767–80.

6. Effect of intensive diabetes management on macrovascular events and risk factors in the Diabetes Control and Complications Trial. Am J Cardiol. 1995;75(14): 894–903.
7. Stokes 3rd J, Kannel WB, Wolf PA, Cupples LA, D'Agostino RB. The relative importance of selected risk factors for various manifestations of cardiovascular disease among men and women from 35 to 64 years old: 30 years of follow-up in the Framingham Study. Circulation. 1987;75(6 Pt 2):V65–73.
8. Margolis DJ, Malay DS, Hoffstad OJ, Leonard CE, MaCurdy T, López de Nava K, et al. Prevalence of diabetes, diabetic foot ulcer, and lower extremity amputation among Medicare beneficiaries, 2006 to 2008: Data Points #1. 17 Feb 2011. Data Points Publication Series [Internet]. Rockville, MD: Agency for Healthcare Research and Quality (US); 2011. Available from http://www.ncbi.nlm.nih.gov/books/NBK63602/.
9. Wrobel JS, Mayfield JA, Reiber GE. Geographic variation of lower-extremity major amputation in individuals with and without diabetes in the Medicare population. Diabetes Care. 2001;24(5):860–4.
10. Centers for Disease Control and Prevention (CDC). Prevalence of self-reported cardiovascular disease among persons aged > or =35 years with diabetes – United States, 1997-2005. MMWR Morb Mortal Wkly Rep. 2007;56(43):1129–32.
11. Reiber GE, Vileikyte L, Boyko EJ, del Aguila M, Smith DG, Lavery LA, et al. Causal pathways for incident lower-extremity ulcers in patients with diabetes from two settings. Diabetes Care. 1999;22(1):157–62.
12. Boulton AJ. The diabetic foot: grand overview, epidemiology and pathogenesis. Diabetes Metab Res Rev. 2008;24 Suppl 1:S3–6.
13. Apelqvist J, Larsson J. What is the most effective way to reduce incidence of amputation in the diabetic foot? Diabetes Metab Res Rev. 2000;16 Suppl 1:S75–83.
14. Margolis DJ, Hoffstad O, Nafash J, Leonard CE, Freeman CP, Hennessy S, et al. Location, location, location: geographic clustering of lower-extremity amputation among Medicare beneficiaries with diabetes. Diabetes Care. 2011;34(11):2363–7.
15. McKinlay JB, Marceau LD, Piccolo RJ. Do doctors contribute to the social patterning of disease? The case of race/ethnic disparities in diabetes mellitus. Med Care Res Rev. 2012;69(2):176–93.
16. Maskarinec G, Grandinetti A, Matsuura G, Sharma S, Mau M, Henderson BE, et al. Diabetes prevalence and body mass index differ by ethnicity: the Multiethnic Cohort. Ethn Dis. 2009;19(1):49–55.
17. Cusi K, Ocampo GL. Unmet needs in Hispanic/Latino patients with type 2 diabetes mellitus. Am J Med. 2011;124(10 Suppl):S2–9.
18. Okosun IS, Liao Y, Rotimi CN, Prewitt TE, Cooper RS. Abdominal adiposity and clustering of multiple metabolic syndrome in White, Black and Hispanic Americans. Ann Epidemiol. 2000;10(5):263–70.
19. Mainous 3rd AG, Diaz VA, Koopman RJ, Everett CJ. Quality of care for Hispanic adults with diabetes. Fam Med. 2007;39(5):351–6.
20. LeMaster JW, Chanetsa F, Kapp JM, Waterman BM. Racial disparities in diabetes-related preventive care: results from the Missouri Behavioral Risk Factor Surveillance System. Prev Chronic Dis. 2006; 3(3):A86.
21. Wendel CS, Shah JH, Duckworth WC, Hoffman RM, Mohler MJ, Murata GH. Racial and ethnic disparities in the control of cardiovascular disease risk factors in Southwest American veterans with type 2 diabetes: the Diabetes Outcomes in Veterans Study. BMC Health Serv Res. 2006;6:58.
22. Dunn JE, Link CL, Felson DT, Crincoli MG, Keysor JJ, McKinlay JB. Prevalence of foot and ankle conditions in a multiethnic community sample of older adults. Am J Epidemiol. 2004;159(5):491–8.
23. Hall YN. Racial and ethnic disparities in end stage renal disease: access failure. Clin J Am Soc Nephrol. 2012;7(2):196–8.
24. Feinglass J, Rucker-Whitaker C, Lindquist L, McCarthy WJ, Pearce WH. Racial differences in primary and repeat lower extremity amputation: results from a multihospital study. J Vasc Surg. 2005; 41(5):823–9.
25. Lavery LA, van Houtum WH, Armstrong DG, Harkless LB, Ashry HR, Walker SC. Mortality following lower extremity amputation in minorities with diabetes mellitus. Diabetes Res Clin Pract. 1997; 37(1):41–7.
26. Holman KH, Henke PK, Dimick JB, Birkmeyer JD. Racial disparities in the use of revascularization before leg amputation in Medicare patients. J Vasc Surg. 2011;54(2):420–6, 426.e1.
27. Ridker PM, Cushman M, Stampfer MJ, Tracy RP, Hennekens CH. Plasma concentration of C-reactive protein and risk of developing peripheral vascular disease. Circulation. 1998;97(5):425–8.
28. Beckman JA, Creager MA, Libby P. Diabetes and atherosclerosis: epidemiology, pathophysiology, and management. JAMA. 2002;287(19):2570–81.
29. American Diabetes Association. Peripheral arterial disease in people with diabetes. Diabetes Care. 2003;26(12):3333–41.
30. Veves A, Akbari CM, Primavera J, Donaghue VM, Zacharoulis D, Chrzan JS, et al. Endothelial dysfunction and the expression of endothelial nitric oxide synthetase in diabetic neuropathy, vascular disease, and foot ulceration. Diabetes. 1998;47(3):457–63.
31. Geng YJ, Libby P. Progression of atheroma: a struggle between death and procreation. Arterioscler Thromb Vasc Biol. 2002;22(9):1370–80.
32. Cooper ME. Pathogenesis, prevention, and treatment of diabetic nephropathy. Lancet. 1998;352(9123):213–9.
33. Effects of ramipril on cardiovascular and microvascular outcomes in people with diabetes mellitus: results of the HOPE study and MICRO-HOPE substudy. Heart Outcomes Prevention Evaluation Study Investigators. Lancet. 2000;355(9200):253–9. Erratum in: Lancet 2000;356(9232):860.
34. Cao Z, Hulthén UL, Allen TJ, Cooper ME. Angiotensin converting enzyme inhibition and calcium antagonism

attenuate streptozotocin-diabetes-associated mesenteric vascular hypertrophy independently of their hypotensive action. J Hypertens. 1998;16(6):793–9.
35. Colwell JA, American Diabetes Association. Aspirin therapy in diabetes. Diabetes Care. 2003;26 Suppl 1:S87–8.
36. Murphy TP, Cutlip DE, Regensteiner JG, Mohler ER, Cohen DJ, Reynolds MR, et al. CLEVER Study Investigators. Supervised exercise versus primary stenting for claudication resulting from aortoiliac peripheral artery disease: six-month outcomes from the claudication: exercise versus endoluminal revascularization (CLEVER) Study. Circulation. 2012;125(1):130–9.
37. Abularrage CJ, Conrad MF, Hackney LA, Paruchuri V, Crawford RS, Kwolek CJ, et al. Long-term outcomes of diabetic patients undergoing endovascular infrainguinal interventions. J Vasc Surg. 2010;52(2):314–22.e1–4.
38. Panayiotopoulos YP, Tyrrell MR, Owen SE, Reidy JF, Taylor PR. Outcome and cost analysis after femorocrural and femoropedal grafting for critical limb ischaemia. Br J Surg. 1997;84(2):207–12.
39. Conte MS. Challenges of distal bypass surgery in patients with diabetes: patient selection, techniques, and outcomes. J Vasc Surg. 2010;52(3 Suppl):96S–103.
40. LaMuraglia GM, Conrad MF, Chung T, Hutter M, Watkins MT, Cambria RP. Significant perioperative morbidity accompanies contemporary infrainguinal bypass surgery: an NSQIP report. J Vasc Surg. 2009;50(2):299–304, 304.e1–4.
41. Meltzer AJ, Shrikhande G, Gallagher KA, Aiello FA, Kahn S, Connolly P, et al. Heart failure is associated with reduced patency after endovascular intervention for symptomatic peripheral arterial disease. J Vasc Surg. 2012;55(2):353–62.
42. Aiello FA, Khan AA, Meltzer AJ, Gallagher KA, McKinsey JF, Schneider DB. Statin therapy is associated with superior clinical outcomes after endovascular treatment of critical limb ischemia. J Vasc Surg. 2012;55(2):371–80.
43. Gallagher KA, Meltzer AJ, Ravin RA, Graham A, Shrikhande G, Connolly PH, et al. Endovascular management as first therapy for chronic total occlusion of the lower extremity arteries: comparison of balloon angioplasty, stenting, and directional atherectomy. J Endovasc Ther. 2011;18(5):624–37. Erratum in: J Endovasc Ther. 2011;18(6):A-5.
44. Rutherford RB, Baker JD, Ernst C, Johnston KW, Porter JM, Ahn S, et al. Recommended standards for reports dealing with lower extremity ischemia: revised version. J Vasc Surg. 1997;26(3):517–38. Erratum in: J Vasc Surg 2001;33(4):805.
45. Norgren L, Hiatt WR, Dormandy JA, Nehler MR, Harris KA, Fowkes FG, TASC II Working Group. Inter-Society Consensus for the Management of Peripheral Arterial Disease (TASC II). J Vasc Surg. 2007;45(Suppl S):S5–67.
46. Conte MS, Geraghty PJ, Bradbury AW, Hevelone ND, Lipsitz SR, Moneta GL, et al. Suggested objective performance goals and clinical trial design for evaluating catheter-based treatment of critical limb ischemia. J Vasc Surg. 2009;50(6):1462–73.e1–3.
47. Sprengers RW, Teraa M, Moll FL, de Wit GA, van der Graaf Y, Verhaar MC; JUVENTAS Study Group; SMART Study Group. Quality of life in patients with no-option critical limb ischemia underlines the need for new effective treatment. J Vasc Surg. 2010;52(4):843–9, 849.e1.
48. Landry GJ. Functional outcome of critical limb ischemia. J Vasc Surg. 2007;45(Suppl A):A141–8.
49. Svensson H, Apelqvist J, Larsson J, Lindholm E, Eneroth M. Minor amputation in patients with diabetes mellitus and severe foot ulcers achieves good outcomes. J Wound Care. 2011;20(6):261–2, 264, 266 passim.
50. Barshes NR, Menard MT, Nguyen LL, Bafford R, Ozaki CK, Belkin M. Infrainguinal bypass is associated with lower perioperative mortality than major amputation in high-risk surgical candidates. J Vasc Surg. 2011;53(5):1251–9.e1.
51. Driver VR, Fabbi M, Lavery LA, Gibbons G. The costs of diabetic foot: the economic case for the limb salvage team. J Vasc Surg. 2010;52(3 Suppl):17S–22. Erratum in: J Vasc Surg. 2010;52(6):1751.
52. LoGerfo FW, Gibbons GW, Pomposelli FB Jr, Campbell DR, Miller A, Freeman DV, Quist WC. Trends in the care of the diabetic foot. Expanded role of arterial reconstruction. Arch Surg. 1992;127(5):617–20; discussion 620–1.
53. Gibbons GW, Marcaccio Jr EJ, Burgess AM, Pomposelli Jr FB, Freeman DV, Campbell DR, et al. Improved quality of diabetic foot care, 1984 vs 1990. Reduced length of stay and costs, insufficient reimbursement. Arch Surg. 1993;128(5):576–81.
54. Fitzgerald RH, Mills JL, Joseph W, Armstrong DG. The diabetic rapid response acute foot team: 7 essential skills for targeted limb salvage. Eplasty. 2009;9:e15.
55. Rogers LC, Andros G, Caporusso J, Harkless LB, Mills Sr JL, Armstrong DG. Toe and flow: essential components and structure of the amputation prevention team. J Vasc Surg. 2010;52(3 Suppl):23S–7.

The Pathogenesis of Diabetic Atherosclerosis

Jeffrey J. Siracuse and Elliot L. Chaikof

Keywords
Diabetes • Atherosclerosis • Hyperlipidemia • Insulin resistance • Reactive oxygen species

Introduction

Patients with diabetes mellitus (DM) have an over tenfold risk for cardiovascular disease in their lifetime [1]. In the United States, 77% of diabetes-related hospital admissions are for cardiovascular complications. A key feature of diabetes contributing to this is the development of an accelerated atherosclerosis [2]. Cardiovascular disease is one of the most morbid complications of DM with men and women being equally at risk, essentially eliminating the protection against cardiovascular disease characteristic of premenopausal women. DM predisposes to higher rates of coronary artery disease (CAD), cerebral vascular disease, and peripheral arterial disease (PAD). Aggressive blood sugar control has been shown to decrease some cardiovascular sequelae in diabetics, particularly in type I DM; however it does not eliminate all risk and intensive glycemic control for type II diabetics has not proven to be beneficial and may even be detrimental [1, 3].

CAD is the most morbid cardiovascular complication of DM with a two- to fourfold increased risk [4]. Compared to cardiovascular disease in nondiabetics, diabetic patients have a greater overall coronary plaque burden and a higher rate of multivessel disease. The proportion of stenotic segments is directly proportional to the duration of disease [5]. In combination, these factors place diabetic patients at greater risk for myocardial infarction (MI). In fact, diabetics without a prior MI are at equal risk for MI as nondiabetics with a prior MI. After MI, complications and death are higher in DM. The increased risk also extends to those undergoing cardiac procedures. After percutaneous coronary intervention (PCI), diabetic patients are at both higher risk for death and need for reintervention [6]. Diabetic patients who undergo coronary artery bypass grafting (CABG) are at higher risk for both complications and death, particularly in those with insulin-dependent type II DM, with no benefit seen in those who have had tight postoperative glycemic control [7, 8].

J.J. Siracuse, M.D. (✉) • E.L. Chaikof, M.D., Ph.D.
Department of Surgery, Beth Israel Deaconess Medical Center, Harvard Medical School, 330 Brookline Ave., Boston, MA 02215, USA
New York-Presbyterian Hospital, Columbia University and Weill Cornell Medical Centers, 630 West 168th Street, New York, NY 10032, USA
e-mail: Jes9061@nyp.org

Similarly to CAD, DM also carries a two- to fourfold increased risk of PAD. The distribution of lower extremity lesions in DM shows a higher propensity of atherosclerotic disease in the deep femoral artery, as well as in all vessels below the knee. Not surprisingly, DM is the leading risk factor for on-traumatic lower extremity amputations and diabetic patients have a higher frequency of infrageniculate arterial interventions [4, 9]. In the presence of DM, occlusive lesions are more common than stenoses [10]. Diabetic patients do not have a higher risk of graft failure, death, or cardiovascular complications after lower extremity bypass, nor do they have higher rates of failure after peripheral percutaneous intervention [10–12]. DM also increases the risk of extracranial cerebral vascular disease with a threefold increased risk of stroke and a greater rate of post-stroke complications, including recurrent stroke and death [4]. Diabetics undergoing carotid endarterectomy (CEA) are more likely to be younger and have concurrent CAD compared to nondiabetics. However, DM is not an independent predictor of perioperative MI, stroke, or death [13].

The effects of diabetes on the vasculature are quite extensive as diabetes affects not only the endothelium and smooth muscle cells, but also platelets, lipoproteins, local vasoactive substance production and function, clotting factors, triglycerides, as well as local arterial response to hypoxia and new collateral vessel formation [4]. The pathogenesis of diabetic atherosclerosis involves not only the direct effects of chronic hyperglycemia, but also insulin resistance, nonesterified free fatty acid (NEFA) production, dyslipidemia, hypercoagulability, and impaired response to injury [4, 14]. It is this widespread dysfunction that makes the side effects so deleterious and the treatment so difficult.

Histology

Arteries are composed of three layers—the tunica intima, media, and adventitia. The tunica intima is the innermost layer with the luminal side being composed of a single layer of endothelial cells. The next layer of the intima consists of an extracellular connective tissue matrix composed primarily of proteoglycans and collagen. Surrounding the intima is an internal elastic lamina that is composed of elastic cells of varying thickness depending on the vessel size. The tunica media is the next layer composed of primarily vascular smooth muscles cells and it is the thickest layer of the blood vessel. This layer is surrounded by the external elastic lamina, which separates the tunica media from the tunica adventitia, the outermost layer of the vessel wall. This layer is mainly composed of collagen with interspersed fibroblasts and vascular smooth muscle cells [15].

The development of diabetes-related atherosclerosis follows the same histologic course as atherosclerosis in nondiabetic patients. This includes endothelial injury, smooth muscle cell proliferation, foam cell development and infiltration, platelet activation, and increased inflammation. Sites of lesions are determined by altered hemodynamic forces and external sources of injury to the endothelial cells. Increased endothelial permeability leads to the retention of deleterious low-density lipoproteins (LDL) that interact with the underlying extracellular matrix (ECM). This interaction retains the LDL in the vessel wall where it can undergo oxidation by reactive oxygen species (ROS). This oxidized LDL can then stimulate the overlying endothelial cells to upregulate cellular adhesion molecules, chemotactic proteins, growth factors, and inhibit nitric oxide (NO) production. These activities recruit monocytes and macrophages, which interact with highly oxidized aggregated LDL to form foam cells. Pro-inflammatory cytokine production by activated macrophages stimulates proliferation of vascular smooth muscle cells (Fig. 2.1). Intimal smooth muscle cells subsequently produce an ECM that gives rise to a fibrous cap. The resulting complex plaque is vulnerable to destabilization, rupture, and superimposed thrombosis leading to an acute vascular occlusion (Fig. 2.2) [15].

Atherosclerotic plaques in the presence of diabetes generally have increased calcification, necrotic cores, receptors for advanced glycosylation endproducts (RAGE), and macrophage and T-cell infiltration. There is also a higher incidence of healed plaque ruptures and vascular

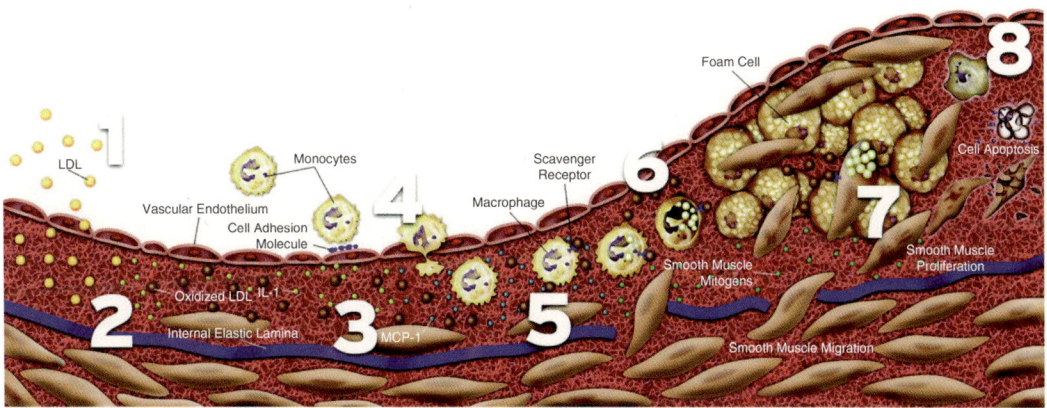

Fig. 2.1 The stages of development of an atherosclerotic plaque. (1) LDL is taken up by the endothelium. (2) Oxidation of LDL by macrophages and VSMCs. (3) Release of growth factors and cytokines. (4) Attraction of additional monocytes. (5) Foam cell accumulation. (6) SMC proliferation. (7, 8) Formation of plaque [reprinted from Faxon DP, Fuster V, Libby P. Atherosclerotic vascular disease conference: Writing Group III: Pathophysiology. Circulation. 2004;109(21):2617–25. With permission from Lippincott Williams & Wilkins]

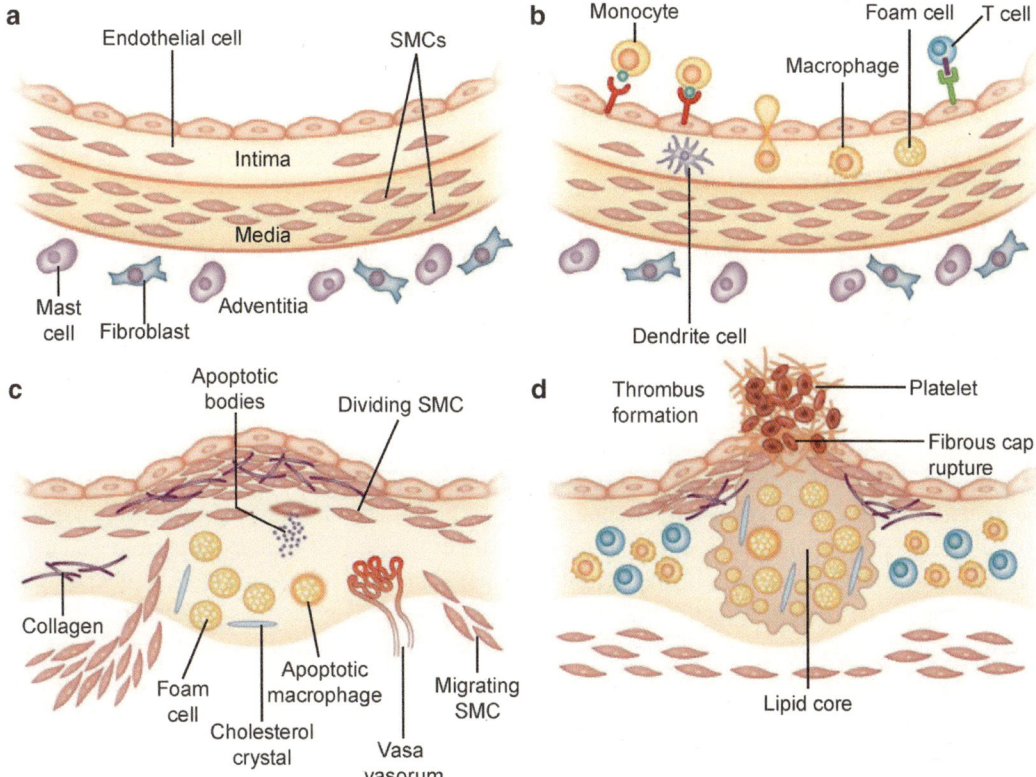

Fig. 2.2 Development of atherosclerotic plaque with superimposed thrombus [reprinted from Libby P, Ridker PM, Hansson GK. Progress and challenges in translating the biology of atherosclerosis. Nature. 2011;473(7347):317–25. With permission from Nature Publishing Group]

remodeling [16]. These features can potentially contribute to the more severe atherosclerosis and a higher incidence of acute adverse events.

Endothelial Cells

Endothelial cells synthesize multiple regulatory substances including NO, prostaglandins, angiotensin, and endothelin-1 (ET-1), and can upregulate adhesion molecules for interactions with neutrophils and platelets. These mediators help regulate vasodilation and vasoconstriction, hemostasis, and inflammation on the vessel surface and within the wall [2, 4]. Nitric oxide (NO) is anti-atherogenic, produced by the action of endothelial nitric oxide synthase (eNOS), and is a key contributor to vasodilation and prevention of platelet aggregation. Endothelial cell injury and dysfunction is thought to be the sentinel event in the development of atherosclerosis [17]. An intact endothelium normally inhibits platelet activation and inflammation by reducing upregulation of platelets and leukocyte adhesion molecules and subsequent migration through the vessel wall, diminishing vascular smooth muscle cell proliferation and migration [4]. Endothelial cells are particularly susceptible to accumulation of glucose seen in hyperglycemia and to many of the secondary side effects of DM including insulin resistance [18].

Vascular Smooth Muscle Cells

Vascular smooth muscle cells primarily comprise the tunica media and are responsible for contraction and relaxation to vary the caliber and pressure of blood vessels. Vessels in higher pressure systems tend to have more smooth muscle cells than those in lower pressure systems. Contraction and relaxation are primarily regulated by the sympathetic nervous system. Autonomic function is altered in DM resulting in abnormal vasodilation and vasoconstriction in response to local factors. The medial layer of smooth muscle cells proliferates into intimal lesions and atherosclerotic plaques develop with smooth muscle cells as the source of collagen to strengthen the plaque [4].

Monocytes

Monocyte activation and transformation into macrophages are a key step in the atherosclerotic and inflammatory process. One of the earliest events in the pathogenesis of atherosclerosis is lipid accumulation in monocytes through uptake of modified or oxidized low-density lipoprotein (LDL) leading to the foam cell infiltration in the arterial wall [15]. Activation of macrophages with subsequent release of smooth muscle growth regulatory molecules in diabetic lesions contributes to vascular smooth muscle cell proliferation [19].

Hyperglycemia

Hyperglycemia increases the production of reactive oxygen species (ROS) as a consequence of mitochondrial dysfunction, which in turn promotes atherosclerotic lesion formation by upregulation of protein kinase C (PKC), activation of the hexosamine and polyol pathways, and accumulation of advanced glycation endproducts (AGE) with upregulation of RAGE receptors. In many tissues, glucose uptake is mediated by insulin-independent glucose transporters (GLUT). Therefore, a rise in intracellular glucose concentrations parallels serum levels [20].

Mitochondria

Mitochondrial dysfunction is one of the initial pathophysiologic events observed in hyperglycemia. Increased glycolysis during aerobic metabolism in the setting of hyperglycemia generates nicotinamide adenine dinucleotide (NADH) and pyruvate. Pyruvate is then transported into the mitochondria where it enters the tricarboxylic acid (TCA) cycle generating three molecules of carbon dioxide, four molecules of NADH, and one molecule of flavin adenine dinucleotide (FADH$_2$). In mitochondria, NADH and FADH$_2$ donate electrons for the generation of adenosine triphosphate (ATP) through oxidative phosphorylation in the electron transport chain (ETC). The ETC progresses sequentially through four

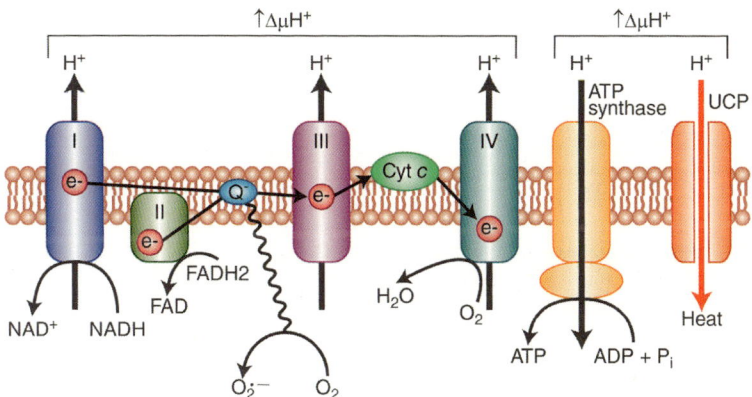

Fig. 2.3 Production of superoxide by the mitochondrial electron-transport chain. Hyperglycemia causes an increase in electron donors from the TCA cycle generating a high mitochondrial membrane potential by pumping protons across the mitochondrial inner membrane. This inhibits electron transport at complex III, increasing the half-life of free-radical intermediates of coenzyme Q (ubiquinone), which reduce O_2 to superoxide [reprinted from Brownlee M. Biochemistry and molecular cell biology of diabetic complications. Nature. 2001;414(6865): 813–20. With permission from Nature Publishing Group]

inner-membrane-associated enzyme complexes, along with cytochrome C, and the mobile carrier Coenzyme Q. NADH has the greatest potential to generate ATP as it donates electrons to complex I, while $FADH_2$ donates electrons to complex II. Electrons from both of these complexes are subsequently passed to coenzyme Q, complex III, cytochrome C, complex IV, and finally to oxygen, which is then reduced to water. The voltage generated across the inner mitochondrial membrane drives the synthesis of ATP. Elevated glucose levels increases glycolysis and, thereby, enhances electron donation to the ETC. An increase in electron flux raises the voltage across the membrane and generates a higher membrane potential eventually reaching a threshold where transport at complex III is blocked, increasing electron donation to O_2 at coenzyme Q, generating ROS, specifically superoxide (O^-) (Fig. 2.3) [18, 20].

Reactive Oxygen Species

ROS promotes atherosclerosis by blocking eNOS synthase, further increasing the production of other ROS, especially superoxide anion (O_2^-), in endothelial cells and vascular smooth muscle cells [4]. Superoxide initially reacts with NO to form peroxynitrite ($ONOO^-$), a potent oxidant that selectively inhibits prostacyclin (PGI_2) by nitrating and disrupting PGI_2 synthase's iron-thiolate center. PGI_2 inactivation causes the buildup of its precursor, prostaglandin endoperoxide (PGH_2), which induces vasoconstriction and endothelial dysfunction. In addition, PGH_2 promotes the conversion of PGI_2 to thromboxane A_2 (TxA_2) by TxA_2 synthase. Both of these events activate the thromboxane (TP) receptor causing platelet aggregation, as well as vascular smooth muscle cell activation, apoptosis, and expression of pro-inflammatory adhesion molecules, including intercellular adhesion molecule-1 (ICAM-1), vascular cell adhesion molecule-1 (VCAM-1), and endothelial-leukocyte adhesion molecule (ELAM-1).

Peroxynitrite is also responsible for uncoupling eNOS by targeting its zinc tetrathiolate cluster. Its interaction with zinc releases it from the tetrahedral conformation and disulfide bonds then form between the two monomers. This disrupts the catalytic activities of eNOS, decreasing NO synthesis and increasing production of ROS. Tetrahydrobiopterin (BH4), an important factor in eNOS function, is also targeted and interrupted by peroxynitrite [21]. Superoxide also inactivates the glycolytic enzyme glyceraldehyde-3-phosphate dehydrogenase (GAPDH), which induces vascular injury through four main pathways described below.

Protein Kinase C Pathway

Increased intracellular hyperglycemia causes de novo synthesis of diacylglycerol (DAG), an intracellular lipid messenger, through increased synthesis of the glycolytic intermediate glyceraldehyde-3-phosphate. DAG activates protein kinase C (PKC), a serine/threonine-related protein kinase, downstream in both endothelial and smooth muscle cells. There are multiple PKC isoforms; however, the most notable in the pathogenesis of diabetic atherosclerosis are PKC-β and PKC-γ.

Hyperglycemia-induced PKC upregulation increases endothelial cell permeability, depresses NO production, and increases production of vasoconstrictors, such as ET-1 and TxA_2. PKC also contributes to the hypercoagulable and pro-inflammatory state seen in DM by upregulating plasminogen activator inhibitor type 1 (PAI-1) and nuclear factor-κB (NF-κB), respectively, in endothelial and smooth muscle cells. PKC can increase ROS levels by activation of membrane-associated nicotinamide adenine dinucleotide phosphate (NAD(P)H)-dependent oxidases and by inhibition insulin-stimulated production of eNOS [18, 20, 22].

Hexosamine Pathway

Inhibition of GAPDH by superoxide also diverts the glycolytic upstream metabolite fructose-6-phosphate into the hexosamine pathway. Fructose-6-phosphate is converted by glutamine:fructose-6 phosphate amidotransferase (GFAT) to glucosamine-6 phosphate and subsequently to uridine diphosphate N-acetylglucosamine (UDP-GlcNAc), which is a precursor for proteoglycans, glycolipids, and glycoproteins [18, 20]. In hyperglycemia, UDP-GlcNAc serves as a substrate for protein O-GlcNAcylation. Post-translation O-GlcNAcylation and subsequent ubiquitation and degradation of atheroprotective proteins in the vasculature, such as eNOS and A20, tip the balance toward heightened atherogenesis while increasing the transcription of proatherogenic proteins, such as thrombospondin-1 [14, 23]. O-GlcNAcylation of the transcription factor Sp1 increases its transactivation and the downstream expression of Sp1-dependent expression of both transforming growth factor-β (TGFβ) and PAI-1, both of which contribute the development of vascular disease through basement membrane thickening and increased thrombosis [14, 18, 20, 22, 23].

Advanced Glycation Endproducts

AGEs are formed intracellularly in vascular endothelial and smooth muscle cells during hyperglycemia by nonenzymatic post-translational modification. The first step is glycation of intracellular proteins by both glucose and glucose-derived compounds. Methylglyoxal-derived AGE, the primary intracellular AGE induced by hyperglycemia, is formed by modification of glyceraldehyde-3-phosphate, which accumulates secondary to ROS inhibition of GAPDH. AGEs cause dysfunction by modification of intracellular and extracellular proteins, the latter of which may serve as ligands for transmembrane RAGE receptors of the immunoglobulin superfamily present on endothelial cells, smooth muscle cells, macrophages, and lymphocytes. Their upregulation results in generation of further ROS and a pro-inflammatory, procoagulable state through upregulation of NF-κB, tissue factor, and VCAM-1 [18, 20, 24]. RAGE upregulation is seen in diabetic atherosclerotic plaques and infarcted cardiac tissue [24].

Polyol Pathway

Aldo-keto reductase reduces a variety of carbonyl compounds to their respective sugar alcohols or polyols. During hyperglycemia, glucose and glucose-derived compounds, such as glyceraldehyde 3-phosphate, are converted to sorbitol by

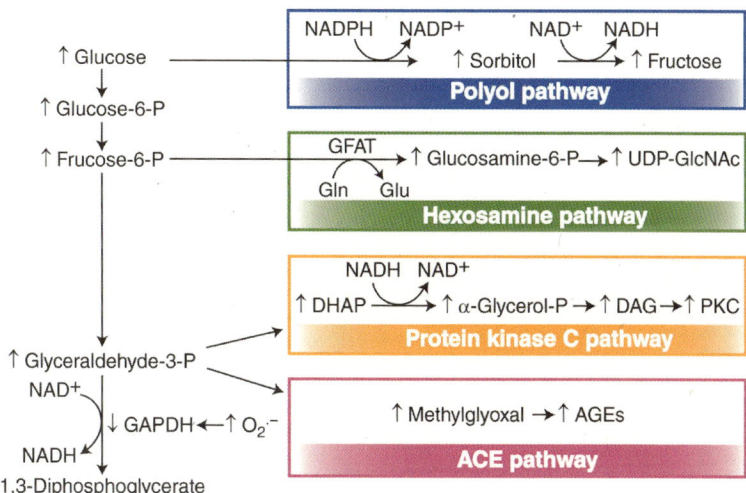

Fig. 2.4 Four pathways of hyperglycemia-induced injury through superoxide overproduction [reprinted from Brownlee M. Biochemistry and molecular cell biology of diabetic complications. Nature. 2001;414(6865):813–20. With permission from Nature Publishing Group]

aldose reductase, which is then oxidized to fructose by sorbitol dehydrogenase (SDH) with NAD$^+$ as a cofactor. Increased ROS increases oxidative stress by consumption of NADPH, a cofactor required for regeneration of reduced glutathione (GSH) and an important scavenger of ROS. The subsequent conversion of sorbitol to fructose generates an additional NADH, further contributing to the overall oxidative state (Fig. 2.4) [18, 22].

Insulin Resistance

Obesity and a sedentary lifestyle are both predisposing factors for the development of insulin resistance and type II DM. In insulin resistance, there is an inadequate response by fat, muscle, and liver cells to insulin stimulation. Independent of hyperglycemia, insulin resistance is a risk factor for atherosclerosis. Insulin resistance in the type II diabetic patient is characterized by decreased insulin production, central stimulation for increased oral intake, increased gluconeogenesis in the liver, decreased uptake by peripheral tissues, and increased lipolysis of adipocytes leading to increased nonesterified fatty acid (NEFA) secretion [25, 26]. NEFA can be deposited in and cause dysfunction of skeletal muscle, liver, and pancreatic β cells, all of which contributes to insulin resistance (Fig. 2.5).

Adipose tissue contributes to insulin resistance by releasing NEFA and pro-inflammatory cytokines, such as tumor necrosis factor-α (TNF-α), interleukin-6 (IL-6), and monocyte chemoattractant protein-1 (MCP-1). Decreased skeletal muscle uptake of glucose is a side effect of insulin resistance and a significant contributor to hyperglycemia in type II DM. Increased intracellular NEFA in skeletal muscle is deleterious by competing with glucose for substrate oxidation and by increasing the intracellular content of fatty acid metabolites such as DAG, fatty acyl-coenzyme A (fatty acyl-CoA), and ceramide. In turn, these can activate a serine/threonine kinase cascade leading to serine/threonine phosphorylation of insulin receptor substrate-1 (IRS-1) and insulin receptor substrate-2 (IRS-2), reducing the ability of these receptors to undergo tyrosine phosphorylation and propagate the normal insulin signal. The downstream target of these receptors is phosphatidylinositol 3-kinase (PI3), which normally mediates insulin's physiologic anti-inflammatory signal by decreasing NF-κb

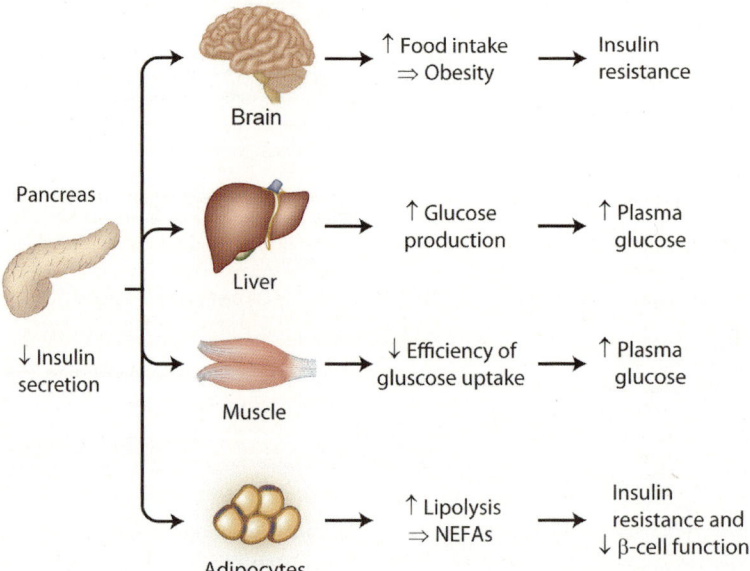

Fig. 2.5 Impaired insulin secretion results in decreased insulin levels and decreased signaling in the hypothalamus, leading to increased food intake and weight gain, decreased inhibition of hepatic glucose production, reduced efficiency of glucose uptake in muscle, and increased lipolysis in the adipocyte, resulting in increased plasma NEFA levels [reprinted from Van Gaal LF, Mertens IL, De Block CE. Mechanisms linking obesity with cardiovascular disease. Nature. 2006;444(7121):875–80. With permission from Nature Publishing Group]

activation, ROS formation, expression of adhesion molecules, and increasing eNOS production [27–29]. PI3 blockade is also associated with decreased uptake of glucose and increased gluconeogenesis in the liver. DAG also has deleterious downstream affects through PKC production. The alternate pathway to PI3, mitogen-activated protein kinase (MAP-kinase), is hyperstimulated when the PI3 pathway is blocked by a compensatory increase in insulin production. This alters insulin's effect from anti-atherogenic to proatherogenic, as unopposed stimulation of the MAP-kinase pathway contributes to vascular hypertrophy, hypertension, increased PAI-1 production, and arrhythmias [28]. Events downstream of insulin-receptor signaling are diminished and the net effect is insulin resistance and diminished uptake of glucose (Fig. 2.6) [30].

The presence of increased adipose tissue is an important contributor to insulin resistance; however it is the distribution of this body fat that plays a key role in determining insulin sensitivity as intraabdominal visceral fat puts one at much higher risk. Even in lean individuals, body fat distribution can markedly affect the degree of insulin resistance if there is increased visceral intraabdominal fat. Mesenteric fat, more than peripheral fat, interferes with insulin's ability to suppress lipolysis leading to higher NEFA production [31–33]. These mesenteric adipocytes tend to be larger and contribute to a proinflammatory environment in DM type II by increasing interferon-γ (IFNγ) expression, macrophage attraction, and upregulation of MCP-1 and NF-κb [29, 34]. Differences in adipocytes, combined with the proximity of the liver to intraabdominal fat, result in greater exposure to NEFAs in liver than in peripheral tissues. In fact, the liver can be insulin resistant at a time when the peripheral tissues are not. Increased delivery of NEFA to the liver also increases gluconeogenesis, as well as production of very low-density lipoprotein (VLDL) [35].

β cells, which contain insulin, are also affected by insulin resistance as they are unable to fully compensate for impaired insulin uptake. β-cell dysfunction can exist in obese individuals with high central fat even in the presence of normoglycemia.

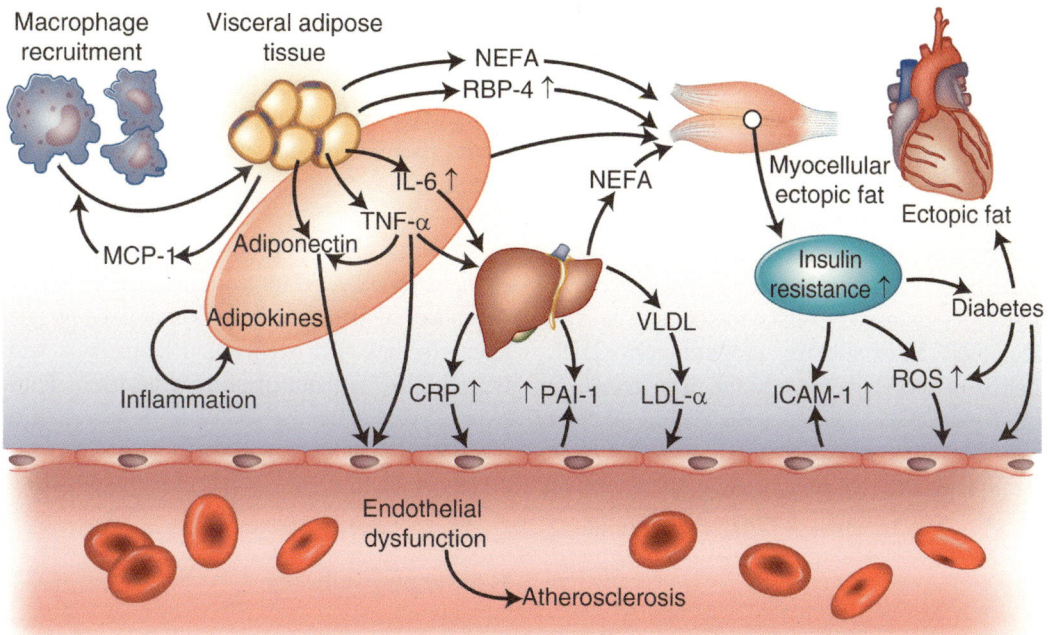

Fig. 2.6 Intraabdominal fat contributes to insulin resistance and cardiovascular dysfunction through cytokine (IL-6, TNF-α, and adiponectin), NEFA and retinol binding protein 4 (RBP-4) production [reprinted from Kahn SE, Hull RL, Utzschneider KM. Mechanisms linking obesity to insulin resistance and type 2 diabetes. Nature. 2006;444(7121):840–6. With permission from Nature Publishing Group]

The β-cell is unable to produce insulin rapidly enough in response to high glucose levels. Insulin resistance further contributes to this effect by NEFA inhibiting insulin mRNA expression and insulin secretion. There are also half as many β cells in type II DM due to hyperglycemia-related toxicity. Impaired insulin secretion leads to decreased signaling in the hypothalamus, leading to increased food intake and weight gain, decreased inhibition of hepatic glucose production, reduced efficiency of glucose uptake in muscle, and increased lipolysis of mesenteric adipocytes with higher NEFA levels. An increase in body weight and NEFA production further contributes to insulin resistance [25].

Hyperlipidemia

The lipid profile generally seen in DM is one of elevated triglycerides, low high-density lipoproteins (HDL), and higher levels of small dense LDL particles. Increased fatty acid transport to the liver stimulates the formation and secretion of VLDL [35]. The enzyme cholesterol ester transfer protein (CETP) catalyzes the transfer of triglycerides from VLDL to HDL in exchange for HDL cholesterol esters. These HDL enriched in triglycerides are an ideal substrate for hepatic lipase, whose activity is augmented in insulin-resistant states and type II DM, leading to increased breakdown of HDL particles. HDL levels are decreased and what HDL remains is functionally impaired, decreasing both its anti-inflammatory and antioxidant properties. Furthermore, glycation of apolipoprotein A-I (ApoA-I), a protein that is integral to the structure and function of HDL, disrupts the lipid–apoprotein interaction causing its disassociation from HDL. ApoA-I is renally excreted and the resultant HDL has reduced receptor binding activity [36–38].

In the presence of insulin resistance LDL levels are unchanged due to decreased production and catabolism. Their uptake is decreased because of a reduction in the number of LDL receptors and their affinity for these receptors. LDL undergoes CETP-mediated exchange of VLDL triglycerides for LDL cholesterol esters. Hydrolysis of triglyceride-rich LDL generates small dense LDL particles that have increased affinity for LDL receptors, preferentially react with intimal proteoglycans, and are more likely to be taken up by macrophages to form foam cells. The proportion of oxidized LDL is also increased in DM due to glycation, increased triglyceride content, and the decreased anti-oxidative properties of HDL. Oxidative modification of LDL also results in rapid uptake by macrophages, leading to foam cell formation, increased cytokine production, and upregulation of cellular adhesion molecules in the endothelium, further contributing to inflammation and atherosclerosis [36, 38].

Endothelin-1

ET-1 is a potent vasoconstrictor that stimulates proliferation of smooth muscle cells and promotes fibrosis and inflammation leading to thrombosis and plaque formation in the vessel wall. ET-1 interacts with two distinct G-protein-coupled receptor subtypes—ET_A and ET_B. The upregulation of ET_A receptors and downregulation of ET_B receptors contribute to vascular dysfunction and atherosclerosis observed in DM [38]. ET_A receptors, which are localized mainly on smooth muscle cells and are responsible for vasoconstriction, proliferation, and ROS formation in response to ET-1. ET_B receptors are located on endothelial cells where they mediate vasodilatation via the release of NO and prostacyclin (PGI_2). Plasma ET-1 levels are elevated in patients with both type I and type II DM. Elevated ET-1 levels have been linked to microalbuminuria and elevated glycosylated hemoglobin (HbA1c).

Platelet Aggregation

Increased platelet aggregation in DM is due to increased systemic production of isoprostanes, including TxA_2, increased responsiveness to platelet-activating factors (PAF) such as epinephrine and ADP, and impaired production of PGI_2 and NO. DM also causes increased glycoprotein expression on the platelet surface, which increases platelet aggregation and platelet interaction with fibrin. Hyperglycemia can also upregulate PKC and generate ROS in platelets causing further dysfunction.

Whereas many of these pathophysiologic changes probably result from the metabolic consequences of insulin resistance, increased platelet reactivity has also been found in patients with type I DM without insulin resistance. Thus, hyperglycemia alone accounts for at least part of the altered platelet response due to AGE-related effects on platelet surface receptors [4, 39, 40].

Hypercoagulability

Independent of platelet dysfunction, diabetes induces a hypercoagulable state. Increased levels of PAI-1 decrease fibrinolytic activity and tissue factor, as well as factors VII and XIII are increased. There is also a relative decrease in antithrombin III and protein C. Many of these abnormalities also correlate with the presence of hyperglycemia and proinsulin split products. Von Willebrand's factor and factor VIII are also both increased, possibly due to endothelial dysfunction (Fig. 2.7) [4, 41].

Response to Injury

Endothelial progenitor cells (EPC) and vascular endothelial growth factor (VEGF) are important components in the vascular response to hypoxia and injury and are both impaired in DM.

Endothelial Progenitor Cells

Vascular injury and tissue ischemia trigger cytokine-mediated release of endothelial progenitor cells (EPC) from bone marrow into the peripheral circulation where they contribute to angiogenesis and repair areas of injured endothelium. Low EPC levels are generally associated

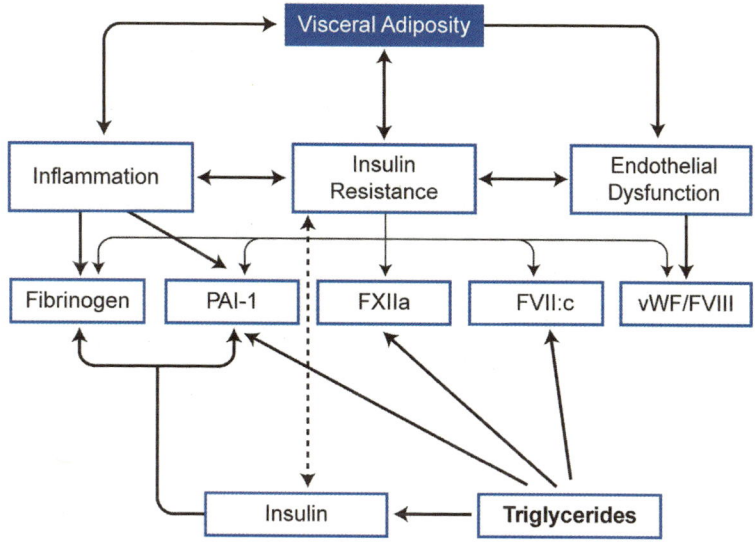

Fig. 2.7 Multifactorial causes of hypercoagulability in diabetes [reprinted from Grant PJ. Diabetes mellitus as a prothrombotic condition. J Intern Med. 2007;262(2):157–72. With permission from John Wiley & Sons, Inc.]

with higher cardiovascular complications and mortality. Tissue ischemia is considered to be the strongest stimulus for EPC release and occurs through activation of hypoxia-inducible pathways particularly upregulation of hypoxia inducible factor (HIF)-1. HIF-1 is a heterodimer consisting of two subunits that dimerizes in the nucleus under hypoxic conditions, which allows it to act as a transcription factor with cofactor p300. The glycolytic metabolite, methylglyoxal, can modify p300, forming an AGE, which decreases HIF-1-mediated gene transactivation. HIF-1 is also decreased due to ROS production and decreased NO. Decreased EPC levels in DM are thought to arise from decreased mobilization, proliferation, and survival as well as functional impairment (Fig. 2.8) [42–44].

Angiogenesis

A key feature of diabetes is poor collateral circulation. Angiography demonstrates fewer collateral vessels in diabetic patients as compared to those without diabetes, which may contribute to a poor outcome after an acute occlusive event and difficulty healing lower extremity wounds. VEGF levels are diminished in the myocardium and lower extremity wounds in DM likely due to inhibition of HIF-1-mediated VEGF expression [20, 44].

Conclusions

Atherosclerosis is a major contributor to the morbidity and mortality observed in DM. The development of atherosclerosis is not only a result of hyperglycemia, but also from the secondary insulin resistance, dyslipidemia, hypercoagulability, altered secretion and function of local regulatory substances, and impaired response to injury. Strict glucose control alone is insufficient and a multifaceted approach targeting all mechanisms is required. A better understanding of these complex pathways is required to improve treatment and outcomes.

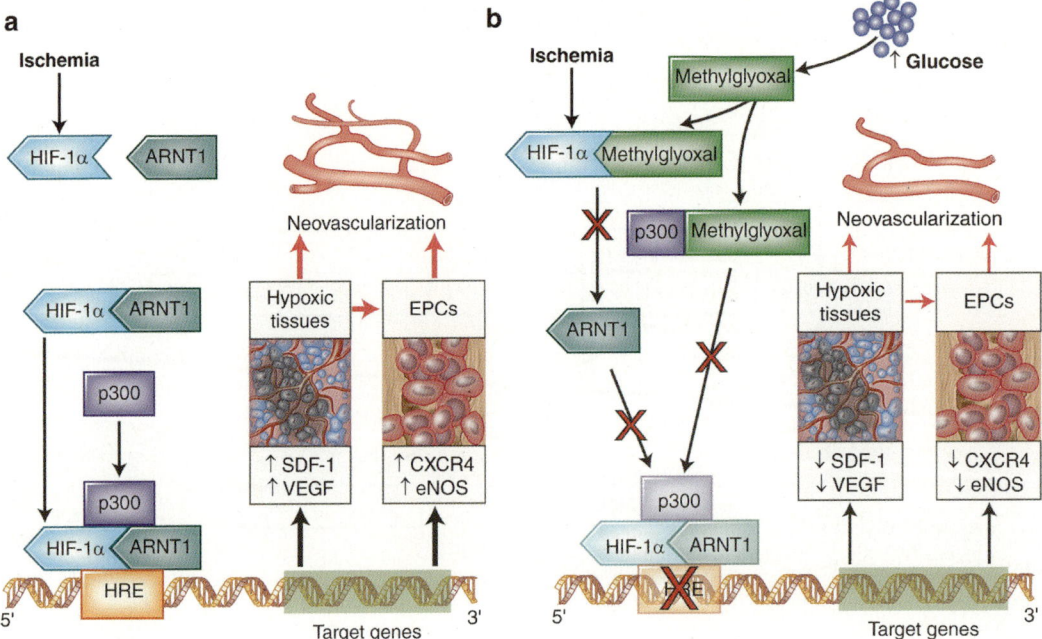

Fig. 2.8 Hyperglycemia inhibits HIF-1 upregulation of genes required for neovascularization [reprinted from Giacco F, Brownlee M. Oxidative stress and diabetic complications. Circ Res. 2010;107(9):1058–70. With permission from Lippincott Williams & Wilkins]

References

1. Nathan DM, Cleary PA, Backlund JY, Genuth SM, Lachin JM, Orchard TJ, et al. Diabetes Control and Complications Trial/Epidemiology of Diabetes Interventions and Complications (DCCT/EDIC) Study Research Group. Intensive diabetes treatment and cardiovascular disease in patients with type 1 diabetes. N Engl J Med. 2005;353(25):2643–53.
2. Faxon DP, Fuster V, Libby P, Beckman JA, Hiatt WR, Thompson RW, et al. American Heart Association. Atherosclerotic vascular disease conference: Writing Group III: pathophysiology. Circulation. 2004;109(21):2617–25.
3. ACCORD Study Group, Gerstein HC, Miller ME, Genuth S, Ismail-Beigi F, Buse JB, et al. Long-term effects of intensive glucose lowering on cardiovascular outcomes. N Engl J Med. 2011;364(9):818–28.
4. Beckman JA, Creager MA, Libby P. Diabetes and atherosclerosis: epidemiology, pathophysiology, and management. JAMA. 2002;287(19):2570–81.
5. Gao Y, Lu B, Sun ML, Hou ZH, Yu FF, Cao HL, et al. Comparison of atherosclerotic plaque by computed tomography angiography in patients with and without diabetes mellitus and with known or suspected coronary artery disease. Am J Cardiol. 2011;108(6):809–13.
6. Mathew V, Gersh BJ, Williams BA, Laskey WK, Willerson JT, Tilbury RT, et al. Outcomes in patients with diabetes mellitus undergoing percutaneous coronary intervention in the current era: a report from the Prevention of REStenosis with Tranilast and its Outcomes (PRESTO) trial. Circulation. 2004;109(4):476–80.
7. Kubal C, Srinivasan AK, Grayson AD, Fabri BM, Chalmers JA. Effect of risk-adjusted diabetes on mortality and morbidity after coronary artery bypass surgery. Ann Thorac Surg. 2005;79(5):1570–6.
8. Carson JL, Scholz PM, Chen AY, Peterson ED, Gold J, Schneider SH. Diabetes mellitus increases short-term mortality and morbidity in patients undergoing coronary artery bypass graft surgery. J Am Coll Cardiol. 2002;40(3):418–23.
9. Jude EB, Oyibo SO, Chalmers N, Boulton AJ. Peripheral arterial disease in diabetic and nondiabetic patients: a comparison of severity and outcome. Diabetes Care. 2001;24(8):1433–7.
10. Paraskevas KI, Baker DM, Pompella A, Mikhailidis DP. Does diabetes mellitus play a role in restenosis and patency rates following lower extremity peripheral arterial revascularization? A critical overview. Ann Vasc Surg. 2008;22(3):481–91. Review.
11. Hamdan AD, Saltzberg SS, Sheahan M, Froelich J, Akbari CM, Campbell DR, et al. Lack of association of diabetes with increased postoperative mortality and

cardiac morbidity: results of 6565 major vascular operations. Arch Surg. 2002;137(4):417–21.
12. Akbari CM, Pomposelli Jr FB, Gibbons GW, Campbell DR, Pulling MC, Mydlarz D, et al. Lower extremity revascularization in diabetes: late observations. Arch Surg. 2000;135(4):452–6.
13. Akbari CM, Pomposelli FB Jr, Gibbons GW, Campbell DR, Freeman DV, LoGerfo FW. Diabetes mellitus: a risk factor for carotid endarterectomy? J Vasc Surg. 1997;25(6):1070–5; discussion 1075–6.
14. Shrikhande GV, Scali ST, da Silva CG, Damrauer SM, Csizmadia E, Putheti P, et al. O-glycosylation regulates ubiquitination and degradation of the anti-inflammatory protein A20 to accelerate atherosclerosis in diabetic ApoE-null mice. PLoS One. 2010;5(12):e14240.
15. Lusis AJ. Atherosclerosis. Nature. 2000;407(6801): 233–41.
16. Virmani R, Burke AP, Kolodgie F. Morphological characteristics of coronary atherosclerosis in diabetes mellitus. Can J Cardiol. 2006;22(Suppl B):81B–4.
17. Deanfield J, Donald A, Ferri C, Giannattasio C, Halcox J, Halligan S, et al. Working Group on Endothelin and Endothelial Factors of the European Society of Hypertension. Endothelial function and dysfunction. Part I: Methodological issues for assessment in the different vascular beds: a statement by the Working Group on Endothelin and Endothelial Factors of the European Society of Hypertension. J Hypertens. 2005;23(1):7–17.
18. Brownlee M. Biochemistry and molecular cell biology of diabetic complications. Nature. 2001; 414(6865):813–20.
19. Suzuki LA, Poot M, Gerrity RG, Bornfeldt KE. Diabetes accelerates smooth muscle accumulation in lesions of atherosclerosis: lack of direct growth-promoting effects of high glucose levels. Diabetes. 2001;50(4):851–60.
20. Giacco F, Brownlee M. Oxidative stress and diabetic complications. Circ Res. 2010;107(9):1058–70.
21. Zou MH, Cohen R, Ullrich V. Peroxynitrite and vascular endothelial dysfunction in diabetes mellitus. Endothelium. 2004;11(2):89–97.
22. Madonna R, De Caterina R. Cellular and molecular mechanisms of vascular injury in diabetes – part II: cellular mechanisms and therapeutic targets. Vascul Pharmacol. 2011;54(3–6):75–9.
23. Du XL, Edelstein D, Rossetti L, Fantus IG, Goldberg H, Ziyadeh F, et al. Hyperglycemia-induced mitochondrial superoxide overproduction activates the hexosamine pathway and induces plasminogen activator inhibitor-1 expression by increasing Sp1 glycosylation. Proc Natl Acad Sci USA. 2000; 97(22):12222–6.
24. Yan SF, Ramasamy R, Schmidt AM. The RAGE axis: a fundamental mechanism signaling danger to the vulnerable vasculature. Circ Res. 2010;106(5):842–53.
25. Kahn SE, Hull RL, Utzschneider KM. Mechanisms linking obesity to insulin resistance and type 2 diabetes. Nature. 2006;444(7121):840–6.
26. Fujimoto WY. The importance of insulin resistance in the pathogenesis of type 2 diabetes mellitus. Am J Med. 2000;108(Suppl 6a):9S–14.
27. Dandona P, Aljada A, Mohanty P, Ghanim H, Hamouda W, Assian E, et al. Insulin inhibits intranuclear nuclear factor kappaB and stimulates IkappaB in mononuclear cells in obese subjects: evidence for an anti-inflammatory effect? J Clin Endocrinol Metab. 2001;86(7):3257–65.
28. Montagnani M, Golovchenko I, Kim I, Koh GY, Goalstone ML, Mundhekar AN, et al. Inhibition of phosphatidylinositol 3-kinase enhances mitogenic actions of insulin in endothelial cells. J Biol Chem. 2002;277(3):1794–9.
29. Muntoni S, Muntoni S. Insulin resistance: pathophysiology and rationale for treatment. Ann Nutr Metab. 2011;58(1):25–36.
30. Dresner A, Laurent D, Marcucci M, Griffin ME, Dufour S, Cline GW, et al. Effects of free fatty acids on glucose transport and IRS-1-associated phosphatidylinositol 3-kinase activity. J Clin Invest. 1999;103(2):253–9.
31. McLaughlin T, Lamendola C, Liu A, Abbasi F. Preferential fat deposition in subcutaneous versus visceral depots is associated with insulin sensitivity. J Clin Endocrinol Metab. 2011;96(11):E1756–60.
32. Steinberg HO, Tarshoby M, Monestel R, Hook G, Cronin J, Johnson A, et al. Elevated circulating free fatty acid levels impair endothelium-dependent vasodilation. J Clin Invest. 1997;100(5):1230–9.
33. Inoguchi T, Li P, Umeda F, Yu HY, Kakimoto M, Imamura M, et al. High glucose level and free fatty acid stimulate reactive oxygen species production through protein kinase C-dependent activation of NAD(P)H oxidase in cultured vascular cells. Diabetes. 2000;49(11):1939–45.
34. Zhang H, Potter BJ, Cao JM, Zhang C. Interferon-gamma induced adipose tissue inflammation is linked to endothelial dysfunction in type 2 diabetic mice. Basic Res Cardiol. 2011;106(6):1135–45.
35. Ginsberg HN. Insulin resistance and cardiovascular disease. J Clin Invest. 2000;106(4):453–8. Review. No abstract available.
36. Vergès B. Lipid modification in type 2 diabetes: the role of LDL and HDL. Fundam Clin Pharmacol. 2009;23(6):681–5.
37. Morgantini C, Natali A, Boldrini B, Imaizumi S, Navab M, Fogelman AM, et al. Anti-inflammatory and antioxidant properties of HDLs are impaired in type 2 diabetes. Diabetes. 2011;60(10):2617–23.
38. Ergul A. Endothelin-1 and diabetic complications: focus on the vasculature. Pharmacol Res. 2011; 63(6):477–82.
39. Vinik AI, Erbas T, Park TS, Nolan R, Pittenger GL. Platelet dysfunction in type 2 diabetes. Diabetes Care. 2001;24(8):1476–85.
40. Capodanno D, Patel A, Dharmashankar K, Ferreiro JL, Ueno M, Kodali M, et al. Pharmacodynamic effects of different aspirin dosing regimens in type 2

diabetes mellitus patients with coronary artery disease. Circ Cardiovasc Interv. 2011;4(2):180–7.
41. Grant PJ. Diabetes mellitus as a prothrombotic condition. J Intern Med. 2007;262(2):157–72.
42. Georgescu A, Alexandru N, Constantinescu A, Titorencu I, Popov D. The promise of EPC-based therapies on vascular dysfunction in diabetes. Eur J Pharmacol. 2011;669(1–3):1–6.
43. Avogaro A, Albiero M, Menegazzo L, de Kreutzenberg S, Fadini GP. Endothelial dysfunction in diabetes: the role of reparatory mechanisms. Diabetes Care. 2011;34 Suppl 2:S285–90.
44. Thangarajah H, Yao D, Chang EI, Shi Y, Jazayeri L, Vial IN, et al. The molecular basis for impaired hypoxia-induced VEGF expression in diabetic tissues. Proc Natl Acad Sci USA. 2009;106(32):13505–10.

Diabetes Mellitus and Peripheral Vascular Disease

Matthew J. Freeby

Keywords

Diabetes mellitus • Hemoglobin A1C • Management • Action in Diabetes and Diamicron Modified Release Controlled Evaluation • Action to Control Cardiovascular Risk in Diabetes • Veterans Affairs Diabetes Trial • Normoglycemia in Intensive Care Evaluation-Survival using Glucose Algorithm Regulation • United Kingdom Prospective Diabetes Study • Diabetes Control and Complications Trial

Diabetes Mellitus and Peripheral Vascular Disease

Diabetes mellitus results when the pancreas is unable to meet insulin requirements to maintain euglycemia. In patients with type 2 diabetes mellitus (T2DM), insulin resistance typically precedes beta cell dysfunction and hyperglycemia. Type 1 diabetes (T1DM) is an autoimmune process whereby insulin-producing beta cells are destroyed leading to insulin deficiency. Diabetes is a common disease—approximately 11.3% of the US population over the age of 20 years has overt hyperglycemia (CDC diabetes fact sheet, 2011). In people over the age of 65 years, almost 27% have diabetes. Even more staggering, approximately 79 million people over the age of 20 years have prediabetes; this makes up 35% of the US population (50% of those over the age of 65 years).

It is not only common, but complications related to its presence can be devastating. Diabetes is associated with cardiovascular disease; there is a two- to fourfold increased risk of cardiac-related death. Hypertension, renal disease, blindness, neuropathy, and depression are also more frequently diagnosed.

Diabetes is also commonly associated with PVD. At least 20–30% of patients with PVD have diabetes [1–3] and it is the most common cause of non-traumatic lower extremity amputation. More than 60% of these amputations occur in people with hyperglycemia. Diabetes duration [4] and poor control [5] increase the risk for peripheral vascular disease. It has been estimated that with every 1% increase in hemoglobin A1C, peripheral vascular disease risk increases by 28%.

M.J. Freeby, M.D. (✉)
Department of Medicine, Columbia University,
1150 St. Nicolas Ave., New York, NY 10032, USA
e-mail: mf2314@columbia.edu

Morbidity and Mortality in Patients with PVD and Diabetes Mellitus

Patients with peripheral vascular disease are at high risk for procedural-related death and comorbid complications. Diabetes mellitus increases risk.

Multiple studies have shown that diabetes can have deleterious effects. In a large study published in 2002, Axelrod et al. assessed vascular surgery outcomes in a Veteran's Administration cohort; a total of 7,871 patients with diabetes were compared to 8,164 patients without diabetes [6]. Patients underwent aortic reconstruction, lower extremity bypass, carotid endarterectomy (CEA), or major amputation between 1997 and 1999. The risk of death was higher in those with diabetes as compared to controls without diabetes (3.9% vs. 2.6%, $P=0.001$). Once adjusted for comorbid conditions, mortality rates were not significantly different. Cardiovascular complications were higher in patients with diabetes (3.3% vs. 2.6%, $P=0.01$), even after adjusting for comorbid conditions. Diabetes diagnosis was found to increase the length of hospital stay by as much as 38%, even after adjusting for comorbidities.

Other studies have also shown negative effects related to diabetes diagnosis, including mortality rates. The New York Carotid Artery Study evaluated 9,308 patients undergoing endarterectomy; patients were at higher risk of death or cardiovascular complication when diabetes was present (odds ratio 1.5, 95% confidence interval 1.10–2.18) [7]. The Vascular Study Group of New England evaluated 2,306 lower extremity bypass procedures by database review; patients with diabetes were at increased risk of death (hazard ratio 1.5; 95% confidence interval 1.1–2.1) [8].

Complication rates may be affected by the type of procedure performed. Recent data suggest that diabetes increases stroke or death in patients receiving CEA, but not carotid artery stenting (CAS) [9]. Parlani et al. evaluated a database of patients undergoing carotid revascularization for primary carotid stenosis from 2001 to 2009. A total of 2,196 procedures (1,116 by CEA and 1,080 by CAS) were performed (average age 71.3 years); 28.7% of subjects were diagnosed with diabetes. It was a predictor of stroke or death rates in the CEA group (odds ratio 2.83; 95% confidence interval 1.05–7.61; $P=0.04$), but not in those undergoing CAS ($P=0.72$). Six-year survival rates were not significantly different between those with and without diabetes mellitus (76.0% versus 80.8%, $P=0.15$).

Diabetes Reduces Successful Revascularization

Diabetes may also reduce the likelihood for successful revascularization. In patients with chronic critical limb ischemia undergoing revascularization, those with diabetes were less likely to have sustained clinical success [10]. After a 1-year follow-up, sustained clinical revascularization was better in patients without diabetes (hazard ratio 0.48; 95% confidence interval 0.29–0.72; $P=0.001$). Additionally, cumulative 1-year mortality trended higher in patients with diabetes (hazard ratio 1.45; 95% confidence interval 0.98–2.17; $P=0.064$).

In a second study, Bakken et al. examined the consequences of endovascular treatment of the superficial femoral artery (SFA) in patients with and without diabetes mellitus [11]. Endovascular treatment (balloon angioplasty ± adjuvant stenting) was performed in 437 patients (525 limbs) in patients averaging 66 years of age. Patients with insulin-dependent diabetes mellitus had lower assisted primary patency ($P<0.01$) and higher incidence of re-stenosis ($P=0.04$). Limb salvage was also significantly worse for patients with diabetes and critical limb ischemia (non-insulin-dependent diabetes, $P=0.01$; insulin-dependent diabetes, $P=0.02$).

The Impact of Diabetes Control on PVD

Complication risk in patients with PVD may also be affected by the level of diabetes control. Dronge and colleagues published a retrospective observational study of 490 patients undergoing major noncardiac surgery between 2000 and 2003 [12]. In addition to patient age, wound class, operative length, and American Society of Anesthesiologists class, preoperative A1C was significantly associated with postoperative infection risk. An A1C of less than 7% was associated with a significant reduction in postoperative infections (odd ratio 2.13; confidence interval 1.23–3.70; $P=0.007$).

Prediabetes Impacts Outcomes in PVD

Prediabetes may also increase comorbidity and death rates in those with PVD. Van Kuijk and colleagues reported an increased risk of death in patients with impaired glucose tolerance (IGT) as compared to their nondiabetic counterparts (hazard ratio 2.06; 95% confidence interval 1.03–4.12) [13]. In this study, 404 patients without known diabetes or glucose intolerance underwent oral glucose tolerance testing (OGTT) prior to vascular surgery. Of the 404 patients studied, 104 were diagnosed with IGT and 43 with overt diabetes. Patients with IGT or diabetes were at higher risk for cardiovascular events (hazard ratio 2.77; 95% confidence interval 1.83–4.20). In a second study evaluating IGT, O'Sullivan and colleagues found higher 30-day mortality rates in patients with A1C levels between 6 and 7% preoperatively compared to those with A1C values less than 6% [14].

Multiple studies have identified diabetes mellitus as an independent risk factor complicating peripheral vascular disease-associated morbidity and mortality. Even more so, mild elevations in glucose, or a prediabetes state may increase complications. By identifying these patients, risk status may be stratified and possibly altered.

Diagnosis

Diabetes diagnosis is clearly defined and likely critical in assessing patients with peripheral vascular disease. Impairments in glucose tolerance increase infection and cardiovascular complication rates; hyperglycemia also reduces rates of successful revascularization. Ensuring diagnosis, and ultimately treatment, may reduce associated risks.

In many instances, the diagnosis of diabetes is clear. A patient will complain of typical diabetes-related symptoms, such as polyuria, polydipsia, and weight loss. Glucose levels may be overtly elevated and a diagnosis can be made. For others, the diagnosis may not be so clear. Endocrine organizations, including the American Diabetes Association (ADA), Endocrine Society, and American Association Clinical Endocrinologists (AACE) have set forth diagnostic guidelines for the diagnosis of diabetes (see Fig. 3.1). Previously, diagnosis was based on plasma glucose levels

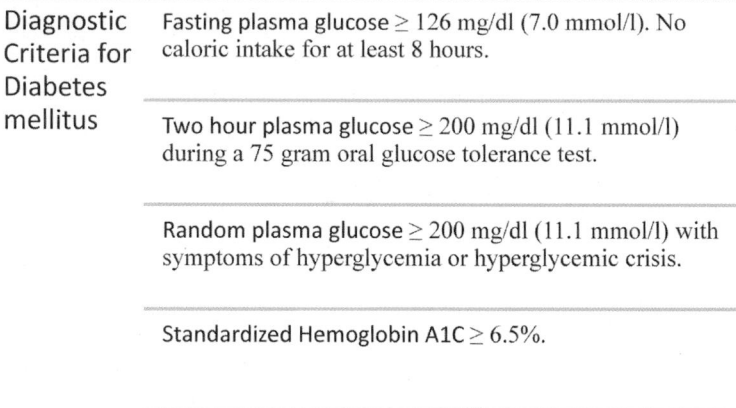

Fig. 3.1 Diabetes diagnostic criteria (adapted from [15, 45])

alone [15]. More recently, a hemoglobin A1C value has been added as a diagnostic tool. At this time, diabetes mellitus is defined by fasting plasma glucose levels (FPG) greater than or equal to 126 mg/dl (7.0 mmol/l) or 2-h plasma glucose levels greater than or equal to 200 mg/dl (11.0 mmol/l) during an oral glucose tolerance test. Diabetes is also diagnosed by random plasma glucose of 200 mg/dl or more in the setting of classic symptoms. In 2009, the ADA, International Diabetes Federation (IDF), and European Association for the Study of Diabetes (EASD) recommended using an A1C of greater than or equal to 6.5% for diabetes diagnosis. For fasting and random glucose values, as well as A1C, testing should be repeated at least once to confirm diagnosis.

The European Society of Cardiology (ESC) and American College of Cardiology (ACC) have made specific recommendations for the patient with peripheral vascular disease undergoing procedure. The ESC recommends screening FPG or OGTT, while the ACC recommends FPG, not OGTT. Whether screened via fasting plasma levels or OGTT, it is important to remember that glucose testing in some form will help to screen subjects at risk.

Diabetes Management

In clinical practice, the vast majority of patients with vascular disease and hyperglycemia have T2DM. Therefore, the management reviewed in this chapter will primarily focus on T2DM. Patients with T1DM are less commonly treated in general practice; it is important to consult a diabetes specialist who can treat patients with T1DM.

Diabetes Therapy in the Outpatient Setting

There are multiple T2DM treatment modalities, including lifestyle modifications, as well as oral and injectable medications. To provide the proper foundation, the ADA recommends that all patients with diabetes undergo self-management education (DMSE) [15]. DMSE has been shown to be an effective tool that equips patients with knowledge and skills to effectively self-manage and cope with day-to-day diabetes-related activities.

In patients with T2DM, the initial therapeutic tool should include dietary and exercise modifications. Patients with diabetes will likely benefit from medical nutrition therapy (MNT). The ADA recommends MNT be provided by a registered dietitian familiar with the components of diabetes [15]. General recommendations include modest weight loss to reduce insulin resistance in those who are overweight or obese. Additionally, a calorie-restricted diet lower in carbohydrates and fat, or a Mediterranean diet may be effective in glycemic control and weight loss. The most proper mix of carbohydrate, protein, and fat should be adjusted to the individual [15]. The benefits of MNT have been studied extensively. Randomized and non-randomized trials have shown clinically significant reductions in A1C values using MNT [16, 17]. In these studies, the average A1C may decrease up to 2% over a 3–6-month period.

In patients without contraindications, exercise is advised. The ADA recommends that patients with T2DM perform at least 150 min/week of moderate-intensity aerobic exercise [15]. In one study, glycemic control improved during an 8-week structured exercise intervention in subjects with T2DM. A1C dropped by an average of 0.66%; body mass index did not change [18]. The American College of Sports Medicine and ADA have copublished a joint position statement summarizing the benefits of exercise in people with T2DM [19].

In patients with T2DM, the EASD and ADA published consensus guidelines for the initiation and adjustment of diabetes therapy [20]. Although patients' needs, comorbidities, and contraindications may vary, the algorithm is a useful guide to treatment. It is likely that many patients with peripheral vascular disease will have contraindications to various diabetes medications; therefore, it may be important to consult a diabetes specialist or physician skilled in diabetes care.

In the majority of patients, dietary and exercise modifications may not be adequate. Medications

Intervention • Examples	A1c Reduction	Benefits	Side Effects	Contraindications
Biguanide • Metformin	1.5%	•No hypoglycemia •No weight gain •CVD events reduction	•GI (diarrhea, bloating, nausea) •Lactic Acidosis	•Renal dysfunction •Decompensated heart failure
Sulfonylurea • Glipizide • Glicazide • Glyburide • Glimepiride	1.5%	•Well-tolerated •Fast-acting	•Hypoglycemia •Weight gain	•Renal dysfunction (glyburide, relative with others) •Liver dysfunction (glyburide, relative with others)
Meglitinides • Repaglinide • Nateglinide	0.5-1.5%	•Well-tolerated •Fast-acting	•Hypoglycemia •Weight gain	•Severe renal impairment •Concurrent gemfibrozil therapy
Insulin • Long-Acting • Short Acting • Mixed-Analogues	1.5-3.5%	•Well-tolerated	•Hypoglycemia •Weight gain	•None
α-Glucosidase Inhibitors • Acarbose • Miglitol	0.5-0.8%	•Non-systemic •Weight neutral	•Gastrointestinal (bloating, flatulence)	•Gastrointestinal impairments (i.e. inflammatory bowel disease or colonic ulceration) •Serum creatinine > 2 mg/dl
Thiazolidinediones (TZDs) • Pioglitazone • Rosiglitazone	0.5-1.4%	•No hypoglycemia •Increase HDL and decrease triglycerides (pioglitazone)	•Weight gain •Heart failure •Bone fracture •Edema •Bladder cancer (Pioglitazone) •Cardiovascular (Rosiglitazone)	•Active liver disease •Class III/IV heart failure •Cardiovascular disease
GLP-1 Agonists • Exenatide • Liraglutide	0.5-1.0%	•Weight loss	•GI (nausea, vomiting) •Acute pancreatitis (possible) •Medullary thyroid cancer in animal models (liraglutide)	•Renal Impairment •Gastroparesis
DPP-4 Inhibitors • Sitagliptin • Saxagliptin • Linagliptin	0.6-0.9%	•No hypoglycemia •Weight neutral	•Acute Pancreatitis •Upper respiratory illness	•Serious hypersensitivity
Amylin Analogue • Pramlintide	0.5-0.7%	•Weight loss	•Gastrointestinal (nausea, vomiting) •Hypoglycemia	•Gastroparesis

Fig. 3.2 Medications used to treat type 2 diabetes mellitus. *GI* gastrointestinal (adapted from [15, 20])

used in the treatment of T2DM are highlighted in Fig. 3.2, including hemoglobin A1C reductions, other benefits, side effects, and contraindications. According to a joint ADA/EASD statement, metformin should be considered as first-line therapy [20]. Metformin is a biguanide; it activates AMP-kinase activity and decreases hepatic glucose output, thereby lowering fasting glucose levels. Since it does not increase insulin production, hypoglycemia is rarely seen in metformin.

Additionally, it has shown some cardiovascular benefit, which was noted in the United Kingdom Prospective Diabetes Study (UKPDS) [21]. As a monotherapy, metformin typically lowers A1C levels by about 1.5% [22]. It is usually well tolerated; gastrointestinal complaints, including nausea, bloating, and diarrhea, are the most common side effects. Contraindications to its use include renal and liver dysfunction, or decompensated heart failure, which may increase the risk for lactic acidosis. Although it is a rare event, lactic acidosis is a potentially fatal complication. In patients undergoing radiologic studies that necessitate the use of contrast, metformin should be held prior to and for 48 h after the study to reduce renal dysfunction risk.

Second-line therapy typically includes sulfonylureas, or insulin. Sulfonylureas include first- (i.e., glyburide) and second-generation (i.e., glipizide, glicazide, and glimepiride) formulations. These medications lower glucose levels by promoting insulin secretion, independent of food intake. A1C levels typically drop by about 1.5% [23]. Sulfonylureas may cause hypoglycemia, which can be severe and prolonged [20]. Although sulfonylureas were initially implicated with increased cardiovascular mortality in the University Group Diabetes Program (UGDP) [24], subsequent studies such as UKPDS 33 and Action in Diabetes and Diamicron Modified Release Controlled Evaluation (ADVANCE) [25, 26] failed to substantiate this earlier research. The meglitinide class of medications is sulfonylurea-like in nature, but binds to separate sites within the sulfonylurea receptor [27]. In turn, meglitinides have a shorter half-life, and may reduce the risk of postprandial hypoglycemia [28]. Examples of these medications include repaglinide and nateglinide; they lower hemoglobin A1C by approximately 1.5%.

Although many patients and health care providers are hesitant to use insulin, the ADA and EASD recommend early implementation in the diabetes care plan. Insulin is administered subcutaneously and can be given in varying formulations that modify its pharmacokinetics, or delivery time. Long-acting insulin (i.e., NPH, glargine, or detemir) is typically used first; shorter-acting insulin analogues (i.e., aspart, glulisine, or lispro) may be used if glucose levels are not well controlled on basal insulin alone. Mixed insulin analogues (i.e., aspart protamine suspension/aspart insulin 70/30 or lispro protamine suspension/lispro insulin 75/25) are a combination of long- and short-acting insulin formulations. Insulin is safe and rapidly effective; it can increase the risk of hypoglycemia.

Other therapies include α-glucosidase inhibitors, thiazolidinediones, glucagon-like peptide-1 agonists, dipeptidyl peptidase-4 (DPP-4) inhibitors, and amylin analogues. These agents are less studied, more expensive, and/or have increased side effects as compared to the medications previously reviewed. When deciding on a regimen, benefits, side effects, contraindications, and patient preference must be taken into account. Therefore, these medications can and should be considered when treating the patient with peripheral vascular disease.

Medications in the class of α-glucosidase inhibitors (i.e., acarbose, miglitol) reduce the rate of polysaccharide digestion in the proximal small intestine and therefore reduce postprandial glucose excursions. They are typically less effective than other medications used in T2DM; A1C levels drop approximately 0.5–0.8% [29]. Although they lack hypoglycemia risk, α-glucosidase inhibitors work by causing malabsorption. Therefore, bloating, gas production, and flatulence are common side effects. Approximately 25–40% of subjects undergoing clinical trials discontinued these medications due to their side effects [30].

Thiazolidinediones (TZDs or glitazones) modulate the peroxisome proliferator-activated receptor-γ (PPAR-γ). TZDs include pioglitazone and rosiglitazone. These medications increase muscle, fat, and liver sensitivity to insulin and appear to have durable effects on glucose control [31]. They typically lower A1C values by approximately 0.5–1.4% [32]. Although TZDs do not increase the risk of hypoglycemia, their side-effect profile may limit use. Side effects include weight gain, fluid retention, peripheral edema, a twofold increased risk of heart failure, and in women, significantly increased fracture risk [20].

Rosiglitazone may increase the risk for myocardial infarction [33], while pioglitazone demonstrated no improvement or worsening of cardiovascular disease in the Prospective Pioglitazone Clinical Trial in Macrovascular Events (PROactive) trial [34]. More recently, long-term pioglitazone use of more than 2 years has been weakly associated with bladder cancer risk [35]. More studies are needed to confirm this risk.

Two classes of medications, glucagon-like peptide-1 (GLP-1) agonists and dipeptidyl peptidase-4 inhibitors, work via the incretin pathway. GLP-1 and gastrointestinal peptide (GIP) are released after ingestion of food products. In people with T2DM, the levels of these hormones are abnormally low. GLP-1 agonists and DPP-4 inhibitors increase GLP-1 and/or GIP levels, and in turn, increase insulin and reduce glucagon levels when food is eaten. GLP-1 agonists (i.e., exenatide and liraglutide) lower A1C levels by 0.5–1% [36], while DPP-4 inhibitors (i.e., linagliptin, saxagliptin, sitagliptin, and vildagliptin) reduce A1C by approximately 0.6–0.9% [37]. Both classes rarely evoke hypoglycemia. GLP-1 agonists can cause gastrointestinal disturbances, including nausea, vomiting, or diarrhea; they are also associated with 2–3 kg weight loss in the first 6 months of use, which is not necessarily related to gastrointestinal side effects. The DPP-4 inhibitors are usually well tolerated. Both medications may be associated with a small risk of acute pancreatitis; GLP-1 agonists may also increase thyroid cancer risk, but further studies are required.

The amylin agonist, pramlintide is a synthetic analogue of the naturally occurring beta cell hormone. Pramlintide has been shown to slow gastric emptying and inhibit glucagon secretion, thereby reducing after meal glucose excursions. It is given subcutaneously and lowers hemoglobin A1C values by 0.5–0.7% [38]. Similar to GLP-1 agonists, pramlintide may cause gastrointestinal side effects such as nausea in approximately 30% of patients; the side effect usually subsides over time. This class of medication may also cause a 1–1.5 kg weight loss over a 6-month period.

Diabetes Mellitus: An Innocent Marker or Modifiable Risk Factor?

Patients with diabetes mellitus are at increased risk for micro- and macrovascular complications [21]. Early studies demonstrated that long-term glucose control reduces microvascular (retinopathy, nephropathy, and neuropathy) complication risk [21, 25]. Macrovascular complications, such as heart attack and stroke, are less correlated but may also be improved by diabetes management [39]. Shorter-term outcomes in patients hospitalized or in the ICU have also been evaluated. Most studies in surgical patients are generalized to multiple specialties.

Diabetes Therapy and Outcomes in the Intensive Care Unit

The majority of data evaluating diabetes treatment in the surgical patient is centered on care received in the ICU. The first, large randomized study was published by Van den Berghe and colleagues in 2001 [40]. The group prospectively randomized 1,548 adults admitted to the surgical ICU who were receiving mechanical ventilation. Patients were randomly assigned to intensive insulin therapy, titrating glucose levels to 80–110 mg/dl (4.4–6.1 mmol/l) versus conventional control. The conventional arm was activated when glucose levels reached greater than 215 mg/dl (11.9 mmol/l); the levels were then titrated to 180–200 mg/dl (10.0–11.1 mmol/l) in this group. If patients required treatment, both arms used intravenous insulin infusion. The results were overwhelmingly in favor of intensive insulin therapy; mortality, infection, ventilatory support, renal impairment or dialysis requirement, and critical illness polyneuropathy demonstrated improved outcomes in those treated to stricter glucose targets. ICU mortality was reduced from 8% in the conventional arm to 4.6% in the intensive arm ($P<0.04$). Overall in-hospital mortality was reduced in the intensive management arm by 34% (10.9% conventional vs. 7.2% intensive, $P=0.01$). The reduction in ICU septicemia was also significantly reduced (7.8% vs. 4.2%, $P=0.03$).

Unfortunately, the findings are have not been corroborated in multiple follow-up studies [41]. The largest trial to date, Normoglycemia in Intensive Care Evaluation-Survival using Glucose Algorithm Regulation (NICE-SUGAR) showed no improvement of intensive treatment as compared to conventional therapy in 6,100 randomly assigned ICU patients [42]. In this mixed study of surgical and medical ICU patients, subjects were randomly assigned to target glucose levels between 81 and 108 mg/dl (4.5–6.0 mmol/l) (intensive treatment) vs. 180 mg/dl (10.0 mmol/l) (conventional treatment). Both treatment groups used intravenous insulin infusion to treat, if required. Approximately 63% of subjects studied were medical ICU patients; 37% were surgical. The results differed from the first Van den Berghe study [40]. Mortality rates at 90 days were higher in the intensively treated group (27.5% vs. 24.9%, $P=0.02$). The treatment effect did not differ for surgical or nonsurgical patients ($P=0.10$). Intensive control did not improve median number days in the ICU or hospital, infection risk, number of days of mechanical ventilation, or renal-replacement therapy. Significant hypoglycemia (glucose ≤ 40 mg/dl, or 2.2 mmol/l) was more common in the intensively treated group (6.8% vs. 0.5%, $P<0.001$). Future research is required to better understand targets and treatment. Recent studies, such as the NICE-SUGAR trial, have tightened glucose control in conventional treatment arms. Therefore, it is important to remember that although recent recommendations have been loosened, intravenous insulin infusion is still recommended at relatively strict glucose targets (threshold > 180 mg/dl, or 10.0 mmol/l) [15].

Diabetes Therapy in the Hospitalized, Non-ICU Patient

In most hospitalized patients, insulin therapy is the mainstay of treatment. Hospitalized patients typically suffer from multiple comorbidities and changes in food intake and health status. Renal dysfunction and cardiac abnormalities are also common. Therefore, oral therapeutics may be contraindicated or suboptimal. Additionally, insulin therapy allows the clinician a method to better adjust to changing glycemic needs and reduce any potential side-effect profile. In those patients requiring insulin therapy, regular insulin sliding scale (RISS) was a commonly used practice in the past. Studies have demonstrated that RISS is inferior to basal–bolus therapy.

In recent studies, hospitalized surgical patients have shown benefits of basal–bolus insulin therapy over conventional insulin sliding scale regimens (RISS). In the *RA*ndomized Study of *B*asal *B*olus Insulin Therapy in the *I*npatient Management of Patients with *T*ype 2 Diabetes (RABBIT-2) trial [43], researchers compared the effects of two insulin regimens on outcomes in patients hospitalized for general surgery procedures. In this multicenter randomized study of 211 general surgery patients, the authors compared postoperative complications and safety of basal–bolus insulin glargine and glulisine to regular insulin sliding scale. Mean glucose levels were reduced in the basal–bolus regimen compared to RISS (145 ± 32 mg/dl vs. 172 ± 47 mg/dl, $P<0.01$). More importantly, there were improvements in the composite outcome (postoperative wound infection, pneumonia, bacteremia, and respiratory and acute renal failure) with basal–bolus insulin therapy (RISS 24.3% vs. basal–bolus therapy 8.6%, $P=0.003$). Although hypoglycemia frequency, as defined by glucose < 70 mg/dl, was increased in basal–bolus therapy, there were no differences in significant hypoglycemia.

Recommendations

Management Goals in Nonhospitalized Patients

Glycemic goals for patients with diabetes are now based on a combination of glucose levels and comorbid conditions. The UKPDS and Diabetes Control and Complications Trial (DCCT) were pivotal studies published in the late

Glycemic Targets for the Non-Hospitalized Patient with Diabetes Mellitus	Hemoglobin A1C < 7% (ADA) or < 6.5% (AACE)*
	Preprandial capillary plasma glucose 70-130 mg/dl (ADA) or < 110 mg/dl (AACE)*
	Peak postprandial capillary plasma glucose < 180 mg/dl (ADA) or < 140 mg/dl (AACE)*

Fig. 3.3 Glycemic targets in nonhospitalized patients. *Asterisk*: Goals should be individualized to cardiovascular disease, comorbid conditions, reduced life expectancy, and individual patient considerations. (*AACE* American Association of Clinical Endocrinologists, *ADA* American Diabetes Association) (adapted from [15, 45, 49])

1990s and early 2000s that formed the basis of treatment guidelines [21, 25, 44]. In short, improved A1C values reduce microvascular complication risk; cardiovascular disease is reduced over longer periods in patients with T1DM. Expert committees representing the ADA and AACE (American Association of Clinical Endocrinologists) publish guidelines annually. Figure 3.3 represents the latest outpatient guidelines for diabetes therapy [15, 45]. Generally, hemoglobin A1C is targeted to less than 7% (or 6.5% AACE), but should be individualized to each patient (Level of Evidence B). For patients with cardiovascular disease, shortened life expectancy, advanced microvascular complications, or hypoglycemia unawareness, less stringent glycemic targets may be more appropriate [15].

The recommendations for individualized care have been updated in recent years because of findings in large randomized trials. The results of the Action to Control Cardiovascular Risk in Diabetes (ACCORD) trial altered targets for patients with cardiovascular disease [46]. In the ACCORD trial, 10,251 patients with diabetes between the ages of 40 and 79 years with history of a cardiovascular event or significant cardiovascular risk were randomized to treatment. Glucose levels were targeted to standard therapy (A1C 7–7.9%) or intensive glucose control (A1C<6%). In this trial, subjects attained hemoglobin A1C levels of 6.4% and 7.5% for intensive and standard therapy, respectively. The study was halted early due to an increased rate of mortality in the intensive treatment arm (1.41% vs. 1.14% per year; 257 vs. 203 deaths over a 3.5-year follow-up, $P=0.04$). There was a nonsignificant reduction in the primary outcome (nonfatal myocardial infarction, stroke, or cardiovascular death) in the intensively treated subjects compared to the conventional arm (hazard ratio 0.90; 95% confidence interval 0.78–1.04, $P=0.16$). This was primarily due to a reduction in nonfatal myocardial infarctions in those treated intensively. Exploratory analyses were unable to find an explanation for the increased mortality risk.

Other studies, such as the ADVANCE and Veteran Affairs Diabetes Trial (VADT), also showed no significant reduction in cardiovascular outcomes with intensive glucose control [26, 47]. These trials targeted hemoglobin A1C levels to less than 6 or 6.5% in their intensive arms versus 7–8.5% for conventional treatment. The ADVANCE trial demonstrated no significant reduction in macrovascular events for those treated to A1C targets of ≤6.5% versus a standard glucose-lowering strategy (hazard ratio 0.94, 95% confidence interval 0.84–1.06; $P=0.32$). Total events (micro- or macrovascular) were greater in the standard control group as compared to the intensively treated group (hazard ratio 0.90; 95% confidence interval; $P=0.013$). In the VADT, 1,791 military veterans (mean age, 60.4 years) with T2DM were randomly assigned to intensive or standard glucose control [47]. After a median 5.6-year follow-up, median A1C levels were 8.4% in the standard care group and 6.9% in those intensively treated. The primary outcome of VADT was first occurrence of a major cardiovascular event or surgery for vascular disease. There was no statistically significant difference between the groups for primary outcome (hazard ratio 0.88; 95% confidence interval 0.74–1.05; $P=0.14$).

Due to these most recent studies, hemoglobin A1C levels for patients with known cardiovascular disease, or at high risk for cardiovascular disease, should be targeted individually [15]. It is important to remember that microvascular event rates are reduced by intensive glucose management. Cardiovascular events and hypoglycemia may increase with strict control.

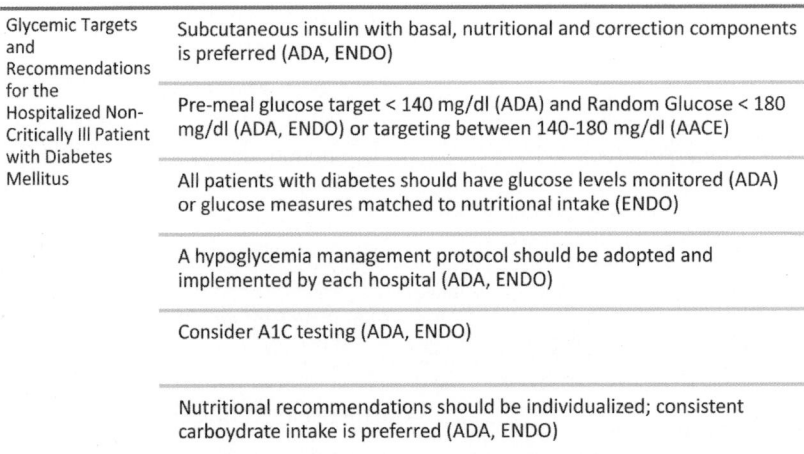

Fig. 3.4 Recommendations for diabetes care in the hospital (*AACE* American Association of Clinical Endocrinologists, *ADA* American Diabetes Association, *ENDO* Endocrine Society) (adapted from [15, 45, 50])

Management Goals for the Hospitalized Patient with Diabetes Mellitus

Guidelines are also published for the patient hospitalized in the ICU [15]. Insulin therapy should be initiated at glucose thresholds of no greater than 180 mg/dl (10.0 mmol/l) based on recent studies (Level of Evidence A). Once insulin therapy is started, a glucose range of 140–180 mg/dl (7.8–10.0 mmol/l) is targeted (Level of Evidence A). In selected patient populations, more stringent goals (glucose target 110–140 mg/dl or 6.1–7.8 mmol/l) may be appropriate, if significant hypoglycemia is prevented (Level of Evidence C). Additionally, it is recommended that physicians and hospitals use intravenous insulin protocols that have demonstrated efficacy and safety in achieving the desired glucose targets (Level of Evidence E).

For non-critically ill patients, less specific recommendations are provided; there is not a strong body of evidence for specific glucose targets in this population [15]. It is recommended that premeal glucose targets are generally less than 140 mg/dl (7.8 mmol/l) with random glucose less than 180 mg/dl (10.0 mmol/l) (Level of Evidence E) or between 140 and 180 mg/dl [45]. Glucose targets can be more or less stringent based on patient stability and comorbidities. Figure 3.4 outlines recommendations for diabetes therapy in the hospitalized non-critically ill patient. In addition to specific targets, glucose monitoring should be initiated immediately for patients known to have diabetes or who might be at higher risk (Level of Evidence B). Patients should receive scheduled subcutaneous insulin with basal, nutritional, and correction components (basal–bolus therapy) and be monitored for hypoglycemia. Hospital systems should have hypoglycemia management protocols in place. Medical nutrition therapy should be individualized to the patient to provide adequate calories to meet metabolic demands. Therefore, a specific meal plan is not endorsed; carbohydrate consistency is preferred to facilitate diabetes treatment with prandial insulin. Finally, hospitalized patients with diabetes should be managed by an individual who has been appropriately trained. Specialists trained in diabetes may reduce hospital stay, improve glycemic control, and improve outcomes [48].

Diabetes mellitus is a common finding in the patient with peripheral vascular disease. It is important to consider diagnosis and the implications for care in all patients being treated in the clinic or hospital, especially those with PVD.

References

1. Hirsch AT, et al. Peripheral arterial disease detection, awareness, and treatment in primary care. JAMA. 2001;286(11):1317–24.
2. Beks PJ, et al. Peripheral arterial disease in relation to glycaemic level in an elderly Caucasian population: the Hoorn study. Diabetologia. 1995;38(1):86–96.
3. Marso SP, Hiatt WR. Peripheral arterial disease in patients with diabetes. J Am Coll Cardiol. 2006;47(5): 921–9.
4. Adler AI, et al. UKPDS 59: hyperglycemia and other potentially modifiable risk factors for peripheral vascular disease in type 2 diabetes. Diabetes Care. 2002;25(5):894–9.
5. Selvin E, et al. Meta-analysis: glycosylated hemoglobin and cardiovascular disease in diabetes mellitus. Ann Intern Med. 2004;141(6):421–31.
6. Axelrod DA, et al. Perioperative cardiovascular risk stratification of patients with diabetes who undergo elective major vascular surgery. J Vasc Surg. 2002;35(5):894–901.
7. Halm EA, et al. Risk factors for perioperative death and stroke after carotid endarterectomy: results of the new york carotid artery surgery study. Stroke. 2009;40(1):221–9.
8. Goodney PP, et al. Factors associated with death 1 year after lower extremity bypass in Northern New England. J Vasc Surg. 2010;51(1):71–8.
9. Parlani G, et al. Diabetes is not a predictor of outcome for carotid revascularization with stenting as it may be for carotid endarterectomy. J Vasc Surg. 2012;55(1): 79–89.
10. Dick F, et al. Surgical or endovascular revascularization in patients with critical limb ischemia: influence of diabetes mellitus on clinical outcome. J Vasc Surg. 2007;45(4):751–61.
11. Bakken AM, et al. Impact of diabetes mellitus on outcomes of superficial femoral artery endoluminal interventions. J Vasc Surg. 2007;46(5):946–58; discussion 958.
12. Dronge AS, et al. Long-term glycemic control and postoperative infectious complications. Arch Surg. 2006;141(4):375–80; discussion 380.
13. van Kuijk JP, et al. Preoperative oral glucose tolerance testing in vascular surgery patients: long-term cardiovascular outcome. Am Heart J. 2009;157(5):919–25.
14. O'Sullivan CJ, et al. Haemoglobin A1c (HbA1C) in non-diabetic and diabetic vascular patients. Is HbA1C an independent risk factor and predictor of adverse outcome? Eur J Vasc Endovasc Surg. 2006; 32(2):188–97.
15. American Diabetes Association. Standards of medical care in diabetes – 2011. Diabetes Care. 2011;34 Suppl 1:S11–61.
16. Gaetke LM, Stuart MA, Truszczynska H. A single nutrition counseling session with a registered dietitian improves short-term clinical outcomes for rural Kentucky patients with chronic diseases. J Am Diet Assoc. 2006;106(1):109–12.
17. Franz MJ, et al. Effectiveness of medical nutrition therapy provided by dietitians in the management of non-insulin-dependent diabetes mellitus: a randomized, controlled clinical trial. J Am Diet Assoc. 1995;95(9):1009–17.
18. Boule NG, et al. Effects of exercise on glycemic control and body mass in type 2 diabetes mellitus: a meta-analysis of controlled clinical trials. JAMA. 2001;286(10):1218–27.
19. Colberg SR, et al. Exercise and type 2 diabetes: the American College of Sports Medicine and the American Diabetes Association: joint position statement. Diabetes Care. 2010;33(12):e147–67.
20. Nathan DM, et al. Medical management of hyperglycemia in type 2 diabetes: a consensus algorithm for the initiation and adjustment of therapy: a consensus statement of the American Diabetes Association and the European Association for the Study of Diabetes. Diabetes Care. 2009;32(1):193–203.
21. Effect of intensive blood-glucose control with metformin on complications in overweight patients with type 2 diabetes (UKPDS 34). UK Prospective Diabetes Study (UKPDS) Group. Lancet. 1998;352(9131):854–65.
22. Bailey CJ, Turner RC. Metformin. N Engl J Med. 1996;334(9):574–9.
23. Groop LC. Sulfonylureas in NIDDM. Diabetes Care. 1992;15(6):737–54.
24. The University Group Diabetes Program. A study of the effects of hypoglycemic agents on vascular complications in patients with adult-onset diabetes. V. Evaluation of pheniformin therapy. Diabetes. 1975;24(Suppl 1):65–184.
25. Intensive blood-glucose control with sulphonylureas or insulin compared with conventional treatment and risk of complications in patients with type 2 diabetes (UKPDS 33). UK Prospective Diabetes Study (UKPDS) Group. Lancet. 1998;352(9131):837–53.
26. Patel A, et al. Intensive blood glucose control and vascular outcomes in patients with type 2 diabetes. N Engl J Med. 2008;358(24):2560–72.
27. Malaisse WJ. Pharmacology of the meglitinide analogs: new treatment options for type 2 diabetes mellitus. Treat Endocrinol. 2003;2(6):401–14.
28. Damsbo P, et al. A double-blind randomized comparison of meal-related glycemic control by repaglinide and glyburide in well-controlled type 2 diabetic patients. Diabetes Care. 1999;22(5):789–94.
29. Van de Laar FA, et al. Alpha-glucosidase inhibitors for type 2 diabetes mellitus. Cochrane Database Syst Rev. 2005;(2):CD003639.
30. Chiasson JL, et al. Acarbose treatment and the risk of cardiovascular disease and hypertension in patients with impaired glucose tolerance: the STOP-NIDDM trial. JAMA. 2003;290(4):486–94.
31. Kahn SE, et al. Glycemic durability of rosiglitazone, metformin, or glyburide monotherapy. N Engl J Med. 2006;355(23):2427–43.

32. Yki-Jarvinen H. Thiazolidinediones. N Engl J Med. 2004;351(11):1106–18.
33. Singh S, Loke YK, Furberg CD. Long-term risk of cardiovascular events with rosiglitazone: a meta-analysis. JAMA. 2007;298(10):1189–95.
34. Dormandy JA, et al. Secondary prevention of macrovascular events in patients with type 2 diabetes in the PROactive Study (PROspective pioglitAzone Clinical Trial In macroVascular Events): a randomised controlled trial. Lancet. 2005;366(9493):1279–89.
35. Lewis JD, et al. Risk of bladder cancer among diabetic patients treated with pioglitazone: interim report of a longitudinal cohort study. Diabetes Care. 2011;34(4):916–22.
36. Buse JB, et al. Effects of exenatide (exendin-4) on glycemic control over 30 weeks in sulfonylurea-treated patients with type 2 diabetes. Diabetes Care. 2004;27(11):2628–35.
37. Raz I, et al. Efficacy and safety of the dipeptidyl peptidase-4 inhibitor sitagliptin as monotherapy in patients with type 2 diabetes mellitus. Diabetologia. 2006;49(11):2564–71.
38. Riddle M, et al. Pramlintide improved glycemic control and reduced weight in patients with type 2 diabetes using basal insulin. Diabetes Care. 2007;30(11):2794–9.
39. Nathan DM, et al. Intensive diabetes treatment and cardiovascular disease in patients with type 1 diabetes. N Engl J Med. 2005;353(25):2643–53.
40. van den Berghe G, et al. Intensive insulin therapy in the critically ill patients. N Engl J Med. 2001;345(19):1359–67.
41. Wiener RS, Wiener DC, Larson RJ. Benefits and risks of tight glucose control in critically ill adults: a meta-analysis. JAMA. 2008;300(8):933–44.
42. Finfer S, et al. Intensive versus conventional glucose control in critically ill patients. N Engl J Med. 2009;360(13):1283–97.
43. Umpierrez GE, et al. Randomized study of basal-bolus insulin therapy in the inpatient management of patients with type 2 diabetes undergoing general surgery (RABBIT 2 surgery). Diabetes Care. 2011;34(2):256–61.
44. The effect of intensive treatment of diabetes on the development and progression of long-term complications in insulin-dependent diabetes mellitus. The Diabetes Control and Complications Trial Research Group. N Engl J Med. 1993;329(14):977–86.
45. Handelsman Y, et al. American Association of Clinical Endocrinologists Medical Guidelines for Clinical Practice for developing a diabetes mellitus comprehensive care plan. Endocr Pract. 2011;17 Suppl 2:1–53.
46. Gerstein HC, et al. Effects of intensive glucose lowering in type 2 diabetes. N Engl J Med. 2008;358(24):2545–59.
47. Duckworth W, et al. Glucose control and vascular complications in veterans with type 2 diabetes. N Engl J Med. 2009;360(2):129–39.
48. Moghissi ES, et al. American Association of Clinical Endocrinologists and American Diabetes Association consensus statement on inpatient glycemic control. Diabetes Care. 2009;32(6):1119–31.
49. Vigersky RA. A review and critical analysis of professional societies' guidelines for pharmacologic management of type 2 diabetes mellitus. Curr Diab Rep. 2012;12(3):246–54.
50. Umpierrez GE, et al. Management of hyperglycemia in hospitalized patients in non-critical care setting: an endocrine society clinical practice guideline. J Clin Endocrinol Metab. 2012;97(1):16–38.

Diabetic Neuropathy

4

Francesco Tecilazich, Thanh L. Dinh, and Aristidis Veves

Keywords

Diabetes mellitus • Diabetic chronic complications • Pathogenesis • Peripheral neuropathy • Autonomic neuropathy • Diabetic neuropathy diagnosis • Diabetic neuropathy management

Introduction

Diabetic neuropathy is a chronic and devastating complication of diabetes mellitus (DM), characterized by the progressive loss of somatic and autonomic nerve fibers [1]. Diabetic neuropathy (DN) is the most common peripheral neuropathy in the Western world and leads to significant morbidity and impact on quality of life of patients. As the nervous system is the most dependent tissue on glucose and oxygen, DM can potentially affect any part of the nervous system.

Epidemiology

As the Western lifestyle has spread globally, DM type 2 (T2DM) has become an epidemic [2]. Furthermore, it is estimated that by 2025, 400 million subjects worldwide will be affected by DM with a prevalence projected of 4.4% [3]. Since diabetic neuropathy affects approximately 30–50% of all the diabetic patients, it is reasonable to assume that there will be a subordinate dramatic increase also of diabetic neuropathy. Diabetic peripheral neuropathy (DPN) is the most frequent neurological complication of DM and the most common form of neuropathy in the developed world [4]. It is usually referred to as diabetic neuropathy since at least 50% of patients with DM have clinically manifest DPN. Diabetic neuropathy accounts for more admissions to the hospital than all the other complications of DM combined together. Diabetic neuropathy is the principal key factor in the pathogenesis of foot ulcerations and wound healing impairment in subjects with DM. In the United States alone, diabetic foot ulcerations are responsible annually of 65,000 amputations, representing a total cost of 4 billion dollars per year [5].

F. Tecilazich, M.D. • A. Veves, M.D., M.Sc., D.Sc. (✉)
Microcirculation Lab, Joslin Beth Israel Deaconess Foot Center, Harvard Medical School, 1 Deaconess Rd., Boston, MA 02215, USA
e-mail: aveves@bidmc.harvard.edu

T.L. Dinh, D.P.M.
Division of Podiatry, Beth Israel Deaconess Medical Center, Harvard Medical School, Boston, MA, USA

The incidence and prevalence of neuropathy in T1 and T2 DM is difficult to compare. The Diabetes Control and Complication Trial (DCCT) and the United Kingdom Prospective Diabetes Study (UKPDS) used different time intervals and methods for defining neuropathy. In the DCCT neuropathy was defined as abnormal nerve conduction in at least two nerves. According to this definition 15–30% of subjects with well-controlled DM developed neuropathy after 5 years (vs. 40–52% of standard care patients) [6]. In contrast, in the UKPDS neuropathy was defined as abnormal biothesiometer readings in both toes. 19% of patients with tightly controlled DM presented these alterations after 6 years (vs. 21% of standard care treated patients) [7]. Finally, data on impaired fasting glycemia (IFG) are controversial and therefore it is not possible to determine if this dysglycemia increases the risk of diabetic sensory or autonomic neuropathies [8–10].

Pathophysiology

Neurons require constant glucose supply in order to fulfill their requirements and their glucose uptake depends on the extracellular glucose concentration. Chronic hyperglycemia leads to neuropathy by determining intraneuronal hyperglycemia, and secondary glucose neurotoxicity responsible of neuronal damage. The molecular mechanisms responsible for glucose neurotoxicity include polyol pathway abnormalities, nonenzymatic glycation, activation of protein kinase C (PKC), and oxidative stress as possible mediators.

Polyol Pathway Abnormalities

Abnormally high concentrations of glucose cause the glucose to enter the polyol (sorbitol) pathway. In the first of the two reactions, aldose-reductase (AR) catalyzes the reduction of glucose to sorbitol. Since Hexokinase has higher affinity for glucose than AR, in the peripheral nerves minor amounts of glucose are converted to sorbitol while most of it is phosphorylated to glucose-6-phosphate. The second reaction is the oxidation of sorbitol to fructose by the enzyme sorbitol dehydrogenase. In the presence of high glucose concentrations, substantial amounts of sorbitol are synthesized since hexokinase becomes quickly saturated. This happens prototypically in the peripheral nerves due to the insulin-independent uptake of glucose [11]. Because of sorbitol's low plasma-membrane permeability, the polyol pathway activation therefore results in an intraneuronal increase of sorbitol (with subsequent direct tissue toxicity or osmotic stress), fructose (which is a ten times more potent glycation agent than glucose), and reactive oxygen species. Of note, AR utilizes NADPH as a cofactor and this will no longer be available as a reducing equivalent for synthesizing nitric oxide and recycling glutathione. The latter reaction is catalyzed by glutathione disulfide reductase which uses reducing equivalents from NADPH to reconvert glutathione to reduced glutathione, the depletion of which causes an increased risk of oxidative stress [12]. The reduced bioavailability of nitric oxide is instead considered an important key factor of endoneural hypoxia, an important and early pathogenic factor in diabetic neuropathy [13].

Nonenzymatic Glycation

Nonenzymatic glycation of proteins exposed to high glucose concentrations determines the formation of the advanced glycosylated end-products (AGEs). Simplifying, the first reaction of this reactions is the formation of a Schiff base by direct addition of open-chain glucose to the lysine groups on proteins. This Schiff base then undergoes a slow, spontaneous Amadori rearrangement to form a stable product, the AGE. These aberrant molecules alter the structure and function of intra- and extracellular proteins by forming covalent cross-links; AGE also induce cellular responses by binding to their receptors (RAGE), localized in the peripheral nerve, both on the endothelial and the Schwann cells [14]. Increased AGE levels are known to be responsible for the increased vascular permeability of diabetes.

[15]. In animal models of DM the prevention of AGE accumulation, with drugs such as aminoguanidine, reduced the development of DN. Several clinical studies support the role of glycation in the pathogenesis of diabetic neuropathy and other diabetic complications. [16, 17] Moreover, a bioptic study showed that AGE was localized to the endoneurium, perineurium and microvessels in diabetic subjects with DN. Interestingly, the loss of axons correlated with intensity of the axonal AGE expression. [18]

Oxidative Stress

Oxidative stress results from an imbalance between the production and the endogenous neutralization of reactive oxygen species (ROS) [19]. ROS are generated from the electron transport chains in the mitochondria and by activated phagocytes, but the mechanisms underlying the increased levels of ROS and the impaired activity of oxidant scavengers (such as superoxide dismutase) in DM are multifold and not completely understood [19]. Increased ROS levels lead to increased peroxidation of lipid membranes, proteins, and DNA with alteration of cellular function and structure. Oxidative stress causes a series of changes in endothelial cell function and gene expression in diabetes, contributing to the development of its neuropathic complications. In addition, oxidative stress increases the levels of endothelin-1 via increase of nuclear factor-κB and angiotensin II by upregulating the renin–angiotensin system. These two molecules are potent vasoconstrictors and possible cofactors to the decreased nerve blood flow, and subsequent endoneurial hypoxia, that contributes to functional and morphological nerve changes in both patients and animal models [13, 20].

Protein Kinase C

PKC includes a superfamily of isoenzymes that includes approximately ten isoforms. These cytoplasmic kinases are key players in intercellular signal transduction for hormones and cytokines, and their activation results in the phosphorylation of intracellular proteins. Elevated glucose concentrations have been shown to increase the activation in particular of PKCβ. PKCβ is in fact preferentially expressed in vascular endothelial cells exposed to hyperglycemia or free fatty acids and is activated in animal models of diabetes. PKC is thought to contribute to DN by a neurovascular mechanism and thereby impairing the nerve blood flow and conduction velocity. However its role in endothelial function remains controversial, since there is contradicting evidence on its role in the pathogenesis of vascular dysfunction in patients with type 2 diabetes. Some authors reported that inhibition of PKCβ determined improvement of the vascular function in both the micro- and macrocirculations; others showed instead that the same inhibition did not affect the endothelium-dependent vasodilation in T2DM. [21–24]

Classification

DN can either be classified according to its clinical presentation or to the underlying pathogenic mechanisms. In this chapter we will describe the two more used clinical classifications. The first was suggested by Watkins and schematically distinguishes diabetic neuropathies in three groups based both on their natural course and on their relationship with duration and control of DM [25]. The first is the gradually progressive group, that includes sensory and autonomic neuropathies and in which severity is related to duration of disease. The second group is the remissive one and includes mononeuropathies, radiculopathies, and the acute painful neuropathies. These neuropathies have an acute onset and are not related to duration of DM. Finally, the third group is represented by the pressure palsies, more frequent but not specific to DM and that are not associated to the duration of DM.

Another very useful and used classification was initially proposed by Bruyn and Garland [26]. This classification distinguishes the patient's clinical involvement in symmetrical or asymmetrical (Table 4.1). Subsequently, Low and Suarez

Table 4.1 Classification of diabetic neuropathy

Symmetrical neuropathies
Distal sensory and sensory-motor neuropathy
Large fiber neuropathy
Small fiber neuropathy
Chronic inflammatory demyelinating polyradiculopathy
Asymmetrical neuropathies
Proximal asymmetric mononeuropathy (or diabetic amyotrophy)
Nerve entrapment syndromes
Truncal radiculopathy
Cranial mononeuropathy
Chronic inflammatory demyelinating polyradiculopathy

have modified this classification as it can be oversimplifying since the syndromes tend to overlap [27]. According to this classification, diabetic neuropathy is subcategorized in seven major types: distal symmetric polyneuropathy, proximal asymmetric mononeuropathy (or diabetic amyotrophy), nerve entrapment syndromes, truncal radiculopathy, cranial mononeuropathy, chronic inflammatory demyelinating polyradiculopathy, and autonomic neuropathy.

Distal Symmetrical Neuropathy

Distal symmetrical neuropathy can be either sensory or motor and may involve small or large fibers [28]. Most of the patients generally present with symmetrical distal sensory-motor polyneuropathy, and they frequently present both small and large fiber neuropathy, as they belong to the spectrum of the same condition. Clinically, peripheral sensory neuropathy manifests as pain, numbness, and reduced touch and vibration sensation, especially at the limbs, in a stocking distribution. Motor neuropathy causes atrophy of the intrinsic muscles of the foot (so-called "intrinsic minus foot").

Small Fiber Neuropathy

Small fiber neuropathy generally is a painful neuropathy that occurs in the early stages of DM. Initially the clinic presentation is dominated by C-fiber type pain and allodynia and cramps, and later substituted by hypoalgesia and impaired warm thermal perception, associated with defective autonomic function (postural hypotension, gastrointestinal symptoms, and erectile dysfunction). Even though not all patients suffer from pain, most patients refer to different types of diabetic neuropathic pain, such as tingling, burning, prickling, shooting, and also aching pain. Diabetic neuropathic pain may also present nocturnal exacerbation, sometimes interfering with the patient's ability to rest and therefore causing sleep deprivation. Some patients present with late-onset restless leg syndrome. Patients may also have distal and "length-dependent" symptoms, like numbness "tightness" and "coldness". However, these symptoms can also be patchy or asymmetrical.

Muscle strength and reflexes are preserved. Electrophysiologically, the sensory conduction velocity may be normal with reduced amplitude, while the motor is less affected. It is classified as acute or chronic painful neuropathy, based on the presence of pain for less or more than 6 months, respectively. Histologically, there is loss of nerve fibers staining with PGP 9.5 in the skin; however, only rarely the medical examination and the electromyography (EMG) are positive for signs of nerve damage.

Large Fiber Neuropathy

Large fibers are myelinated and rapidly conducting fibers that serve motor function, vibration perception, position sense, and cold thermal sensation. The first clinical sign of large fiber neuropathy is impairment in the vibration perception, followed by Aδ-type pain (dull sensation, eventually cramp-like). The clinical picture will also show depressed tendon reflexes and pes equinus (due to shortening of the Achilles tendon) with atrophy of the intrinsic muscles of the foot. Large fibers tend to be affected first in DM because of their length, and even though the symptoms are generally minimal, the electromyography abnormalities are readily detected.

The differential diagnosis of DPN can be challenging. Neuropathy can be also secondary to other metabolic diseases, such as amyloidosis, uremia, and porphyria; vitamin deficiencies, such as B1, B6, and B12; drugs and chemicals, like alcohol, cytotoxic agents, chlorambucil, nitrofurantoin, and isoniazid; neoplastic disorders; infective or inflammatory diseases, such as Guillain–Barré syndrome and Lyme borreliosis; and genetic disorders, such as Charcot–Marie–Tooth disease and hereditary sensory neuropathies.

Proximal Asymmetric Mononeuropathy

This uncommon condition affects generally the lower extremity muscles and has been initially described as diabetic amyotrophy in 1955 [29]. Clinically the patient reports severe continuous pain at the lower limb, associated with leg weakness. The clinical examination shows unilateral atrophy of the proximal muscles of the leg, with functional impairment. It is important to exclude other causes of muscle wasting, such as malignancies. The treatment is supportive and palliative, aiming to control pain. It has been reported that pain generally tends to settle after 1 year [30].

Cranial Mononeuropathy

The most frequently affected cranial nerve is the third and is characterized by unilateral orbital pain, ptosis, and ophthalmoplegia associated with frontal headache. Cranial mononeuropathy has been suggested to be secondary to ischemia. Other causes responsible for oculomotor nerve palsy, such as malignancies or aneurysms, have always to be excluded. The prognosis is generally good with spontaneous resolution within 3 months.

Nerve Entrapment Syndromes

Nerve entrapment syndromes (or pressure neuropathies) are generally localized at the upper extremities (carpal tunnel syndrome and ulnar nerve entrapment) and more rarely at the lower limbs (common peroneal entrapment that causes foot drop). Patients experience paresthesia and pain that is exacerbated during the night and that can be irradiated to the forearm. Carpal tunnel syndrome refers to the involvement of the median nerve and is characterized by the reduction in sensation in the median territory of the hand and wasting of the bulk muscle in the thenar eminence. The ulnar nerve may undergo pressure damage in the ulnar groove at the elbow. This causes reduction in sensation in the ulnar territory of the hand and wasting of the dorsal interossei muscles.

The diagnosis of pressure neuropathies relies on electrophysiological tests that show nerve conduction abnormalities. The treatment is surgical, with good initial response, even though the relapse rate is higher than in the nondiabetic population. [31]

Truncal Radiculopathy

Truncal radiculopathy is a rare diabetic mononeuropathy affecting the truncal nerves. It is a primarily sensory neuropathy characterized by acute pain and sensory impairment distributed in a dermatomal pattern at the thorax or abdomen. The major diagnostic goal is to exclude other causes of compression of nerve roots, preferably with MRI of the spine. The prognosis is generally good, as the symptoms tend to resolve within months.

Chronic Inflammatory Demyelinating Polyradiculopathy

Chronic Inflammatory demyelinating polyradiculopathy (CIDP) is an immune-mediated disorder. Its incidence is higher in both T1 and T2 DM subjects than in nondiabetic subjects [32]. Clinically, CIPD can resemble DPN even though a severe, rapid, and progressive polyneuropathy should always alert the clinician. Intravenous immune globulins, corticosteroids, and plasma exchange have been shown good results and are the most widely adopted medications for the treatment of CIPD [33].

Autonomic Neuropathy

Autonomic neuropathy may affect systems like the cardiovascular, metabolic, gastrointestinal, genitourinary, and the peripheral. In contrast to the very high prevalence of alterations of the autonomic nervous system, patients rarely present symptomatic autonomic neuropathy. Interestingly enough, the mortality rate among these patients tends to be higher than among those without symptoms [34].

Cardiovascular Autonomic Neuropathy

Cardiovascular autonomic neuropathy (CAN) is the impairment of the autonomic control of the cardiac system. In contrast with the proven beneficial effects of tight metabolic control on progression of peripheral neuropathy [6], evidence on positive effects of glycemic control on autonomic dysfunction is less strong. Clinical manifestations of CAN range from mild exercise intolerance, resting tachycardia, silent myocardial infarction, and cardiac denervation syndrome to sudden cardiac death. The greater perianesthesia hemodynamic instability present in diabetic subjects affected by CAN is co-responsible for the poorer surgical outcomes of these patients [35].

Orthostatic Hypotension

Orthostatic hypotension is defined as a symptomatic fall in systolic or diastolic blood pressure ≥ 20 or 10 mmHg, respectively, upon change of body position from supine to standing. It is secondary to defective contraction of resistance vessels in the standing position, abnormal reduction in blood volume, or diminished cardiac output in the standing position. In diabetes, it is believed to be secondary to cardiac denervation and to impaired function of the sympathetic vasomotor fibers of resistance vessels causing reduced vascular tone. A blunted increase of plasma norepinephrine (hypoadrenergic orthostatic hypotension) is usually present [36].

Gastrointestinal

Diabetic subjects present a higher incidence of gastrointestinal (GI) symptoms compared to the general population [37]. GI disturbances in diabetic subjects are of multifactorial origin; the etiological factors possibly involved in their pathogenesis are hyperglycemia, hypokalemia, microvascular disease, hormonal dysregulation, increased susceptibility to infections, and autonomic neuropathy. Through the interaction with the enteric nervous system, the autonomic system controls the motor, sensory, and secretory functions of the gut. GI dysfunctions may be present at every level of the gut; however, the most frequent and important manifestation is the gastroduodenal dysfunction (better known as gastroparesis diabeticorum). It is an electromechanical disorder of the stomach and upper small bowel that can affect postprandial glucose concentrations and should always be considered in case of unexplained hypoglycemia in insulin treated diabetic subjects [38]. Patients present with both fasting and postprandial nausea and vomiting, sometimes associated with epigastric pain and dyspepsia. In severe cases, patients might present signs of malnutrition or bleeding secondary to Mallory–Weiss tears caused by repeated bouts of vomiting. Other GI alterations are esophageal delayed transit, diarrhea (possibly complicated by bacterial overgrowth and disordered secretion), and fecal incontinence (result of internal anal sphincter tone instability).

Genitourinary

Urogenital complications are frequently diagnosed in diabetic subjects, and include bladder and sexual dysfunctions. Clinical manifestations of bladder dysfunction range from reduced urinary flow and incomplete bladder emptying (with subsequent recurrent urinary tract infections, such as cystitis) secondary to detrusor hypocontractility to bladder desensitization and absent detrusor contractility with overflow incontinence. Autonomic neuropathy causes instead irritative symptoms such as pollakiuria, nycturia, and incontinence.

Besides decreased libido, sexual disorders in men are represented primarily by erectile dysfunction (ED) but also by ejaculatory and orgasmic problems. ED is the inability to attain and/or maintain a penile erection for sexual activity. Among diabetic subjects, its prevalence is estimated from 35 to 90%, the variance is probably explained from the different diagnostic criteria used in the studied populations [39]. Since penile erection is a neurovascular event, psychological factors, alterations in the nervous and vascular systems, as well as in the smooth muscles, collagen, and endothelial cells of the corporal erectile tissue determine ED. ED is an important predictor of cardiovascular events and that it is independently associated with silent coronary artery disease, suggesting the need to perform an exercise ECG before starting a treatment for ED [40].

Female sexual dysfunction includes decreased libido (associated with episodes of depression), disorders in genital arousal, delayed or absent orgasm, and dyspareunia. The prevalence FSD and associated risk factors in diabetic women however are less clear than in men [41].

Sudomotor

Sudomotor dysfunction is common; initially there may be hyperhidrosis of the feet, but later it may result in anhidrosis and vasomotor alterations with subsequent dryness of the skin that becomes more prone to fissurations and subsequent ulcerations [42]. Diabetic subjects affected by cervical sympathetic denervation can experience gustatory sweating. This excessive facial sweating happens during meals, especially if spicy, when salivation is induced upon cholinergic stimulation. The proposed mechanism in fact is aberrant re-innervation of sympathetically denervated sweat glands with misdirected cholinergic parasympathetic fibers (physiologically from minor petrus nerve to parotid gland). [43]

Encephalopathy

Diabetic encephalopathies are diabetic complications of the central nervous system (CNS). These conditions are characterized by functional impairment of cognition, disturbances in cerebral signal conduction, neurotransmission, and synaptic plasticity. They can be classified in primary (related to impaired insulin action and hyperglycemia) and in secondary (due to diabetic vascular disease). The pathophysiological mechanisms responsible for changes in the CNS are substantially the same as in the peripheral and autonomic systems. Impaired insulin action plays a key role since insulin has direct and indirect neurotrophic actions. Moreover, there is growing evidence of the link between diabetes, particularly type 2, and dementia, both Alzheimer's disease (AD) and vascular dementia [44], apparently via insulin receptor signaling alterations [45]. Impaired insulin action seems to alter amyloid deposition that leads to formation of amyloid plaques, one of the characteristic hallmarks of neurodegeneration in AD.

Nerve–Axon Reflex Vasodilation

Pain and trauma, like other stress conditions, stimulate the adjacent C fibers to secrete neuropeptides (like Substance P, Neuropeptide Y, Neurotensin, Calcitonin gene-related peptide, and Histamine) via the activation of C-nociceptive nerve fibers. This protective mechanism, known as nerve–axon reflex vasodilation (NARV), depends on the existence of an intact neurogenic vascular response, as the secreted molecules affect vessel homeostasis causing vasodilation and increased vessel permeability. NARV's vasodilation is equal to one-third of the maximal vasodilatory capacity and has been shown to be impaired in both diabetic patients with and without neuropathy [46], with the largest reduction in neuropathic feet. Because of the NARV impairment, the diabetic neuropathic patients present a reduced hyperemic response in their injured feet [47] that become functionally ischemic (Fig. 4.1).

Hypoglycemia and the Nervous System

Hypoglycemia can cause coma and death. Paraphysiologically, hypoglycemia triggers a sequence of metabolic, neural, and clinical responses [48]. The activation of the autonomic nervous system determines on the one hand the clinical manifestations of hypoglycemia (namely tremor, palpitations, hunger, anxiety, diaphoresis, and paresthesia) and on the other hand the

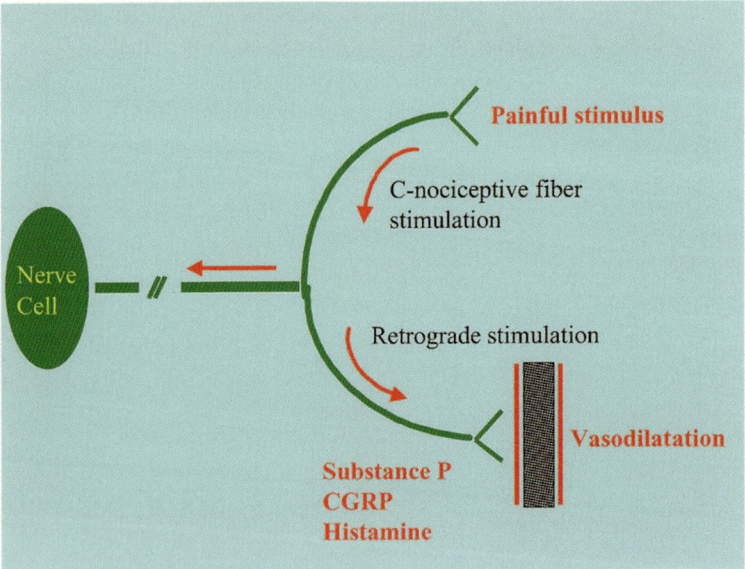

Fig. 4.1 The nerve–axon reflex. The C-nociceptive fibers stimulation determines retrograde activation of the adjacent fibers that release active vasodilators (such as histamine, SP, and CGRP). The final result is hyperemia during injury or inflammation

increase of glucose concentration by decreasing insulin secretion and by stimulating the secretion of glucagon, catecholamines, cortisol, growth hormone, and pancreatic polypeptide. Hypoglycemia unawareness and unresponsiveness are two life-threatening aspects of decreased glucose homeostatic counter-regulation. Interestingly enough, even though the autonomic nervous system plays a pivotal role in this mechanism, subjects affected by diabetic autonomic neuropathy do not seem to have impaired hypoglycemic counter-regulation per se. However, autonomic neuropathy further attenuates the already decreased activation of the autonomic nervous system following recent antecedent hypoglycemia [49]. This phenomenon is referred to as hypoglycemia induced autonomic failure and is frequently observed in diabetic subjects in tight glycemic control [50].

Diagnosis

Diagnosis of diabetic neuropathy therefore relies on neurological symptom score (NSS), nerve disability score (NDS), and on electromyography (EMG). There are different subcategories of disease and the presentation itself can profoundly vary based on which nerves and which class of fibers are affected. A comparison of scored symptoms and signs and clinical neurophysiological studies against morphometric and teased fiber studies of the sural nerve demonstrated that the former three provide sensitive and reliable measures of severity of neuropathy. [51] The NSS and NDS are known to be valid and sensitive and are extensively used in clinical practice. NSS consists of 17 items: eight focusing on muscle weakness, five on sensory disturbances, and four on autonomic symptoms. It is based on scoring of the present or absent selected neuropathy symptoms, such as pain or discomfort, burning, numbness or tingling, fatigue, cramping, or aching. The NSS test considers also type, severity, position, exacerbation, and eventual reduction of the symptoms are considered. Since all questions are verbal, to try to reduce measurement biases the operator should perform the test without "leading the witness". The NDS was pioneered by Dr. Dyck at the Mayo Clinic [52]. This score consists of 35 items, it examines on the left and right hemisomas the cranial nerves, muscle weakness, tendon reflexes, and sensation. The examination should be preferably performed by a neurologist with special training and experience in the field of peripheral neuropathy. This renders it a very useful tool in research, but on the other hand, it limits its role in clinical practice. Several modified NDS tests have been elaborated, some of which can be performed also by nonspecialists [53–55]. Of note, the 10-g monofilament and the Achilles tendon reflex are good tools for predicting the development of foot ulcers, but are not sensitive in detecting early stage neuropathy [56].

Therapy

There are still limited options for the treatment of diabetic neuropathy. Ideally therapies should be directed at preventing or arresting the progressive loss of nerve function, and on the other hand they should improve symptoms, possibly with minimal side effects. There is abundant evidence that achieving a good glycemic control is fundamental in the management of diabetic neuropathy, as discussed before; in fact hyperglycemia plays an important role in the pathogenesis of neuropathy. The evidence that improvement of glycemic control is beneficial on neuropathic pain is instead limited to small studies [57]. However, an elegant study by Boulton et al. has shown that glycemic fluctuations itself are detrimental to neuropathic pain [58].

Pain Management

The most widely used drugs for pain control are tricyclic antidepressants (TCAs), anticonvulsants, opioids, and N-methyl-D-aspartate (NMDA) Receptor Antagonists.

Tricyclic Antidepressants
TCAs are heterocyclic chemical compounds used primarily for the treatment of depression. They are a class of drugs that includes medications with selective serotonin reuptake inhibitors, such as amitriptyline (the most extensively prescribed TCA), and balanced serotonin and norepinephrine reuptake inhibitors, like duloxetine (only TCA drug to receive FDA approval for PDN) [59]. The mechanism of action of TCAs in neuropathic pain is probably multimodal with contribution of monoamine reuptake inhibition and blockade of NMDA receptors (which mediate hyperalgesia and allodynia) as well as sodium channels. Patients undergoing TCA treatment must be carefully monitored for possible side effects, such as drowsiness and lethargy, and particularly for the anticholinergic side-effect postural hypotension.

Anticonvulsants
Anticonvulsants, such as gabapentin, phenytoin, and carbamazepine, have been used in the management of neuropathic pain for many years [60]. Limited evidence is available on the usefulness of phenytoin and carbamazepine, meanwhile gabapentin and pregabalin have shown to be effective in the management of pain in diabetic neuropathies. Both gabapentin and its higher-potency and higher-effective analog pregabalin are structurally related to the neurotransmitter gamma-aminobutyric acid (GABA) and act also as ligands for the auxiliary-associated protein alpha-2-delta subunit of voltage-gated calcium channels. Their mechanism of action is GABA independent and secondary to the inhibition of the calcium flux into NMDA activated neurons. Recently other newer anticonvulsants, like lamotrigine, sodium valproate, and topiramate, have shown to be effective in the management of neuropathic pain [54].

Opioids
The use of opioids in the treatment of patients with neuropathic pain remains controversial. However, in a randomized control trial the use of tramadol, a weak synthetic non-narcotic opioid-like centrally acting analgesic, has shown to be useful in the management of neuropathic pain [61]. Moreover, oxycodone has shown to be effective in controlling neuropathic pain. Of note, oxycodone is about twice as potent and has lower incidence of side effects than morphine.

NMDA Receptor Antagonists
This class of medications induce dissociative anesthesia and include ketamine and dextromethorphan.

Besides being used for postoperative pain reduction, these medications are popular as recreational drugs for their dissociative, hallucinogenic, and euphoriant properties. In a multicenter, open-label study the NMDA Receptor Antagonist dextromethorphan, in combination with quinidine, demonstrated to significantly impact on pain intensity and relief rating scales, and patients' assessments of sleep and pain intensity [62].

Antiarrhythmics

Mexiletine is a class 1B antiarrhythmic and is a structural analog of lignocaine. Mexiletine has been successfully used to control neuropathic pain; however, regular ECG monitoring is necessary during treatment [63]. Long-term use of mexiletine is not recommended and its use should be limited to patients that have failed to respond to other treatments.

Topical Treatments

Topical therapy with capsaicin, lidocaine, and nitrate has been used with limited effects on diabetic neuropathy. Capsaicin is an alkaloid, the "hot" ingredient of red chili peppers, and reduces pain by depleting nociceptive C fibers of Substance P. Lidocaine dampens the peripheral nociceptor sensitization by blocking the sodium channel. Isosorbide dinitrate and glyceryl trinitrate have shown a significant reduction in pain and burning discomfort. Even though the local application of all these molecules has shown somewhat positive efficacy, further studies are needed since these studies are small and single-centered [64, 65].

Treatments Targeting Pathogenic Mechanisms

Numerous interventions that have targeted pathogenic mechanisms have been tested, including drugs directed against metabolic dysfunction (AR inhibitors, inhibitors of glycation, antioxidants), microvascular insufficiency (PKC inhibitors, vascular endothelial growth factors and vasodilators), autoimmunity (intravenous immunoglobulins), and nerve regeneration (neurotrophins). However, none of these interventions has gained so far acceptance in clinical practice.

Aldose Reductase Inhibitors

Over 32 randomized controlled trials, involving almost 5,000 participants, in the past 30 years have tested AR inhibitors (ARI) in treating diabetic neuropathy. The results of ARI agents (like ranirestat, epalrestat, and many others) for DPN treatment remain inconclusive; in fact a meta-analysis involving 879 ARI treated and 909 control (placebo or no treatment) participants showed no overall significant difference between the groups in the treatment of diabetic polyneuropathy [66].

Inhibitors of Glycation

Aminoguanidine has been used to this end; however, owing to its other pharmacological properties (inhibition of nitric oxide synthase and monoamine oxides) its use as an investigative tool in vivo is limited. New glycation inhibitors, such as pyridoxamine, might offer new insights into the effects of macromolecule glycation in nerve dysfunction.

Oxidative Stress

α-Lipoic acid (ALA) is a natural cofactor of the dehydrogenase complex and is a potent lipophilic free radical scavenger antioxidant. Despite initial encouraging results, pivotal studies were negative. The Alpha Lipoic Acid in Diabetic Neuropathy (ALADIN) study, a large multicenter randomized controlled trial, showed that ALA had no effect in controlling neuropathic pain. [67] The effects of another antioxidant, thioctic acid, are currently under study in a four-year randomized clinical multicenter trial (NATHAN, Neurological Assessment of Thioctic Acid in Neuropathy).

PKC Inhibitors

Ruboxistaurin (RBX) mesylate is a PKC inhibitor that specifically inhibits PKC-β overactivation and that has shown to improve neural function in diabetic animals [68]. In a double-blinded randomized clinical trial treatment with RBX in patients with DPN failed to achieve the primary end point of improving quantitative sensory testing for vibration detection threshold among all symptomatic patients. [69]

Vascular Endothelial Growth Factor

The rationale of vascular endothelial growth factor (VEGF) in the treatment of diabetic neuropathy is based on the loss of vasa nervorum. Since VEGF is a potent angiogenetic stimulator, secreted in response to tissue hypoxia, its application could reverse at least partially the dysfunction. In animal models, VEGF gene transfer has shown to improve nerve conduction and nerve blood flow [70]. However, given the detrimental effects of VEGF in the retina in diabetes, testing of this molecule in humans has been not yet tried.

Intravenous Immunoglobulins

Treatment with intravenous immunoglobulins is indicated in peripheral diabetic neuropathies with signs of antineural autoimmunity, especially chronic demyelinating polyneuropathy [71].

Neurotrophic Therapy

Neurotrophic factors modulate gene expression in the neurons, and through this they promote neuronal survival. Reduction in the levels of neurotrophic factors can lead to neuronal apoptosis [72]. Nerve growth factor (NGF) is a member of this class of molecules and its expression has been shown to be suppressed in diabetic neuropathic patients. In animal models the use of recombinant human NGF (rhNGF) restores the levels of this neurotrophin and prevents manifestation of sensory neuropathy [73]. Moreover, 250 subjects with symptomatic small fiber neuropathy showed improved Ad and C fibers function after rhNGF therapy [74]. However, two subsequent large multicenter clinical trials did not demonstrate beneficial effects of rhNGF therapy for diabetic neuropathy.

References

1. Urbancic-Rovan V. Causes of diabetic foot lesions. Lancet. 2005;366(9498):1675–6.
2. Zimmet P, Alberti KG, Shaw J. Global and societal implications of the diabetes epidemic. Nature. 2001;414(6865):782–7.
3. Wild S, Roglic G, Green A, Sicree R, King H. Global prevalence of diabetes: estimates for the year 2000 and projections for 2030. Diabetes Care. 2004;27(5):1047–53.
4. Dyck PJ, Kratz KM, Karnes JL, et al. The prevalence by staged severity of various types of diabetic neuropathy, retinopathy, and nephropathy in a population-based cohort: the Rochester Diabetic Neuropathy Study. Neurology. 1993;43(4):817–24.
5. Apelqvist J, Bakker K, van Houtum WH, Nabuurs-Franssen MH, Schaper NC. International consensus and practical guidelines on the management and the prevention of the diabetic foot. International Working Group on the Diabetic Foot. Diabetes Metab Res Rev. 2000;16 Suppl 1:S84–92.
6. The effect of intensive diabetes therapy on the development and progression of neuropathy. The Diabetes Control and Complications Trial Research Group. Ann Intern Med. 1995;122(8):561–8.
7. Saouaf R, Arora S, Smakowski P, Caballero AE, Veves A. Reactive hyperemic response of the brachial artery: comparison of proximal and distal occlusion. Acad Radiol. 1998;5(8):556–60.
8. Eriksson KF, Nilsson H, Lindgarde F, et al. Diabetes mellitus but not impaired glucose tolerance is associated with dysfunction in peripheral nerves. Diabet Med. 1994;11(3):279–85.
9. Franklin GM, Kahn LB, Baxter J, Marshall JA, Hamman RF. Sensory neuropathy in non-insulin-dependent diabetes mellitus. The San Luis Valley Diabetes Study. Am J Epidemiol. 1990;131(4):633–43.
10. Singh JP, Larson MG, O'Donnell CJ, et al. Association of hyperglycemia with reduced heart rate variability (The Framingham Heart Study). Am J Cardiol. 2000;86(3):309–12.
11. Greene DA, Winegrad AI. In vitro studies of the substrates for energy production and the effects of insulin on glucose utilization in the neural components of peripheral nerve. Diabetes. 1979;28(10):878–87.
12. Brownlee M. Biochemistry and molecular cell biology of diabetic complications. Nature. 2001;414(6865):813–20.
13. Cameron NE, Eaton SE, Cotter MA, Tesfaye S. Vascular factors and metabolic interactions in the pathogenesis of diabetic neuropathy. Diabetologia. 2001;44(11):1973–88.
14. Wada R, Yagihashi S. Role of advanced glycation end products and their receptors in development of diabetic neuropathy. Ann N Y Acad Sci. 2005;1043:598–604.
15. Makita Z, Radoff S, Rayfield EJ, et al. Advanced glycosylation end products in patients with diabetic nephropathy. N Engl J Med. 1991;325(12):836–42.
16. Meerwaldt R, Links TP, Graaff R, et al. Increased accumulation of skin advanced glycation end-products precedes and correlates with clinical manifestation of diabetic neuropathy. Diabetologia. 2005;48(8):1637–44.

17. Garay-Sevilla ME, Regalado JC, Malacara JM, et al. Advanced glycosylation end products in skin, serum, saliva and urine and its association with complications of patients with type 2 diabetes mellitus. J Endocrinol Invest. 2005;28(3):223–30.
18. Misur I, Zarkovic K, Barada A, Batelja L, Milicevic Z, Turk Z. Advanced glycation endproducts in peripheral nerve in type 2 diabetes with neuropathy. Acta Diabetol. 2004;41(4):158–66.
19. Van Dam PS, Van Asbeck BS, Erkelens DW, Marx JJ, Gispen WH, Bravenboer B. The role of oxidative stress in neuropathy and other diabetic complications. Diabetes Metab Rev. 1995;11(3):181–92.
20. Low PA, Lagerlund TD, McManis PG. Nerve blood flow and oxygen delivery in normal, diabetic, and ischemic neuropathy. Int Rev Neurobiol. 1989;31:355–438.
21. Ohara Y, Sayegh HS, Yamin JJ, Harrison DG. Regulation of endothelial constitutive nitric oxide synthase by protein kinase C. Hypertension. 1995;25(3):415–20.
22. Beckman JA, Goldfine AB, Gordon MB, Garrett LA, Creager MA. Inhibition of protein kinase Cbeta prevents impaired endothelium-dependent vasodilation caused by hyperglycemia in humans. Circ Res. 2002;90(1):107–11.
23. Beckman JA, Goldfine AB, Goldin A, Prsic A, Kim S, Creager MA. Inhibition of protein kinase Cbeta does not improve endothelial function in type 2 diabetes. J Clin Endocrinol Metab. 2010;95(8):3783–7.
24. Mehta NN, Sheetz M, Price K, et al. Selective PKC beta inhibition with ruboxistaurin and endothelial function in type-2 diabetes mellitus. Cardiovasc Drugs Ther. 2009;23(1):17–24.
25. Watkins PJ, Edmonds ME. Clinical features of diabetic neuropathy. In: Pickup J, Williams G, editors. Textbook of diabetes, vol. 2. Oxford: Blackwell; 1997. p. 50.51–20.
26. Bruyn GW, Garland H. Neuropathies of endocrine origin. In: Vinken PJ, Bruyn GW, editors. Handbook of clinical neurology, vol. 8. Amsterdam: North Holland Publishing; 1970. p. 29.
27. Low PA, Suarez GA. Diabetic neuropathies. Baillieres Clin Neurol. 1995;4(3):401–25.
28. Bird SJ, Brown MJ. The clinical spectrum of diabetic neuropathy. Semin Neurol. 1996;16(2):115–22.
29. Garland H. Diabetic amyotrophy. Br Med J. 1955;2(4951):1287–90.
30. Coppack SW, Watkins PJ. The natural history of diabetic femoral neuropathy. Q J Med. 1991;79(288):307–13.
31. Clayburgh RH, Beckenbaugh RD, Dobyns JH. Carpal tunnel release in patients with diffuse peripheral neuropathy. J Hand Surg [Am]. 1987;12(3):380–3.
32. Sharma KR, Cross J, Farronay O, Ayyar DR, Shebert RT, Bradley WG. Demyelinating neuropathy in diabetes mellitus. Arch Neurol. 2002;59(5):758–65.
33. Koller H, Kieseier BC, Jander S, Hartung HP. Chronic inflammatory demyelinating polyneuropathy. N Engl J Med. 2005;352(13):1343–56.
34. Watkins PJ. Diabetic autonomic neuropathy. N Engl J Med. 1990;322(15):1078–9.
35. Burgos LG, Ebert TJ, Asiddao C, et al. Increased intraoperative cardiovascular morbidity in diabetics with autonomic neuropathy. Anesthesiology. 1989;70(4):591–7.
36. Hilsted J, Parving HH, Christensen NJ, Benn J, Galbo H. Hemodynamics in diabetic orthostatic hypotension. J Clin Invest. 1981;68(6):1427–34.
37. Bytzer P, Talley NJ, Leemon M, Young LJ, Jones MP, Horowitz M. Prevalence of gastrointestinal symptoms associated with diabetes mellitus: a population-based survey of 15,000 adults. Arch Intern Med. 2001;161(16):1989–96.
38. Horowitz M, Jones KL, Rayner CK, Read NW. 'Gastric' hypoglycaemia – an important concept in diabetes management. Neurogastroenterol Motil. 2006;18(6):405–7.
39. Malavige LS, Levy JC. Erectile dysfunction in diabetes mellitus. J Sex Med. 2009;6(5):1232–47.
40. Gazzaruso C, Giordanetti S, De Amici E, et al. Relationship between erectile dysfunction and silent myocardial ischemia in apparently uncomplicated type 2 diabetic patients. Circulation. 2004;110(1):22–6.
41. Bhasin S, Enzlin P, Coviello A, Basson R. Sexual dysfunction in men and women with endocrine disorders. Lancet. 2007;369(9561):597–611.
42. Tentolouris N, Marinou K, Kokotis P, Karanti A, Diakoumopoulou E, Katsilambros N. Sudomotor dysfunction is associated with foot ulceration in diabetes. Diabet Med. 2009;26(3):302–5.
43. Restivo DA, Lanza S, Patti F, et al. Improvement of diabetic autonomic gustatory sweating by botulinum toxin type A. Neurology. 2002;59(12):1971–3.
44. Ott A, Stolk RP, van Harskamp F, Pols HA, Hofman A, Breteler MM. Diabetes mellitus and the risk of dementia: the Rotterdam Study. Neurology. 1999;53(9):1937–42.
45. Gasparini L, Netzer WJ, Greengard P, Xu H. Does insulin dysfunction play a role in Alzheimer's disease? Trends Pharmacol Sci. 2002;23(6):288–93.
46. Caselli A, Rich J, Hanane T, Uccioli L, Veves A. Role of C-nociceptive fibers in the nerve axon reflex-related vasodilation in diabetes. Neurology. 2003;60(2):297–300.
47. Hernandez C, Burgos R, Canton A, Garcia-Arumi J, Segura RM, Simo R. Vitreous levels of vascular cell adhesion molecule and vascular endothelial growth factor in patients with proliferative diabetic retinopathy: a case-control study. Diabetes Care. 2001;24(3):516–21.
48. Rizza RA, Cryer PE, Gerich JE. Role of glucagon, catecholamines, and growth hormone in human glucose counterregulation. Effects of somatostatin and combined alpha- and beta-adrenergic blockade on plasma glucose recovery and glucose flux rates after insulin-induced hypoglycemia. J Clin Invest. 1979;64(1):62–71.
49. Meyer C, Grossmann R, Mitrakou A, et al. Effects of autonomic neuropathy on counterregulation and

awareness of hypoglycemia in type 1 diabetic patients. Diabetes Care. 1998;21(11):1960–6.
50. Amiel SA, Tamborlane WV, Simonson DC, Sherwin RS. Defective glucose counterregulation after strict glycemic control of insulin-dependent diabetes mellitus. N Engl J Med. 1987;316(22):1376–83.
51. Dyck PJ, Sherman WR, Hallcher LM, et al. Human diabetic endoneurial sorbitol, fructose, and myo-inositol related to sural nerve morphometry. Ann Neurol. 1980;8(6):590–6.
52. Dyck PJ, Karnes J, O'Brien PC, Swanson CJ. Neuropathy Symptom Profile in health, motor neuron disease, diabetic neuropathy, and amyloidosis. Neurology. 1986;36(10):1300–8.
53. Young RJ, Zhou YQ, Rodriguez E, Prescott RJ, Ewing DJ, Clarke BF. Variable relationship between peripheral somatic and autonomic neuropathy in patients with different syndromes of diabetic polyneuropathy. Diabetes. 1986;35(2):192–7.
54. Boulton AJ, Malik RA, Arezzo JC, Sosenko JM. Diabetic somatic neuropathies. Diabetes Care. 2004;27(6):1458–86.
55. Bril V, Perkins BA. Validation of the Toronto Clinical Scoring System for diabetic polyneuropathy. Diabetes Care. 2002;25(11):2048–52.
56. Vinik AI, Newlon P, Milicevic Z, et al. Diabetic neuropathies: an overview of clinical aspects. In: LeRoith D, Taylor SI, Olefsky JM, editors. Diabetes mellitus: a fundamental and clinical text. Philadelphia: Lippincot-Raven; 1996.
57. Archer AG, Watkins PJ, Thomas PK, Sharma AK, Payan J. The natural history of acute painful neuropathy in diabetes mellitus. J Neurol Neurosurg Psychiatry. 1983;46(6):491–9.
58. Oyibo SO, Prasad YD, Jackson NJ, Jude EB, Boulton AJ. The relationship between blood glucose excursions and painful diabetic peripheral neuropathy: a pilot study. Diabet Med. 2002;19(10):870–3.
59. New drug for neuropathic pain. FDA Consum. 2004;38(6):2.
60. Jensen TS. Anticonvulsants in neuropathic pain: rationale and clinical evidence. Eur J Pain. 2002;6(Suppl A):61–8.
61. Harati Y, Gooch C, Swenson M, et al. Double-blind randomized trial of tramadol for the treatment of the pain of diabetic neuropathy. Neurology. 1998;50(6):1842–6.
62. Thisted RA, Klaff L, Schwartz SL, et al. Dextromethorphan and quinidine in adult patients with uncontrolled painful diabetic peripheral neuropathy: a 29-day, multicenter, open-label, dose-escalation study. Clin Ther. 2006;28(10):1607–18.
63. Jarvis B, Coukell AJ. Mexiletine. A review of its therapeutic use in painful diabetic neuropathy. Drugs. 1998;56(4):691–707.
64. Yuen KC, Baker NR, Rayman G. Treatment of chronic painful diabetic neuropathy with isosorbide dinitrate spray: a double-blind placebo-controlled cross-over study. Diabetes Care. 2002;25(10):1699–703.
65. Rayman G, Baker NR, Krishnan ST. Glyceryl trinitrate patches as an alternative to isosorbide dinitrate spray in the treatment of chronic painful diabetic neuropathy. Diabetes Care. 2003;26(9):2697–8.
66. Chalk C, Benstead TJ, Moore F. Aldose reductase inhibitors for the treatment of diabetic polyneuropathy. Cochrane Database Syst Rev. 2007;(4):CD004572.
67. Ziegler D, Hanefeld M, Ruhnau KJ, et al. Treatment of symptomatic diabetic peripheral neuropathy with the anti-oxidant alpha-lipoic acid. A 3-week multicentre randomized controlled trial (ALADIN Study). Diabetologia. 1995;38(12):1425–33.
68. Yamagishi S, Uehara K, Otsuki S, Yagihashi S. Differential influence of increased polyol pathway on protein kinase C expressions between endoneurial and epineurial tissues in diabetic mice. J Neurochem. 2003;87(2):497–507.
69. Vinik AI, Bril V, Kempler P, et al. Treatment of symptomatic diabetic peripheral neuropathy with the protein kinase C beta-inhibitor ruboxistaurin mesylate during a 1-year, randomized, placebo-controlled, double-blind clinical trial. Clin Ther. 2005;27(8):1164–80.
70. Schratzberger P, Walter DH, Rittig K, et al. Reversal of experimental diabetic neuropathy by VEGF gene transfer. J Clin Invest. 2001;107(9):1083–92.
71. Hughes RA, Dalakas MC, Cornblath DR, Latov N, Weksler ME, Relkin N. Clinical applications of intravenous immunoglobulins in neurology. Clin Exp Immunol. 2009;158 Suppl 1:34–42.
72. Srinivasan S, Stevens M, Wiley JW. Diabetic peripheral neuropathy: evidence for apoptosis and associated mitochondrial dysfunction. Diabetes. 2000;49(11):1932–8.
73. Apfel SC, Kessler JA. Neurotrophic factors in the therapy of peripheral neuropathy. Baillieres Clin Neurol. 1995;4(3):593–606.
74. Apfel SC, Kessler JA, Adornato BT, Litchy WJ, Sanders C, Rask CA. Recombinant human nerve growth factor in the treatment of diabetic polyneuropathy. NGF Study Group. Neurology. 1998;51(3):695–702.

Microvascular Changes in the Diabetic Foot

Thomas S. Monahan

Keywords
Diabetes complications • Endothelium • Endothelial dysfunction • Basement membrane • Hyperglycemia • Oxidative stress • Protein kinase C • Ischemia

Introduction

Diabetes has many profound clinical effects in patients with lower extremity arterial insufficiency. As a physician caring for these patients it is important to understand the pathology and how the pathologic events translate into relevant clinical findings. The pathologic processes found in the microvascular circulation in patients with diabetes directly affect the ability to provide adequate gas exchange to interstitial tissues, deliver nutrition and remove waste products, mount a hyperemic response, and respond to injury.

T.S. Monahan, M.D. (✉)
Division of Vascular Surgery, Department of Surgery, University of Maryland Medical Center, University of Maryland School of Medicine, 22 Green St. South, Baltimore, MD 21201, USA
e-mail: tmonahan@smail.unmaryland.edu

Normal Microvascular Structure and Function

Structure

The microcirculation consists of arterioles, venules, and capillaries. The vascular wall typically consists of three distinct layers: the tunica intima comprised of endothelial cells, the tunica media primarily comprised of vascular smooth muscle cells, and the tunica adventitia primarily comprised of connective tissue. The microcirculation differs from the rest of the cardiovascular system in the composition of the vascular wall. The microcirculation is the smallest component of the cardiovascular system. Arterioles and venules generally consist of one to two layers of smooth muscle cells surrounding a single layer of endothelium. Capillaries lack a muscular layer and consist of a single continuous layer of endothelial cells surrounded by a basement membrane. The structure of capillaries allows close regulation of the exchange of oxygen, carbon dioxide, nutrients, and waste products at the tissue level.

Function

The microcirculation serves multiple essential purposes. Arterioles serve as the primary site of vascular resistance. The largest change in blood pressure in the cardiovascular system occurs as blood flows from arteriole to capillary. Hydrostatic capillary pressure is a highly regulated process; capillary hydrostatic pressure is regulated by both arteriole (precapillary) and venule (postcapillary) resistance. Changes in the precapillary, postcapillary, or both pressures significantly affect perfusion at the capillary level. This regulation is normally tightly controlled in skin and muscle tissue. This regulation is evident when contrasting inactive, collapsed capillaries of resting tissue and the flow-mediated dilated capillary beds in metabolically active tissues. Capillary flow is highly regulated and variable due to physiologic demands [1].

Among the myriad functions of blood, circulating blood allows the exchange of oxygen and carbon dioxide at the tissue level; it delivers nutrients and removes waste products. These processes are closely regulated at the level of the microcirculation. Capillary flow and hydrostatic pressure influence capillary exchange with interstitial fluids. When discussing capillary perfusion it is important to understand that flow does not equal pressure. Blood flow (Q) is proportional to perfusion pressure (P) and inversely proportional to resistance (R).

$$Q \alpha \frac{P}{R}.$$

Thus, in a system where resistance varies greatly, flow and pressure are two distinct parameters.

As blood enters the capillary, a portion of its fluid component is exuded from the capillary into the surrounding interstitial tissue. There is a hydrostatic gradient between the pressure of the blood in the capillary and the lower pressure of the adjacent interstitial fluid. Conversely, blood typically has a higher oncotic pressure than interstitial fluid. This gradient tends to draw fluid from the interstitial fluid into the capillary. These forces are referred to as the *Starling forces* (Fig. 5.1) [2]. The regulation of exchange between capillaries and interstitial fluid is significantly influenced by Starling forces; however, the endothelial cells composing capillary walls are more than passive barriers subject to these forces.

The endothelium exerts a tremendous amount of control of the microcirculation. The endothelium lines the entirety of the cardiovascular system and in total weighs about 1 kg in the average adult. The importance of the endothelium was recognized in 1953 when Dr. Palade observed active transport across the endothelium using electron microscopy. Prior to these observations, the endothelium was thought to be a largely passive organ that allowed transport through hypothetical pores [3]. The endothelium participates in active transport, regulates vascular tone, and even influences the structure of the basement membrane.

The structure and function of the microcirculation are deranged in the setting of diabetes mellitus. The nature of the derangements has significant implications for the oxygenation, nutrition, response to injury, and wound healing for patients with diabetes.

Changes in Microvasculature with Diabetes

Structural Changes

Diabetes mellitus has been referred to as "small vessel disease." This is a misconception, which must be dispelled. The origin of this misconception dates back to 1959 when Dr. Goldberg published his observations of periodic acid Schiff (PAS) positive material in the basement membrane of arterioles in amputated limbs of patients with diabetes [4]. A thickened, near occlusive lesion of endothelial cells was noted in the 92 patients with diabetes in this study of 152 amputated limbs. Although thickened basement membranes have been consistently observed in patients with diabetes, the near occlusive nature of the lesion has not been described in subsequent investigations [5, 6]. Perhaps the most compelling was a study of a series of amputated limbs from ten patients with

5 Microvascular Changes in the Diabetic Foot

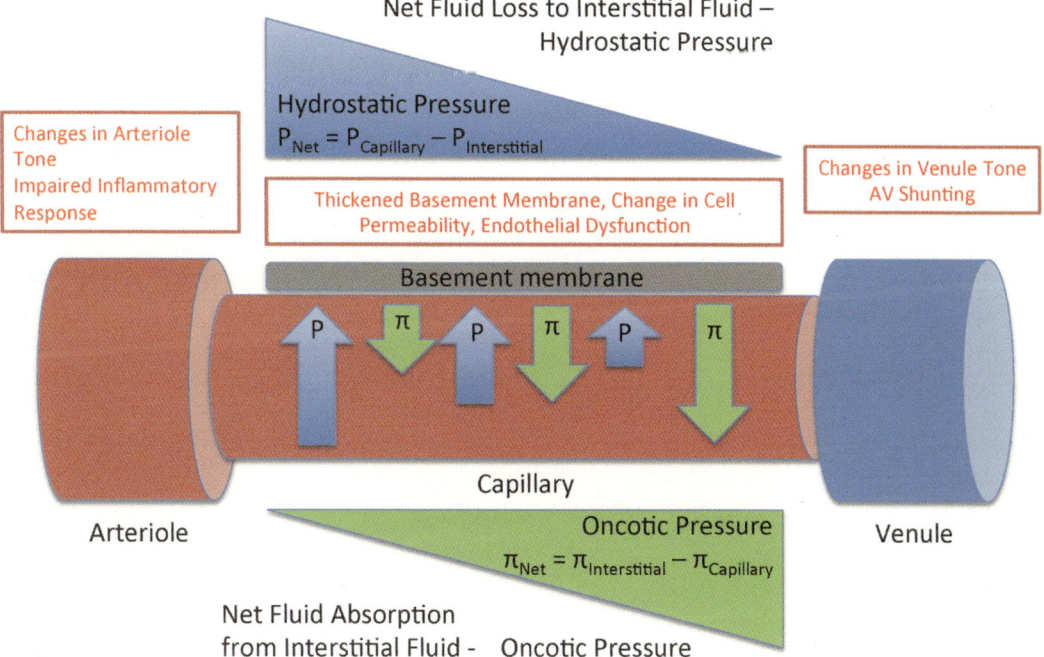

Fig. 5.1 The Starling forces. Hydrostatic force in the capillary is higher than in the adjacent interstitial tissues. Oncotic pressure is higher in the capillary than in the interstitial fluid. Hydrostatic pressures favor the passage of fluid out of the capillary and oncotic pressure favors the flow of fluid into the capillary. Capillary perfusion is tightly regulated. Diabetes can induce changes in arteriole tone, venule tone, arteriovenous shunting, and the microcirculation response to inflammation. All of these factors have an impact on capillary perfusion. Diabetes also induces basement membrane thickening, and changes in endothelial cell permeability. The effects of diabetes significantly impact the function of the microcirculation

diabetes and ten patients without diabetes. The limbs were injected with acrylic plastic (Batson's corrosion solution) and studied for patterns of arterial disease. The distribution of occlusive disease was largely similar between patients with and without diabetes. It was also observed that patients with diabetes had increased amounts of occlusive disease of the tibial vessels and decreased occlusive disease of pedal vessels [6]. Referring to diabetes as "small vessel disease" led to the misconception that patients with diabetes have occlusion of small vessels, and that surgical revascularization is of only limited value.

Observations of the previously described structural changes in the microcirculation in diabetes coupled with measurements of flow and pressure in the microcirculation have led to the formation of a hypothesis for the formation of microcirculation angiopathy. This hypothesis was first described by Parving [7] and then endorsed by other authors. Presently, it is believed that the microcirculation early in diabetes mellitus is characterized by increased flow. The increase in flow results in increased shear stress on the endothelium. The endothelium in turn produces increased extracellular matrix proteins. The end result is a thickened basement membrane and the loss of microcirculation autoregulation [7–11]. Subsequent investigations have demonstrated that the changes of the basement membrane occur at the transcriptional level. Changes in the relative contributions of matrix metalloproteins, inhibitors of matrix metalloproteins, and collagen in the basement membrane have been noted in microarray data—an assessment of mRNA expression—suggesting that the structure of the basement membrane is regulated at least in part at the level of gene expression [12].

Although it is becoming clear that diabetes mellitus does not cause occlusion of the microcirculation, the presence of diabetes results in many physiologic derangements of the microcirculation. Diabetes changes the flow in capillary beds, alters the normal function of endothelium, impacts the response to inflammation, and ultimately affects health and the response to injury of the lower extremity.

Functional Changes

There are multiple physiologic changes that occur in the microcirculation with the onset and continuation of diabetes mellitus. It can be difficult to separate out cause from effect. *The changes that occur in the microcirculation with diabetes can be thought of in broad categories including capillary perfusion, endothelial dysfunction, and perturbation of the nerve–axon reflex.* Obviously these categories are interconnected and allow for significant overlap. Diabetes is a risk factor for the development of peripheral arterial disease. The relationship between diabetes and atherosclerosis is discussed in detail in Chap. 2. Likewise, diabetes is associated with neuropathy. A detailed discussion of diabetes and neuropathy is discussed in Chap. 4. Discussion of neuropathy will be limited to its effect on the microcirculation.

Capillary Perfusion

Lower extremity resting blood flow is often increased in patients with diabetes and neuropathy. On examination, patients frequently have warm extremities and often bounding pulses. Resting hyperemia and hyperperfusion is at least in part due to diminished sympathetic tone resulting in peripheral vasodilation [13]. However, increased perfusion of the lower extremity does not translate directly into increased capillary perfusion.

The observation that patients with diabetes have hyperemic lower extremities lead to the hypothesis that capillary pressure was also increased in patients with diabetes. Patients with diabetes of short duration (less than 1 year), diabetes with incipient nephropathy, and overt nephropathy were compared to age- and sex-matched "healthy" patients. Fingernail bed pressure was measured using a glass micropipette in each cohort. These studies demonstrated a significant increase in capillary pressure in all of the diabetic cohorts compared to the matched control subjects [14]. These observations were consistent with subsequent studies in which Doppler fluximetry was used to quantitate capillary flow in patients with non-insulin-dependent diabetes and normal control subjects. The patients with diabetes had increased capillary flow; however their capillary flow was not augmented by a vasodilation stimulus (heat) as it was in the control subjects [15].

These studies examined the role of the microcirculation in the upper extremities in patients with diabetes. There is a considerable amount of evidence that diabetes affects the skin and muscles of the lower extremity and upper extremity somewhat differently [16, 17]. Other investigators have demonstrated contradictory data—diminished capillary flow and pressure in the lower extremities in patients with diabetes [17–19].

After capillaries are occluded, the normal physiologic response is a subsequent increase in capillary flow resulting in hyperemia—postocclusive reactive hyperemia (PRH). PRH is significantly diminished in all patients with insulin dependent diabetes compared to healthy control subjects. PRH was diminished in both subjects with good metabolic control ($HbA_{1c} < 7.5\%$) and poor metabolic control ($HbA_{1c} > 7.5\%$). However, patients with good metabolic control had no change in the time to peak velocity compared to normal patients. Furthermore, glycemic control was determined to be directly proportional to time to peak flow and inversely proportional to the maximal PRH response. These findings suggest that capillary perfusion is adversely impacted (decreased) by diabetes. Metabolic control significantly affects the degree to which perfusion is affected [19]. More recent studies have demonstrated through the use of intravital capillary video microscopy that not only is flow diminished in PRH, but capillary recruitment is also significantly decreased in patients with insulin-dependent diabetes. Consistent with previous observations, the diminished PRH response observed seems to be due to maximal capillary recruitment at rest, resulting in the inability to mount a hyperemic response to noxious stimuli [17].

Capillary recruitment and perfusion can be changed by changes in arteriolar and venule pressure. Arteriovenous shunting also significantly diminishes capillary perfusion. Both venous pressure and venous pO_2 are significantly increased in patients with diabetes and Charcot foot [20]. In patients with Charcot foot or neuropathy, increased diastolic blood flow was noted and resistance was decreased significantly. These findings taken together strongly argue that in the setting of diabetes, there are shunts that allow oxygen-rich arterial blood to bypass the capillary beds and travel directly to the venous circulation through arteriovenous shunts. These shunts significantly impact the distribution of blood at the tissue level resulting in local malperfusion and impacting the ability of the vascular system to deliver nutrients to the tissues of the lower extremity [11, 13, 21–23].

There has been much study in the effects of diabetes on capillary flow and pressure. The results of various studies often seem to be in opposition to each other. The differences observed between the presented studies likely reflect "snapshot" images of a complex disease at different stages of its progression. Additionally, diabetes is a heterogenous disease and it is difficult to make meaningful comparisons of capillary pressure and flow between a newly diagnosed patient with insulin-dependent diabetes and a patient with multiple comorbidities and long-standing, non-insulin-dependent diabetes. Regardless, there is copious evidence that demonstrates that capillary flow and pressure are significantly changed in diabetes compared to normal physiology. These changes significantly impair the normal exchange of oxygen and carbon dioxide, delivery of nutrition, and the removal of waste products of metabolism. Capillary perfusion can be significantly impaired despite the presence of a warm extremity with palpable pulses.

Endothelial Dependent Vasodilation

Nitric oxide is a potent vasodilator produced by the endothelium. Drs. Furchgott and Zawadzki first described the existence of an endothelium-derived vasodilating agent in 1980. In their landmark paper, they describe the inhibition of acetylcholine-induced vasodilation in rabbit aortas by stripping the endothelium. They hypothesized that there was a substance— endothelium-derived relaxing factor (EDRF)—that was produced in the endothelium and produced significant vasodilation when it acted upon the vascular smooth muscle cells [24]. Subsequent studies elucidated that endothelial cell calcium flux induces the synthesis of nitric oxide through nitric oxide synthase [25]. Nitric oxide diffuses into adjacent vascular smooth muscle cells where it induces relaxation through cyclic GMP-dependent mechanisms.

Blood vessels exhibit both endothelial-dependent and endothelial-independent vasodilation. Using provocative agents specific to one or the other of these systems can assess the relevant contribution of each system. For example, acetylcholine will specifically cause endothelial-dependent vasodilation, whereas sodium nitroprusside will interact directly with smooth muscle cells inducing an endothelium independent vasodilation. It has been clearly and unequivocally demonstrated that endothelial-dependent vasodilation is impaired in patients with diabetes [26].

Endothelial-dependent vasodilation is also significantly impaired in the coronary circulation with minimal atherosclerotic disease as a result of inactivation of endothelial nitric oxide synthase [27, 28]. In fact, endothelial-dependent vasodilation also is significantly impaired in patients with risk factors, but no clinically or radiographically evident disease [29]. Just as endothelial-dependent vasodilation is impaired before the onset of clinically or radiographically evident atherosclerosis, it is also impaired before the onset of the symptoms of diabetes. In fact, transient hyperglycemia alone is adequate to significantly acetylcholine-induced, endothelial-dependent vasodilation in both the macrocirculation and the microcirculation [30].

Nerve–Axon Reflex

Close regulation of microvascular tone is important. Microvascular tone is not only regulated by response to local changes in the vasculature, but rather by an intricate system. This system involves a complex interaction of the cells of the microvasculature, the nervous system, and multiple mediators. An intact nervous system is necessary for maximal microvascular responsiveness to stimuli. In normal subjects, approximately a third of acetylcholine-induced vasodilation is dependent on an intact local nervous system [31]. In the normal system, C-nociceptive fibers are stimulated resulting in an antidromic stimulation of adjacent fibers. These fibers in turn release a variety of mediators including substance P, calcitonin gene-related peptide, and histamine. These mediators further potentiate vasodilation. Taken together this response is known as the Lewis triple flare response [11].

This important response is significantly blunted in patients with diabetes and neuropathy. However, it is interesting to note that in patients with diabetes, but no evidence of neuropathy, the response was not different from patients without diabetes. Although not the major contributor to vasodilation, the nerve–axon response does play a significant role in the regulation of microcirculation tone. The significance of this finding is that patients with neuropathy might be functionally ischemic at the level of the microcirculation without the contribution of the nerve–axon reflex [11, 31].

Vascular Permeability and Oxidative Stress

The endothelium is an active, dynamic organ. Transport across the endothelium is not a passive process governed only by the Starling forces. The integrity of the endothelial cells and gap junctions are necessary to regulate transport between the capillary circulation and the interstitium. Several derangements in endothelial cell biology negatively impact endothelial cell integrity in diabetes. The major stressor is oxidative stress. *Oxidative stress negatively impacts endothelial cell biology through five major pathways: polyol pathway flux, increased formation of advanced glycation end products, increased expression of the receptor for AGEs, activation of protein kinase C, and increased activity of the hexosamine pathway* [32].

Intracellular glucose concentration is regulated in part by the activity of membrane-bound glucose transporters (GLUTs). To maintain intracellular glucose homeostasis, GLUT activity is inversely proportional to extracellular glucose concentration. However, in certain cell types susceptible to damage, such as vascular endothelial cells, glucose transport is proportional to extracellular glucose concentration resulting in intracellular hyperglycemia [33]. As a result of increased intracellular glucose concentrations, there are increased amounts of reactive oxygen species produced by the mitochondria producing other, more reactive, species. It is these species that initiate the pathways resulting in damage to the endothelium [34].

Unused glucose, in the setting of increased intracellular hyperglycemia, results in increased activity of aldose reductase, which reduces glucose to sorbital. Sorbitol is then further oxidized to fructose. This family of aldo-keto reductase enzymes collectively is referred to as the *polyol pathway*. Increased flux through these pathways results in intracellular sorbitol accumulation and excessive consumption of NADPH. Increased sorbitol concentrations also can glycate nitrogens on proteins resulting in the formation of advanced glycation end products (AGEs). These changes greatly impair the cell's ability to generate reactive oxygen species and further exacerbate the ability to control oxidative stress.

Increased amounts of *AGEs* are observed in patients with diabetes. *AGEs cause damage through two main mechanisms, directly affecting a target or through binding with their receptors, receptor of advanced glycation end product (RAGEs)*. In the setting of diabetes, AGEs induce increased formation of extracellular matrix; AGEs are found in this thickened tissue in greater quantities in patients with diabetes. This thickening occurs in many vascular beds of both the macro- and microcirculation including the glomeruli, renal arteries, and aorta [35]. Depending on the site, glycation of a protein can affect its function. It has also been described that AGEs induce a decrease in vascular endothelial growth factor (VEGF), and endothelial nitric oxide synthase [32]. Finally, AGEs can effect changes in transcription through binding with their receptors. *RAGEs expression is also upregulated as a result of intracellular hyperglycemia.* It is established that specific RAGEs induces signaling through (NF)-KB, and p21 ras, activating the myriad of frequently deleterious pathways regulated by these factors. RAGE also directly induces the transcription of many genes including thrombomodulin, tissue factor, and VCAM-I. These changes taken together produce a prothrombotic, inflammatory milieu with increased endothelial cell permeability [32, 36].

The protein kinase C (PKC) pathway is the fourth pathway influenced by intracellular hyperglycemia. PKC is a family of enzymes with 15 isozymes [37]. PKC is classically activated by diacylglycerol (DAG) or intracellular calcium flux. Upon activation, PKC then phosphorylates a variety of downstream effectors. In the setting of intracellular hyperglycemia, the increased concentration of glucose results in increased DAG formation.

The pathologic effects of PKC signaling are predominantly expressed through the β and δ isozymes and cause damage in multiple ways. Stimulation PKC-δ leads to PDGF receptor phosphorylation causing decreased signaling and pericyte apoptosis [38]. PKC-δ has also been shown to induce vascular smooth muscle cell apoptosis via a p53 induction [39]. PKC-β has been implicated in causing decreased nitric oxide production, increases in prostaglandin release, and inhibition of the sodium potassium pump (Na$^+$/K$^+$ ATPase) [40]. The Na$^+$/K$^+$ ATPase is essential to maintain intracellular electrolyte homeostasis. Disruption of this pump increases cellular permeability. Na$^+$/K$^+$ ATPase dysfunction is well described in many cell types in the setting of diabetes [34, 41]. PKC signaling further increases cellular permeability by inducing increases in transcription of vascular permeability factor (VPF) also known as vascular endothelial growth factor (VEGF) [42]. In summary, increased PKC signaling, particularly the β and δ isozymes, results in many deleterious events ultimately affecting cell permeability and the ability of the microcirculation to regulate transport.

A final mechanism by which increased oxidative stress induces cellular damage is through *increasing flux in the hexosamine pathway*. In the setting of intracellular hyperglycemia, a portion of the fructose-6-phosphate shunted to a pathway, which ultimately converts into *N*-acetyl glucosamine. Multiple transcription factors will bind *N*-acetyl glucosamine affecting transcription. Modification of the transcription factor Sp1 results in increased expression of transforming growth factor β (TGF-β) and plasminogen activator inhibitor-1 (PAI-1). Overexpression of TGF-β has a variety of unsalutatory effects including increasing the microvascular protein matrix. PAI-1 is associated with atherothrombotic events [43, 44]. Intracellular hyperglycemia results in increased reactive oxygen species. The generation of increased reactive oxygen species is the proximate event in multiple pathways, which profoundly affect the microcirculation through a series of diverse mechanisms.

In summary, diabetes profoundly impacts the function of the microcirculation in many different manners. These include capillary perfusion, microcirculation vascular tone, capillary permeability, the response to inflammation, and tissue wasting. Because the microcirculation plays such a critical role in maintaining tissue oxygenation and nutrition, these changes have significant clinical repercussions that cannot be overemphasized when caring for patients with diabetes. Moreover, these changes often will have a clinical impact often before other overt signs of diabetes are present.

Clinical Significance of Microvascular Changes in Diabetes

The effect of diabetes on the microcirculation has important clinical significance for practitioners caring for patients with diabetes. *Understanding the effects of diabetes on the microcirculation impacts preventative care, diagnosis of the complications of diabetes, and managing wounds and ultimately has implications for the surgical treatment of complications of diabetes.*

The guidelines for diagnosis, treatment, and goals of therapy for diabetes are well established [45]. Diabetes is thought of as a chronic disease, and many patients have little regard for their glucose control. But in fact, hyperglycemia can have a direct, acute effect on the function of the microcirculation. Endothelium-dependent vasodilation is impaired by hyperglycemia even in patients without diabetes [30]. Additionally, short-term improvement in glycemic control has been demonstrated to result in less arteriovenous shunting in patients with diabetes [46]. Endothelial dysfunction is induced by intracellular hyperglycemia. The initiation of events resulting from endothelial dysfunction begins before overt signs of diabetes are present. These data have important clinical significance for glycemic control in patients with diabetes, but do not yet suffer from the sequelae of diabetes [17].

The association between diabetes and lower extremity neuropathy is well described. This association is covered in great detail in other areas of this book. Neuropathy also has significant implications for the microcirculation and ultimately the response to injury. Patients with diabetes and neuropathy have significantly decreased capillary perfusion compared to patients without neuropathy [11, 13, 47]. Patients with diabetes also have significant impairment of the nerve–axon reflex. Taken together, in diabetes there is a significantly blunted response to injury. The injured tissue does not mount the hyperemic, inflammatory response typical of injury or infection [18]. Patients with diabetes, especially those with neuropathy often have a very benign outward appearance despite extensive injury or infection. A patient with gas gangrene might present with minimal local erythema despite extensive soft tissue destruction (Fig. 5.2). Providers caring for patients with diabetes need to be vigilant and have a high index of suspicion for serious underlying infection.

Wounds in diabetes are often more difficult to heal than in patients without diabetes. Once a wound has formed, there are multiple factors that impair the ability to heal. As previously mentioned, there is impaired capillary perfusion due in part to changes in vascular tone, arteriovenous shunting, and the absence of the nerve–axon response. Diminished capillary flow translates into local tissue hypoxia. Alterations in the capillary permeability and endothelial dysfunction can significantly impair the ability to deliver nutrients to the healing wound [48]. Although much of the damage to the function of the microcirculation cannot be reversed, we know that hyperglycemia potentiates the pathologic processes of diabetes. Maintenance of euglycemia in the setting of ulceration is important to optimize the conditions of wound healing. Finally, patients with diabetes often require increased blood flow to heal a wound than patients without diabetes. Absence of pedal pulses and a nonhealing wound in the setting of diabetes should prompt an arteriogram and assessment for revascularization. Bypass surgery has consistently been demonstrated to greatly improve wound healing and limb salvage in patients with diabetes. In fact, bypass surgery actually improves the function of the microcirculation in patients with diabetes [49]. In conclusion, it is incorrect to call diabetes small vessel disease. Diabetes has multiple deleterious effects and does result in increased atherosclerosis, however the small vessels are often spared making revascularization an important tool for limb salvage.

5 Microvascular Changes in the Diabetic Foot

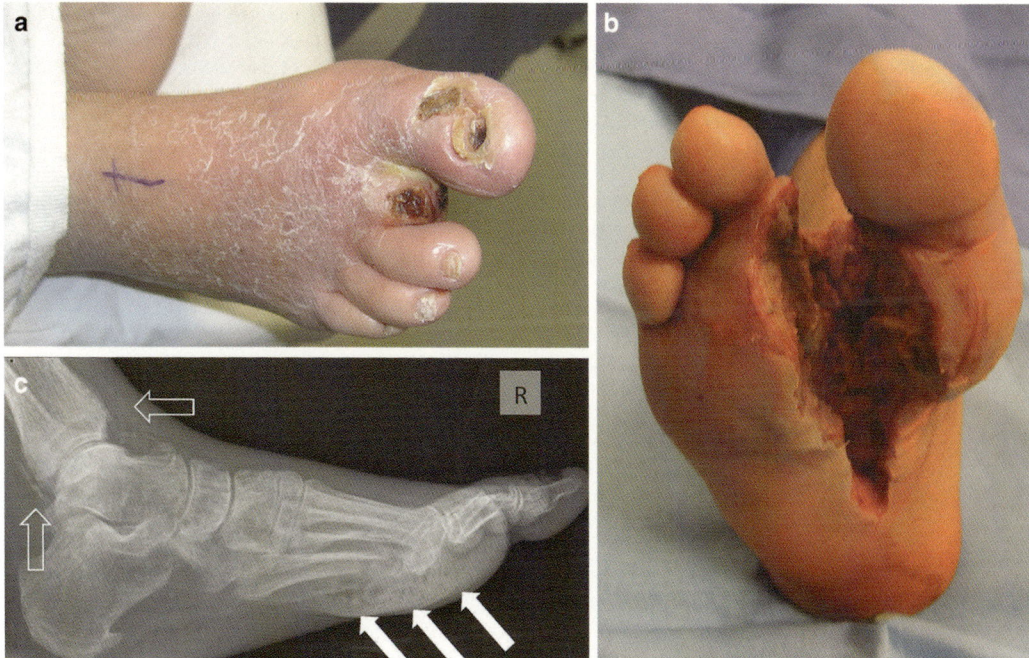

Fig. 5.2 Impaired response to injury. Patients with diabetes frequently do not mount a significant inflammatory response to injury. This patient presented with mild cellulitis after a toe amputation (panel **a**). Despite only having minimal erythema, the patient had gas gangrene (panel **b**—*closed arrows* indicate subcutaneous gas). He ultimately required extensive drainage and debridement (panel **c**)

References

1. Mahy IR, Tooke JE, Shore AC. Capillary pressure during and after incremental venous pressure elevation in man. J Physiol. 1995;485(Pt 1):213–9.
2. Taylor AE. Capillary fluid filtration. Starling forces and lymph flow. Circ Res. 1981;49(3):557–75.
3. Majno G. Maude Abbott Lecture – 1991. The capillary then and now: an overview of capillary pathology. Mod Pathol. 1992;5(1):9–22.
4. Goldenberg S, et al. Nonatheromatous peripheral vascular disease of the lower extremity in diabetes mellitus. Diabetes. 1959;8(4):261–73.
5. Strandness Jr DE, Priest RE, Gibbons GE. Combined clinical and pathologic study of diabetic and nondiabetic peripheral arterial disease. Diabetes. 1964;13:366–72.
6. Conrad MC. Large and small artery occlusion in diabetics and nondiabetics with severe vascular disease. Circulation. 1967;36(1):83–91.
7. Parving HH, et al. Hemodynamic factors in the genesis of diabetic microangiopathy. Metabolism. 1983;32(9):943–9.
8. Zatz R, Brenner BM. Pathogenesis of diabetic microangiopathy. The hemodynamic view. Am J Med. 1986;80(3):443–53.
9. Tooke JE. Microvascular haemodynamics in diabetes mellitus. Clin Sci (Lond). 1986;70(2):119–25.
10. Tooke JE. Microvascular function in human diabetes. A physiological perspective. Diabetes. 1995;44(7):721–6.
11. Schramm JC, Dinh T, Veves A. Microvascular changes in the diabetic foot. Int J Low Extrem Wounds. 2006;5(3):149–59.
12. Baum O, et al. Basement membrane remodeling in skeletal muscles of patients with limb ischemia involves regulation of matrix metalloproteinases and tissue inhibitor of matrix metalloproteinases. J Vasc Res. 2007;44(3):202–13.
13. Archer AG, Roberts VC, Watkins PJ. Blood flow patterns in painful diabetic neuropathy. Diabetologia. 1984;27(6):563–7.
14. Sandeman DD, Shore AC, Tooke JE. Relation of skin capillary pressure in patients with insulin-dependent diabetes mellitus to complications and metabolic control. N Engl J Med. 1992;327(11):760–4.
15. Sandeman DD, et al. Microvascular vasodilatation in feet of newly diagnosed non-insulin dependent diabetic patients. BMJ. 1991;302(6785):1122–3.
16. Jorneskog G, Fagrell B. Discrepancy in skin capillary circulation between fingers and toes in patients with type 1 diabetes. Int J Microcirc Clin Exp. 1996;16(6):313–9.

17. Tibirica E, et al. Impairment of skin capillary recruitment precedes chronic complications in patients with type 1 diabetes. Rev Diabet Stud. 2007;4(2):85–8.
18. Rayman G, et al. Microvascular response to tissue injury and capillary ultrastructure in the foot skin of type I diabetic patients. Clin Sci (Lond). 1995;89(5):467–74.
19. Jorneskog G, Brismar K, Fagrell B. Pronounced skin capillary ischemia in the feet of diabetic patients with bad metabolic control. Diabetologia. 1998; 41(4):410–5.
20. Purewal TS, et al. Lower limb venous pressure in diabetic neuropathy. Diabetes Care. 1995;18(3):377–81.
21. Boulton AJ, Scarpello JH, Ward JD. Venous oxygenation in the diabetic neuropathic foot: evidence of arteriovenous shunting? Diabetologia. 1982;22(1):6–8.
22. Flynn MD, Tooke JE. Diabetic neuropathy and the microcirculation. Diabet Med. 1995;12(4):298–301.
23. Flynn MD, Tooke JE. Aetiology of diabetic foot ulceration: a role for the microcirculation? Diabet Med. 1992;9(4):320–9.
24. Furchgott RF, Zawadzki JV. The obligatory role of endothelial cells in the relaxation of arterial smooth muscle by acetylcholine. Nature. 1980;288(5789): 373–6.
25. Palmer RM, Ashton DS, Moncada S. Vascular endothelial cells synthesize nitric oxide from L-arginine. Nature. 1988;333(6174):664–6.
26. Veves A, et al. Endothelial dysfunction and the expression of endothelial nitric oxide synthetase in diabetic neuropathy, vascular disease, and foot ulceration. Diabetes. 1998;47(3):457–63.
27. Nabel EG, Selwyn AP, Ganz P. Large coronary arteries in humans are responsive to changing blood flow: an endothelium-dependent mechanism that fails in patients with atherosclerosis. J Am Coll Cardiol. 1990;16(2):349–56.
28. Healy B. Endothelial cell dysfunction: an emerging endocrinopathy linked to coronary disease. J Am Coll Cardiol. 1990;16(2):357–8.
29. Vita JA, et al. Coronary vasomotor response to acetylcholine relates to risk factors for coronary artery disease. Circulation. 1990;81(2):491–7.
30. Akbari CM, et al. Endothelium-dependent vasodilatation is impaired in both microcirculation and macrocirculation during acute hyperglycemia. J Vasc Surg. 1998;28(4):687–94.
31. Hamdy O, et al. Contribution of nerve-axon reflex-related vasodilation to the total skin vasodilation in diabetic patients with and without neuropathy. Diabetes Care. 2001;24(2):344–9.
32. Giacco F, Brownlee M. Oxidative stress and diabetic complications. Circ Res. 2010;107(9):1058–70.
33. Kaiser N, et al. Differential regulation of glucose transport and transporters by glucose in vascular endothelial and smooth muscle cells. Diabetes. 1993;42(1):80–9.
34. Brownlee M. The pathobiology of diabetic complications: a unifying mechanism. Diabetes. 2005;54(6): 1615–25.
35. Niwa T, et al. Immunohistochemical detection of imidazolone, a novel advanced glycation end product, in kidneys and aortas of diabetic patients. J Clin Invest. 1997;99(6):1272–80.
36. Schmidt AM, et al. Advanced glycation endproducts interacting with their endothelial receptor induce expression of vascular cell adhesion molecule-1 (VCAM-1) in cultured human endothelial cells and in mice. A potential mechanism for the accelerated vasculopathy of diabetes. J Clin Invest. 1995;96(3): 1395–403.
37. Mellor H, Parker PJ. The extended protein kinase C superfamily. Biochem J. 1998;332(Pt 2):281–92.
38. Geraldes P, et al. Activation of PKC-delta and SHP-1 by hyperglycemia causes vascular cell apoptosis and diabetic retinopathy. Nat Med. 2009;15(11): 1298–306.
39. Ryer EJ, et al. Protein kinase C delta induces apoptosis of vascular smooth muscle cells through induction of the tumor suppressor p53 by both p38-dependent and p38-independent mechanisms. J Biol Chem. 2005;280(42):35310–7.
40. Koya D, et al. Characterization of protein kinase C beta isoform activation on the gene expression of transforming growth factor-beta, extracellular matrix components, and prostanoids in the glomeruli of diabetic rats. J Clin Invest. 1997;100(1): 115–26.
41. Vague P, et al. C-peptide, Na+, K(+)-ATPase, and diabetes. Exp Diabesity Res. 2004;5(1):37–50.
42. Williams B, et al. Glucose-induced protein kinase C activation regulates vascular permeability factor mRNA expression and peptide production by human vascular smooth muscle cells in vitro. Diabetes. 1997;46(9):1497–503.
43. Du XL, et al. Hyperglycemia-induced mitochondrial superoxide overproduction activates the hexosamine pathway and induces plasminogen activator inhibitor-1 expression by increasing Sp1 glycosylation. Proc Natl Acad Sci USA. 2000;97(22):12222–6.
44. Brownlee M. Biochemistry and molecular cell biology of diabetic complications. Nature. 2001;414(6865): 813–20.
45. American Diabetes Association. Standards of medical care in diabetes – 2011. Diabetes Care. 2011;34 Suppl 1:S11–61.
46. Flynn MD, et al. The effect of insulin infusion on capillary blood flow in the diabetic neuropathic foot. Diabet Med. 1992;9(7):630–4.
47. Greenman RL, et al. Early changes in the skin microcirculation and muscle metabolism of the diabetic foot. Lancet. 2005;366(9498):1711–7.
48. Pham HT, Economides PA, Veves A. The role of endothelial function on the foot. Microcirculation and wound healing in patients with diabetes. Clin Podiatr Med Surg. 1998;15(1):85–93.
49. Arora S, et al. Cutaneous microcirculation in the neuropathic diabetic foot improves significantly but not completely after successful lower extremity revascularization. J Vasc Surg. 2002;35(3):501–5.

Diabetic Foot Ulceration and Management

Peter A. Blume, Akhilesh K. Jain, and Bauer Sumpio

Keywords

Diabetic foot • Chronic ulcer • Charcot's foot • Neuropathy • Amputation • Platelet-derived growth factor • Neuropathy

Diabetic Foot Ulceration and Management

An ulcer is defined as a disruption of the skin with erosion of the underlying subcutaneous tissue. Foot ulcers are common in patients with diabetes mellitus with a prevalence as high as 25%. Minor trauma, often footwear related, and exacerbated by prolonged pressure and local infection is a frequent inciting event. It is estimated that 15% of Americans with diabetes will develop manifestations of diabetic foot disease in their lifetime [1, 2]. In this population, the prevalence of lower extremity ulcers ranges from 4 to 10% with an annual incidence of 2–3% [3]. Infection is a frequent (40–80%) and costly complication of these ulcers and presents a major cause of morbidity and mortality. Diabetic foot ulcers and their sequel amputations, besides being the most serious and expensive complications of diabetes, are a major cause of disability, morbidity, and mortality for these patients [1]. Although cancer and trauma can result in amputations, chronic diabetic foot ulcers lead to more than 80% of nontraumatic amputations. A detailed knowledge of the clinical picture, pathogenesis, relevant diagnostic tests, and treatment modalities is essential in planning the optimal treatment strategy for diabetic ulcers. An incorrect or delayed initial diagnosis may increase the risk of serious complications, including permanent disability and amputations.

Lower extremity disease, including peripheral arterial disease, peripheral neuropathy, foot ulceration, or lower extremity amputation, is twice as common in patients with diabetes compared to those without. Lower extremity disease affects 30% of persons with diabetes who are older than 40 years. There are 20 million people in the USA

P.A. Blume, D.P.M., F.A.C.F.A.S. (✉)
Department of Anesthesia, Yale School of Medicine,
508 Blake St., New Haven, CT 06515, USA

Department of Orthopedics and Rehabilitation,
Yale School of Medicine,
508 Blake St., New Haven, CT 06515, USA
e-mail: peter.b@snet.net

A.K. Jain, M.D.
Section of Vascular Surgery, Yale University,
New Haven, CT, USA

B. Sumpio, M.D., Ph.D.
Department of Vascular Surgery, Yale School of Medicine, New Haven, CT, USA

with diabetes of whom 10–15% is at risk for ulceration.

The median time of healing for a diabetic foot ulcer is approximately six months. During this time most patients require multiple hospitalizations to health care facilities for reasons such as infection control, debridement, wound closure, revascularization, and other medical complications. Ulceration and infection of lower extremities are the leading causes of hospitalization in patients with diabetes [3]. Treatment of pedal soft-tissue deficits in the diabetic patient population continues to be a medical and surgical challenge, extending the length of their disability and significantly increasing the cost of medical care. Despite all interventions, only two-thirds of ulcers eventually heal with the remainder resulting in some form of amputation. In 2005, approximately 1.6 million people were living with limb loss and this number is expected to more than double by 2050 [4]. Worldwide, over one million lower extremity amputations are performed annually on people suffering from diabetes and majority of these amputations are preceded by ulcers. Nearly half of all patients who undergo amputation will develop limb-threatening ischemia in the contralateral limb and many will require an amputation of the opposite limb within five years. In 2000, the Centers for Disease Control and Prevention (CDC) released the national diabetes fact sheet which estimated that 12 million Americans were diagnosed with diabetes each year. The estimated annual direct and indirect costs of diabetes treatment in the USA were approximately $174 billion, with one in five diabetes dollars spent on lower extremity care. Similar fact sheet released by CDC for the year 2011 estimated a total of 25.8 million US children and adults diagnosed with diabetes with an estimated prevalence of 8.3%. The total cost of diagnosed diabetes for the year 2007 was $174 billion, of which $116 billion was spent as direct medical costs and $58 billion on indirect costs attributed to disability, loss of productivity, and premature mortality. In the year 2010, about 1.9 million new cases of diabetes were added to the existing pool in the age group of 20 years and older. In 2007, diabetes contributed to a total of 231,404 deaths. More than 60% of nontraumatic lower-limb amputations occur in people with diabetes, which amounted to 65,700 nontraumatic lower-extremity amputations in 2006.

The cost of treating leg ulceration is staggering. Epidemiologic studies from Sweden estimated annual costs of treatment of lower extremity ulcers at $25 million. The average cost of diabetic foot ulcer treatment ranges from $3,609 to $27,721 [5]. As expected, the cost of diabetic foot ulcer care increases as the severity of the wound increases. The average diabetic foot ulcer cost has been reported to be approximately four times higher in patients with peripheral arterial disease ($23,372) compared with patients with neuropathic wounds ($5,218). The greatest expense for diabetic foot ulcers is for therapies that are not effective, because patients with unhealed wounds are more likely to have bone and soft-tissue infections that require hospitalizations [6]. In England, the estimated cost of care for patients with leg ulcers in a population of 250,000 was about $130,000 annually per patient [7]. Items factored into the equation include physician visits, hospital admissions, home health care, wound care supplies, rehabilitation, time lost from work, and jobs lost. Adding to the cost is the chronic nature of these wounds, the high rate of recurrence, and the propensity to become infected.

Preventing ulcerations and/or amputations is critical from both medical and economical standpoints. Due to the fact that chronic ulceration affects a patient's lifestyle and mobility, leg ulcers carry an enormous social cost. One of the indicators of this social cost is health-related quality of life index (HRQOL) which is defined as the sum of the physical, emotional, and social issues in a person's life that may be affected by, or may affect, a health issue. HRQOL may include factors such as physical health, pain, mobility, emotional state, dependence on others, difficulty with usual activities, and living conditions. HRQOL is worse among individuals with diabetes than in individuals without diabetes. There are multiple variables that are associated with a poorer HRQOL in patients with diabetes. There is substantial evidence, however, that the most important variable affecting HRQOL of people with diabetes is the presence of complications of which diabetic foot ulcer is the major factor [8–10]. Diabetic foot ulcers result in significant decrements in quality of life, including decreased mobility, falls, increased dependence on others, loss of employment, reduced income, increased risk of amputation, repetitive trips to the physician or clinic for care, and increased expense. The negative effect of diabetic foot ulcers on HRQOL results in large part from reduced mobility. The loss of mobility directly affects the individual's ability to engage in common everyday tasks and to participate in leisure activity. Deficits related to activities of daily living may also compromise HRQOL. Compromised mobility and the need to keep the foot dressing dry may limit self-care activities, such as bathing, and patients report loss of self-esteem related to altered hygiene patterns. The ability to work may be temporarily or permanently affected by the condition [11]. Employment is often markedly affected by the presence of the diabetic foot ulcer or associated treatment, and financial hardship is a major issue for many patients. Majority (50–79%) of patients with diabetic foot ulcers are unemployed, have retired early, or are unable to work because of the ulcer [12]. Conservative estimates indicate that about ten million workdays are lost in the USA annually secondary to lower extremity ulcers [13, 14]. A report in 1994 focused on the financial, social, and psychological implications of lower extremity lesions in 73 patients [15]. Among the study patients, 68% reported feelings of fear, social isolation, anger, depression, and negative self-image because of the ulcers. In addition, 81% of the patients felt that their mobility was adversely affected. Within the younger, actively working population, there was a strong correlation between lower extremity ulceration and adverse effect on finances, time lost from work, and job loss. In addition, there was a strong correlation between time spent on ulcer care and feelings of anger and resentment.

Despite being one of the most serious and costly complications of diabetes, foot complications can be effectively prevented. By implementing a care strategy that combines prevention, multidisciplinary treatment of foot ulcers, appropriate organization, close monitoring, and education of both healthcare professionals and people with diabetes, it is possible to reduce amputation rates by up to 85%.

Biomechanics of Walking and Diabetic Foot Ulcer Formation

An appreciation of the biomechanics required for walking is essential in understanding the etiology of foot ulcers. The foot is a complicated biologic structure containing 26 bones, numerous joints, and a network of ligaments, muscles, and blood vessels. Gait is a complex set of events that requires triplanar foot motion and control of multiple axes for complete bipedal ambulation [16]. When the heel hits the ground, its outer edge touches down first and the foot is in a supine position, which makes it firm and rigid. The soft tissue structures (muscles, tendons, and ligaments) then relax, allowing the foot to pronate and become less rigid. This enables the foot to flatten, absorb the shock of touchdown, and adapt to uneven surfaces. During midstance, the heel lies below the ankle joint complex, the front and back of the foot are aligned, and the foot easily bears weight. Toward the end of midstance, the soft tissue structures begin to tighten; the foot resupinates and regains its arch. The foot is again firm, acting as a rigid lever for propulsion. As the heel lifts off the ground, it swings slightly to the inside, and the toes push weight off the ground.

Sensory input from the visual and vestibular systems, as well as proprioceptive information from the lower extremities, is necessary to modify learned motor patterns and muscular output to execute the desired action. Various external and internal forces affect foot function [17]. The combination of body weight pushing down and the ground reactive force pushing up creates friction and compressive forces. Shear results from the bones of the foot sliding parallel to their plane of contact during pronation and supination. Foot deformities or ill-fitting footwear enhance pressure points because they focus the forces on a smaller area. When the foot flattens too much or overpronates, the ankle and heel do not align during midstance and some bones are forced to support more weight. The foot strains under the body's weight, causing the muscles to pull harder on these areas, making it more difficult for tendons and ligaments to hold bones and joints in proper alignment. Over time, swelling and pain on the bottom of the foot or near the heel may occur. Bunions can form at the great toe joint, and hammertoe deformities can form at the lesser toes. Abnormal foot biomechanics resulting from limited joint mobility and foot deformities magnify shearing forces, resulting in increased plantar pressure on the foot during ambulation (see Fig. 6.1). This can represent critical causes for tissue breakdown.

Pathology of Diabetic Foot Ulcer Formation

The pathophysiologic mechanisms underlying ulcer formation are multifactorial and include neuropathy, infection, ischemia, and abnormal foot structure and biomechanics. It is not surprising then that the management of the diabetic foot is a complex clinical problem requiring multidisciplinary approach [18, 19].

The Diabetic Foot

Persons with diabetes mellitus are particularly prone to foot ulcers. The American Diabetes Association consensus group found that among persons with diabetes, the risk of foot ulceration was increased among men, patients who had had diabetes for more than 10 years, and patients with poor glucose control or cardiovascular, retinal, or renal complications [20].

Peripheral neuropathy and peripheral vascular disease (PVD) are two major complications of diabetes which play a major role in development of diabetic foot. Development of diabetic foot disease can be attributed to several primary risk factors including neuropathy, ischemia, infection, and immune impairment (Table 6.1). Four foot-related risk factors have been identified in the

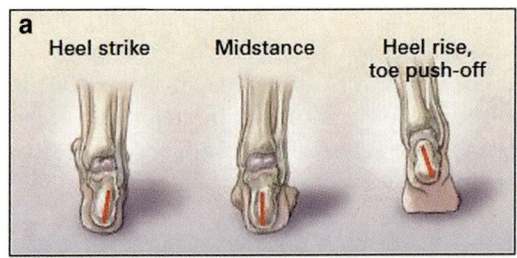
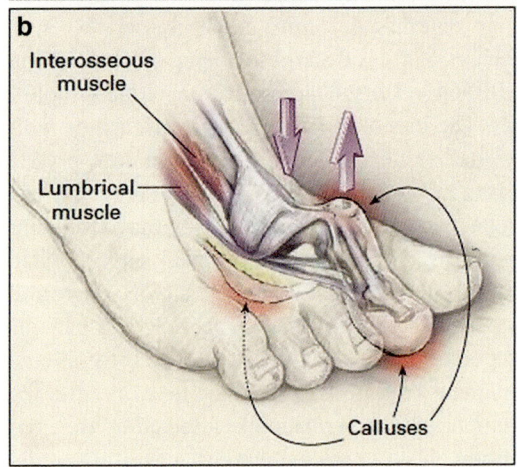
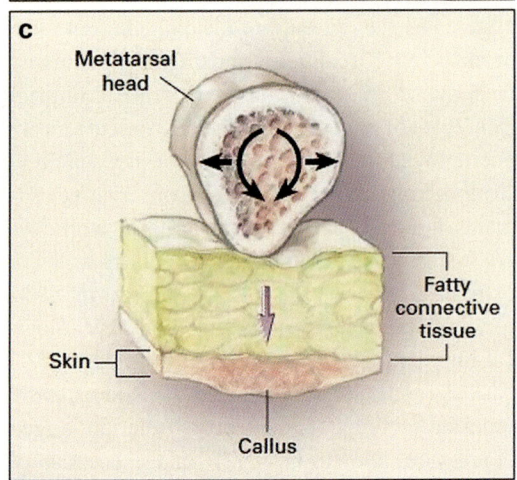

Fig. 6.1 Abnormal biomechanics contributing to pressure ulcer at first metatarso-phalangeal joint

genesis of pedal ulceration: altered biomechanics, limited joint mobility, bony deformity, and severe nail pathology [20].

Neuropathy

This subject will be discussed in detail in Chap. 4; however it is briefly discussed here. Neuropathy is the most common etiology underlying foot

Table 6.1 Risk factors for diabetic ulcers

Primary	Peripheral neuropathy, peripheral vascular disease, infection, immune impairment
Foot related risk factors	Altered biomechanics, limited joint mobility, bony deformity, severe nail pathology
Other factors	Trauma, improperly fitted shoes, impaired vision, venous disease

ulceration and frequently involves the somatic and autonomic fibers. Although there are many causes of peripheral neuropathy, diabetes mellitus is by far the most common. Neuropathy, usually distal sensorimotor polyneuropathy, is present in about 42% of diabetic patients after 20 years [21]. The peripheral neuropathy is thought to result from abnormalities in metabolic pathways, of which there are several hypotheses including deficiencies in sorbitol metabolism via the polyol pathway [22, 23].

Type-A sensory fibers are responsible for light touch, vibration, pressure, proprioception, and motor innervations to the intrinsic muscles of the foot. Type-C sensory fibers detect painful stimuli, noxious stimuli, and temperature. When these fibers are affected, protective sensation is lost which manifests as a distal, symmetric loss of sensation described in a "stocking" distribution and proves to be the primary factor predisposing patients to ulcers and infection [24]. Patients are unable to detect increased loads, repeated trauma, or pain from shearing forces. Injuries such as fractures, ulceration, and foot deformities therefore go unrecognized. Repeat stress to high-pressure areas or bone prominences, which would be interpreted as pain in the nonneuropathic patient, also goes unrecognized. Sensory dysfunction results in increased shearing forces and repeated trauma to the foot [25, 26].

Neurotrophic ulcers typically form on the plantar aspect of the foot at areas of excessive focal pressures. This is most commonly encountered over the bony prominences of the metatarsal heads and the forefoot region due to the requirements of midstance and heel off during the gait cycle (see Fig. 6.1). Several investigators have demonstrated that there is an increase in both static and dynamic foot pressures in a neuropathic foot [27–29].

Three mechanisms frequently play a part in the development of mechanically induced neuropathic ulcerations. The first mechanism is usually the result of a quick traumatic event, like stepping on a sharp object such as a nail or a piece of broken glass, which results in piercing of the skin. The second mechanism is application of chronic low grade pressure as would be seen with wearing an ill-fitting shoe. This creates focal areas of tissue ischemia over a bony prominence such as a bunion or hammer toe. If the pressure is maintained for a significant period of time, this leads to necrosis and ulceration.

The third mechanism involves a force of repetitive, moderate pressure. This accounts for the majority of diabetic plantar ulcers. Repetitive pressure >10 kg/cm acting on the foot during gait will contribute to the formation of this type of ulcer. In the absence of neuropathy, the repetitive pressure beneath prominent areas produces pain that prompts a sensate person to take measures to alleviate the discomfort. Such measures include limping or modification of gait to place weight on a different part of the foot, changing to more comfortable shoes, applying pads, or seeking medical treatment. The loss of protective sensation in the neuropathic patient lets these symptoms go undetected resulting in areas of inflammation and enzymatic autolysis culminating in tissue breakdown and ulceration. The location of this type of ulcer is predictable. Areas of increased pressure are commonly identified by areas of plantar callus formation, which conversely are the areas prone to ulceration in a neuropathic patient. Patients have inadequate protective sensation during all phases of gait; therefore, high loads are undetected due to loss of pain threshold, which results in prolonged and increased forces [25, 28]. These problems manifest as abnormal pressure points, increased shearing, and greater friction to the foot. Because this goes unrecognized in the insensate foot, gait patterns remain unchanged and the stresses eventually cause tissue breakdown and ulceration. To date, high pressures alone have not been shown to cause foot ulceration. Rheumatoid patients with high plantar foot pressures but no sensitivity deficit have almost no evidence of foot ulceration [30]. Loss of protective sensation secondary to neuropathy can rapidly lead to ulceration at these high pressure zones if patient education and preventive measures are not taken.

Motor neuropathy is associated with demyelinization and motor end-plate damage. The distal motor nerves are the most commonly affected, resulting in atrophy of the small intrinsic muscles of the foot. Wasting of lumbrical and interosseous muscles of the foot results in collapse of the arch and loss of stability of the metatarso-phalangeal joints during midstance of the gait. Overcompensation by extrinsic muscles can lead to depression of the metatarsal heads, digital contractures, and cocked-up toes; equinus deformities of the ankle; or a varus hindfoot [31].

Autonomic involvement causes an interruption of normal sweating at the epidermal level and causes arteriovenous shunting at the subcutaneous and dermal level. Hypohidrosis leads to a noncompliant epidermis that increases the risk of cracking and fissuring. Arteriovenous shunting diminishes the delivery of nutrients and oxygen to the tissues making them susceptible to breakdown [32].

Diabetic patients are especially prone to development of a neuro-osteoarthropathy also known as Charcot's foot. This condition is thought to involve autonomic-nerve dysfunction resulting in abnormal perfusion to foot bones leading to their fragmentation and collapse. The resulting "rocker-bottom foot" is prone to tissue breakdown and ulceration (see Fig. 6.2) [1, 28].

Musculoskeletal Deformities

Atrophy of the small muscles within the foot results in nonfunctioning intrinsic foot muscles referred to as an "intrinsic minus foot" [33]. The muscles showing early involvement are the flexor digitorum brevis, lumbricals, and interosseous muscles. This group acts to stabilize the proximal phalanx against the metatarsal head preventing dorsiflexion at the metatarso-phalangeal joint (MTPJ) during midstance in the gait cycle. With progression of the neuropathy, these muscles atrophy and fail to function properly. This causes the MTPJs to become unstable, allowing the long flexors (flexor digitorum longus and flexor hallucis longus) and extensors (extensor digitorum longus and extensor hallucis longus) to act unchecked on the digits. Dorsal contractures develop at the MTPJs with development of hammer digit syndrome, also known as intrinsic minus disease.

The deformity acts to plantar flex the metatarsals, making the heads more prominent and increasing the plantar pressure created beneath them. It also acts to decrease the amount of toe weight bearing during the gait cycle, which also increases pressure on the metatarsal heads. Normal anatomy consists of a metatarsal fat pad located plantar to the MTPJs. This structure helps to dissipate pressures on the metatarsal heads from the ground. When the hammer digit deformity occurs, the fat pad migrates distally and becomes nonfunctional. This results in elevated plantar pressures that increase the risk of skin breakdown and ulceration due to shearing forces [34].

Overpowering by the extrinsic foot muscles also leads to an equinus deformity at the ankle and a varus hindfoot. A cavovarus foot type can develop, leading to decreased range of motion of the pedal joints, an inability to adapt to terrain, and low tolerance to shock. In essence, a mobile adapter is converted to a rigid lever. Pressure is equal to body weight divided by surface area, thus decreasing surface area below a metatarsal head with concomitant rigid deformities and leading to increased forces or pressure to the sole of the foot. When neuropathic foot disease is associated with congenital foot deformities such as long or short metatarsals, a plantar flexed metatarsal, abnormalities in the metatarsal parabola, or a Charcot's foot, there is a higher propensity toward breakdown as a result of increased and abnormal plantar foot pressures [27].

In patients with "flatfoot" deformities, there is often excessive pronation and a hypermobile first ray that leads to an excessive amount of pressure beneath the second metatarsal. In neuropathic patients with this foot type, callus formation and subsequent ulcerations often develop beneath the second metatarsal head. In contrast, patients with a rigid cavus foot commonly ulcerate beneath the

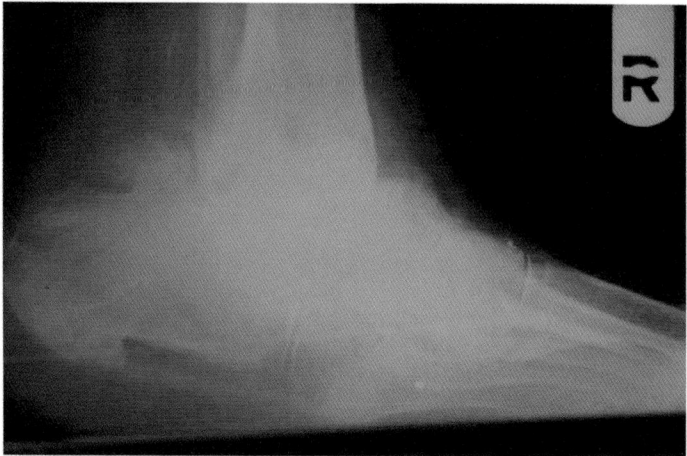

Fig. 6.2 X-ray image of rocker bottom foot with increased propensity to pressure ulcers formation. Also notice the severe soft tissue reaction in the region of talus and navicular bones

heel, the first metatarsal, and/or the fifth metatarsal. In patients with a "rocker-bottom" Charcot deformity, the area beneath the cuboid is an area of increased risk.

Increasing body weight and decreasing the surface area of contact of the foot components with the ground increases pressure. A low pressure but constant insult over an extended period can have the same ulcerogenic effect as high pressure over a shorter period. This is typical of the effect of tight-fitting shoes. If the magnitude of these forces in a given area is large enough, either skin loss or hypertrophy of the stratum corneum (callus) occurs. The presence of callus in patients with neuropathy should raise a red flag because the risk of ulceration in a callused area is increased by two orders of magnitude.

The Impact of Arterial Disease in the Diabetic Population

One of the major factors affecting diabetic foot disease is the development of lower extremity arterial disease [4]. Peripheral arterial disease is estimated to be two to four times more common in persons with diabetes than in others [35]. Compared to general population, diabetics are affected by atherosclerosis at a younger age. Besides this, in diabetics, atherosclerosis tends to progress at a much faster rate and results in higher rates of amputation [36–38]. Its hallmark is the involvement of the tibioperoneal vessels with relative sparing of the pedal vessels. Characteristically, diabetic occlusive lesions spare the arteries above the knee but involve the infrapopliteal arteries with calcific single- or multiple-level disease. In more than 90% of patients, one or more of the large vessels at the ankle and in the foot are spared. In most cases, the peroneal artery in the calf remains patent and is the last of the three crural arteries to occlude prior to which it continues to provide pedal circulation via its terminal branches. Consequently, bypass to a single tibial or peroneal artery or a pedal bypass has the potential to provide good blood flow to the foot. Occlusive lesions affecting the foot and precluding revascularization are not common in diabetic patients [1]. The presence of multisegment disease, the frequency of calcification of both the atherosclerotic lesions and the wall of the arteries involved, and the presence of renal insufficiency are additional challenges often encountered. Incompressibility of extremity arteries makes ankle brachial indices misleading in the assessment of the severity of associated PVD. Segmental volumes plethysmography and toe-brachial index can be used to determine the severity of the PVD. Precise, comprehensive anatomic imaging is the cornerstone of successful revascularization of the ischemic lower extremity in patients with diabetes mellitus. Contrast arteriography has been the mainstay for many years and remains the gold standard due to its superior image resolution and being the only modality used for both diagnosis and treatment. Coexistent renal insufficiency, however, makes conventional angiography impractical in significant percent of diabetic patients. CO_2 angiogram and noninvasive Doppler studies are other alternative imaging options in this patient population.

The incidence of lower extremity ulcers caused by peripheral arterial disease is increasing in Western nations [8, 11]. The general "aging" of the population and better diagnostic techniques may provide possible explanations for this observation. Risk factors for the development of atherosclerotic lesions causing leg ischemia include diabetes mellitus, smoking, hyperlipidemia, hypertension, obesity, and age [20]. Lack of perfusion decreases tissue resilience, leads to rapid death of tissue, and impedes wound healing. Wound healing and tissue regeneration depend on an adequate blood supply to the region. Ischemia due to vascular disease impedes healing by reducing the supply of oxygen, nutrients, and soluble mediators that are involved in the repair process [21].

Purely ischemic diabetic foot ulcers are uncommon, representing only 10–15% of ulcers in patients with diabetes. More commonly, ulcers have a mixed ischemic and neuropathic origin, representing 33% of diabetic foot ulcers [23]. The initiation of an ischemic ulcer usually requires a precipitating factor such as mechanical stress. Ulcers often develop on the dorsum of the foot, over the first and fifth metatarsal heads. A heel ulcer can develop from constant pressure applied while the heel is in a dependent position or during prolonged immobilization and bed rest. Once formed, the blood supply necessary to allow healing of an ulcer is greater than that needed to maintain intact skin. This leads to chronic ulcer development unless the blood supply is improved.

Infection

Patients with diabetes appear to be more prone to various infections than their nondiabetic counterparts [43]. Forty to eighty percent of diabetic foot ulcers have evidence of infection. Several factors increase the risk of development of diabetic foot infections including diabetic neuropathy, peripheral arterial disease, and immunologic impairment. Diabetic state causes impairment in the functioning of polymorphonuclear leukocytes that can manifest as a decrease in migration, phagocytosis, and decreased intracellular activity. Evidence suggests impaired cellular immune response, as well as abnormalities in complement function [44, 45]. Some of the defects appear to improve with control of hyperglycemia [46] underscoring the need for a tight and consistent control of hyperglycemia.

Undiagnosed clean neuropathic foot ulcers often convert to acute infections with abscess and/or cellulitis [47]. Most infections involve soft tissues of the foot but about 20% of the patients develop culture positive osteomyelitis. Presence of peripheral arterial disease, neuropathy, or impaired leukocyte functions may reduce the local inflammatory response and classical signs or symptoms of local infection that makes the diagnosis of infection in a diabetic foot especially challenging.

Diabetic foot infections can be classified into those that are nonthreatening and those that are life or limb threatening. Non-limb-threatening diabetic foot infections are often mild infections associated with a superficial ulcer. They often have less than 2 cm of surrounding cellulitis and demonstrate no signs of systemic toxicity. These infections have on average 2.1 organisms [47]. Aerobic gram-positive cocci are the sole pathogens in 42% of these cases, with the most notable organisms being *Staphylococcus aureus*, coagulase-negative *S. aureus*, and streptococci. These less severe infections can often be managed with local wound care, rest, elevation, and oral antibiotics on an outpatient basis. A foot infection in a diabetic patient can present with a more severe, life- or limb-threatening picture. In these patients, there is usually a deeper ulceration or an undrained abscess, gangrene, or necrotizing fasciitis. Methicillin-resistant *Staphylococcus aureus* (MRSA) is an increasingly common isolate [43]. They tend to have greater than 2 cm of surrounding cellulitis, as well as lymphangitis and edema of the affected limb. These more severe cases generally present with fever, leukocytosis, and hyperglycemia.

In contrast to nondiabetic individuals, complex foot infections in diabetic patients usually involve multiple organisms with complex biofilm environments [48]. Studies report an average of five to eight different species per specimen [49–52]. These included a combination of gram-positive and -negative, as well as aerobic and anaerobic organisms. The most prevalent organisms identified were *S. aureus*, coagulase-negative *Staphylococcus*, group B *Streptococcus*, *Proteus*, *Escherichia coli*, *Pseudomonas*, and *Bacteroides*. Recently, methicillin-resistant *S. aureus* (MRSA) infection has become more common in diabetic foot ulcers and is associated with previous antibiotic treatment and prolonged time to healing [43, 53, 54]. Anaerobic infections with Clostridium are also not uncommon. These patients require immediate hospitalization, broad-spectrum IV antibiotics, and aggressive surgical debridement. Superficial wound cultures are often unreliable, as they may demonstrate organisms responsible for colonization that do not affect the associated infection. Deep wound or bone cultures are the best way to accurately assess the microbiology in a diabetic foot infection and to assess for osteomyelitis.

Associated Cardiovascular Disease in the Diabetic Population

Cardiovascular disease is increased in individuals with type 1 or type 2 DM. The Framingham Heart Study revealed a marked increase in PAD, CHF, CHD, MI, and sudden death (risk increase from one- to fivefold) in DM. The American Heart Association has designated DM as a "CHD risk equivalent." Type 2 diabetes patients without a prior MI have a similar risk for coronary artery-related events as nondiabetic individuals who have had a prior MI. Because of the extremely high prevalence of underlying cardiovascular disease in individuals with diabetes (especially in type 2 DM), evidence of atherosclerotic vascular disease (e.g., cardiac stress test) should be sought in an individual with diabetes who has symptoms suggestive of cardiac ischemia or peripheral or carotid arterial disease. The increase in cardiovascular morbidity and mortality rates appears to relate to the synergism of hyperglycemia with other cardiovascular risk factors. In addition to CHD, cerebrovascular disease is increased in individuals with DM (threefold increase in stroke). Individuals with DM have an increased incidence of CHF. Hypertension can accelerate other complications of DM, particularly cardiovascular disease and nephropathy.

Renal Complications of Diabetes and Diabetic Foot

Diabetic nephropathy is the leading cause of end-stage renal disease (ESRD) in the USA and a leading cause of DM-related morbidity and mortality. Like other microvascular complications, the pathogenesis of diabetic nephropathy is related to chronic hyperglycemia. Almost 44% of patients starting hemodialysis in the USA have diabetes mellitus as their primary diagnosis. Peripheral vascular disease (PVD) remains a major problem in patients with chronic renal insufficiency undergoing dialysis. When compared to general population, PVD not only affects a substantially higher percentage of patients with renal failure, it also has worse outcome with higher rates of amputation. Patients with ESRD have about fourfold increase in foot complications compared to patients without ESRD. The greatest amputation rate is seen in patients with diabetes and those who are older. Of those undergoing amputation only 49% of patients survive 1 year, and the survival rate is only 32.7% at 2 years [39]. Patients with chronic kidney disease and dialysis have more below-knee amputations and above-knee amputations than patients with no renal disease. In a 10-year review of over 1,000 medical records, Lavery et al. identified a 290%

increase in hazard for death for dialysis treatment and a 46% increase for chronic kidney disease (CKD). Subjects with an above-knee amputation had a 167% increase in hazard and below-knee amputation patients had a 67% increase in hazard for death [40]. In one of the largest cohort studies on this subject, review of over 90,000 patients confirmed a strong association between stage of chronic kidney disease and diabetic foot ulcer or lower extremity amputation that is probably not just related to the presence of PVD. Patients with even moderate CKD have increased risk of diabetic foot ulcers and lower extremity amputation, which rises exponentially with the severity of renal disease. Thus, renal disease, higher level of amputation, and advancing age adversely affect survival after a lower-extremity amputation in individuals with diabetes.

Despite the availability of a suitable distal bypass target in a patient with diabetic foot, surgical revascularization and limb salvage can be a challenging task because of comorbid cardiopulmonary, endocrine, and renal pathology. Impaired wound healing and infectious complications occur secondary to uremia, malnutrition, diabetes mellitus, and long-term immunosuppression. Not only is the perioperative mortality up to 10%, the wound complication rate after peripheral revascularization reaches almost 30% in these patients. Majority of amputations (about 60%) following surgical revascularization in patients with diabetic foot and ESRD in fact result from persistent ischemia and uncontrolled foot infection despite a patent bypass [41]. Even with adequate perfusion, failure of tissue healing in patients with ESRD could be explained by associated conditions such as anemia, malnutrition, and depressed immune function. Delayed wound healing occurs with uremia, which reduces formation of granulation tissue in wounds when compared with controls. Diabetes, in addition, results in reduced collagen content in the granulation tissue. Although patients undergoing transplantation are not affected by uremia, they receive immunosuppressive medications that impair wound healing and add to wound complications.

Assessment of the Patient with a Diabetic Foot Ulcer

Accurate diagnosis of the underlying cause of lower extremity ulceration is essential for successful treatment. The etiology of most leg ulcers can be ascertained quite accurately by careful, problem-focused history and physical examination [29]. Diagnostic and laboratory studies are occasionally necessary to establish the diagnosis but are more often performed to guide treatment strategy [42].

History

Arterial insufficiency is suggested by a history of underlying cardiac or cerebrovascular disease, complaints of leg claudication or impotence, or pain in the distal foot when supine (rest pain). Symptoms of arterial insufficiency occur because of inadequate perfusion to the lower extremity relative to its metabolism. Tissue hypoxia and the subsequent increase in concentration of lactic acid produce pain. Patients may complain of pain in the buttocks or calves brought on with activity and relieved with rest (intermittent claudication) or pain in the forefoot aggravated by elevation and relieved by dependency (rest pain). The presence of an extremity ulcer is an easily recognized but late sign of peripheral vascular insufficiency. Patients with lower extremity ulcers resulting from atherosclerotic disease usually have a risk-factor profile that includes: older age, male sex, smoking, diabetes mellitus, hypertension, hypercholesterolemia, and obesity. Patients with leg ulcers and multiple atherosclerotic risk factors often have atherosclerosis in other arterial beds [43].

Up to one-third of patients with diabetes mellitus can have significant atherosclerotic disease, without specific symptoms. Most common complaints are those of neuropathic disease, which include history of numbness, paresthesias, and burning pain in the lower extremities. Patients often report previous episodes of foot ulcers and chronic skin infections.

Physical Examination of the Diabetic Foot

A complete examination can only be performed with the patient supine in an examination gown. The patient's vital signs are recorded and abnormalities noted. The patient's temperature, respiratory rate, heart rate, and blood pressure in both upper extremities should be obtained. Fever may indicate the presence of an infected ulcer, and the presence of tachycardia and tachypnea may support the diagnosis of a septic foot.

A classic look, listen, and feel examination includes inspection of the skin of the extremities, palpation of all peripheral pulses, measurement of ankle-brachial indices, assessment of extremity temperature, auscultation for bruits, and a thorough neurologic examination [29]. Patients with diabetic foot frequently have nonpalpable pedal pulses secondary to coexistent PAD and medial calcinosis and hence bedside Doppler evaluation of pedal signals is essential to have a preliminary assessment of vascular status.

Visual inspection coupled with an accurate history can determine the presence of a chronic vascular condition. The color of the skin is conferred by the blood in the subpapillary layer and varies with the position of the extremity, temperature of the skin, and degree of blood oxygenation. Also in chronic arterial insufficiency, the arterioles are maximally dilated as a compensatory response to the chronic ischemia intensifying color changes. In acute arterial occlusion the venules empty, leading to a chalky white appearance regardless of extremity position. Partial but inadequate perfusion either from an incomplete acute or chronic occlusion allows for pooling of blood in the venules, which may be red in the cold or blue at higher temperatures.

When the extremity is at the level of the heart, the pooled blood masks the color imparted by the arterial flow. Elevation of the extremity above the level of the central venous pressure (rarely >25 cm) allows the pooled venous blood to drain, enabling an accurate assessment of the degree of arterial flow. The normal extremity remains pink, whereas that with arterial insufficiency becomes pallid. Conversely, allowing the extremity to become dependent causes an intense rubor or cyanosis. The time of return of blood to the dependent extremity is a useful marker of the severity of the deficit (normally <20 s). With a diminished nutritional supply to the skin, there is thinning and functional loss of the dermal appendages, evident as dry, shiny, and hairless skin. The nails may become brittle and ridged. Comparison of color and trophic changes between extremities gives a good indication of the severity of the process unless a bilateral deficit is present, in which case the experience of the examiner is required to make an accurate diagnosis.

Skin temperature is a reliable indicator of the blood flow rate in the dermal vessels, though flow is governed primarily by constriction or dilation of the arterioles to maintain a constant core temperature. Nevertheless, the temperature of the skin as a marker of perfusion is useful and can be assessed by lightly palpating the skin with the back of the hand and comparing similar sites from one extremity to the other. An ischemic limb is cool, and demarcation of temperature gives a rough indication of the level of the occlusion. Again, assessment of temperature differences is confounded when both extremities are affected.

Ulcer Evaluation

Specific characteristics of the ulcer such as location, size, depth, and appearance should be recorded during the initial evaluation and with each subsequent follow-up visit to record progress and evaluate the treatment regimen [44] (Table 6.2). Ulcers of the foot should be gently examined with a cotton-tipped probe to establish the presence of a sinus tract. The margins of the ulcer should be undermined to evaluate the extent of tissue destruction. Ulcer extension to tendon, bone, or joint should be sought. A positive probe-to-bone finding has a high predictive value for osteomyelitis and is an extremely sensitive and cost-effective screen (see Figs. 6.3 and 6.4) [45]. In a study involving 132 consecutive patients, Lozano et al. demonstrated that probe-to-bone test has a sensitivity of 98%, specificity of 78%, positive predictive value of 95%, and negative predictive value of 91% ($P<0.001$) when compared

Table 6.2 Classification of diabetic foot ulcers: proposed by Wagner

Grade 0	No ulcer in a high-risk foot
Grade 1	Superficial ulcer involving the full skin thickness but not underlying tissues
Grade 2	Deep ulcer, penetrating down to ligaments and muscle, but no bone involvement or abscess formation
Grade 3	Deep ulcer with cellulitis or abscess formation, often with osteomyelitis
Grade 4	Localized gangrene
Grade 5	Extensive gangrene involving the whole foot

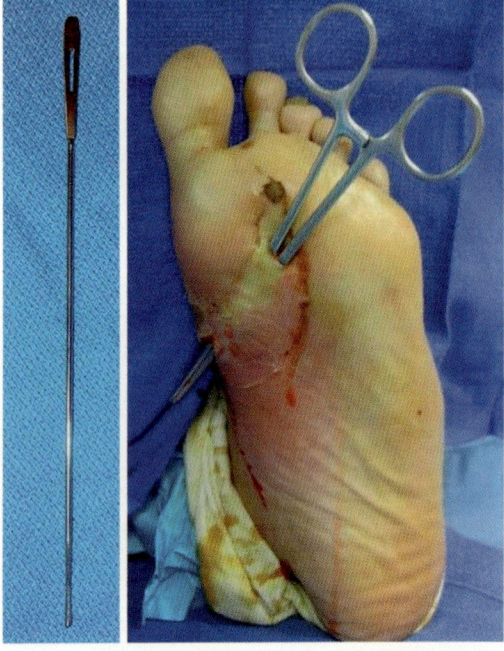

Fig. 6.3 A classic bone probe. Hemostat across a wound, confirming a tunneling, deep space infection

to gold standard of bone histology and culture [46]. Other, although less accurate, indicators of coexisting osteomyelitis in a diabetic foot ulcer include clinical signs of infection, radiography signs of osteomyelitis, and ulcer specimen culture.

Ulcerations caused by ischemia are typically located on the tips of the toes and between the digits. The lesions often appear punched out and are painful but exhibit little bleeding. Ischemic ulcers are characterized by absence of bleeding, pain, and a precipitating trauma or underlying foot deformity. They also often develop on the dorsum of the foot and over the first and fifth metatarsal heads. Ischemic ulcers are uncommon on the plantar surface as the pressure is usually less sustained and the perfusion better. A heel ulcer can develop from constant pressure applied while the heel is in a dependent position or during prolonged immobilization and bed rest. It should not be a surprise that a patient with relatively mild symptoms of arterial insufficiency develops limb-threatening extremity ulcers. This is due to the fact that once an ulcer is present; the blood supply necessary to heal the wound is greater than that needed to maintain intact skin. A chronic ulcer will develop unless the blood supply is improved.

Neuropathic ulcerations typically occur at the heel (Fig. 6.5) or over the metatarsal heads on the plantar surface at pressure points (mal perforans ulcer, Fig. 6.6) but may also occur in less characteristic locations secondary to trauma. They usually are painless. The sensory neuropathy in the diabetic patient may allow the destructive process to go unchecked, with extension into the deep plantar space and minimal appreciation by the patient.

In addition to ulcers, patients may present with varying degrees of tissue loss or frankly gangrenous digits, forefoot, or hindfoot. The presence of dry gangrene is a relatively stable process allowing for a complete vascular evaluation; however, any progression to an infected wet gangrene requires immediate surgical debridement.

Vascular Examination

A handheld Doppler ultrasound should be used in case of inability to easily palpate a given vessel. These can be supplemented with noninvasive vascular tests and other diagnostic tests as necessary for each clinical situation. An ankle-brachial index is an important tool for assessing perfusion to the foot. Patients with an ABI less than 0.6 often experience claudication; patients with an ABI less than 0.3 may complain of rest pain; and in patients with tissue loss, the ABI is often less than 0.5 [47]. In patients with diabetes and renal failure due to calcification of the vessel, ABI may

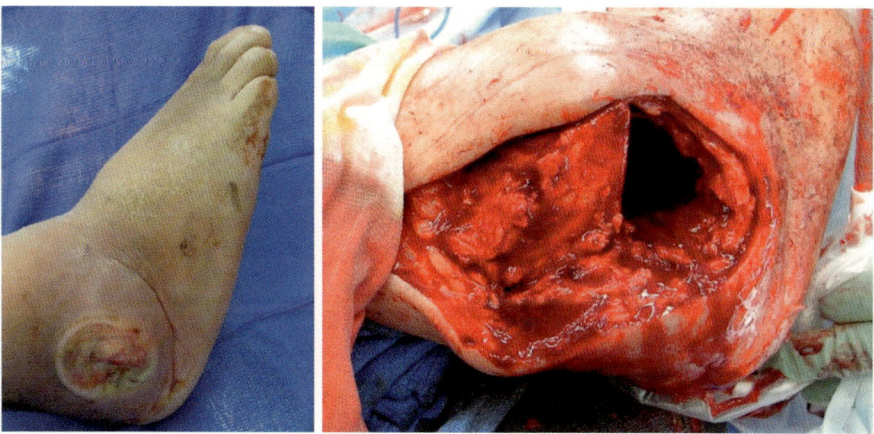

Fig. 6.4 Lateral malleolus ulcer. Inspection does not reveal obvious bone involvement; however it had positive probe to bone test. Debridement revealed necrotic and infected bone which was subsequently confirmed on bone culture

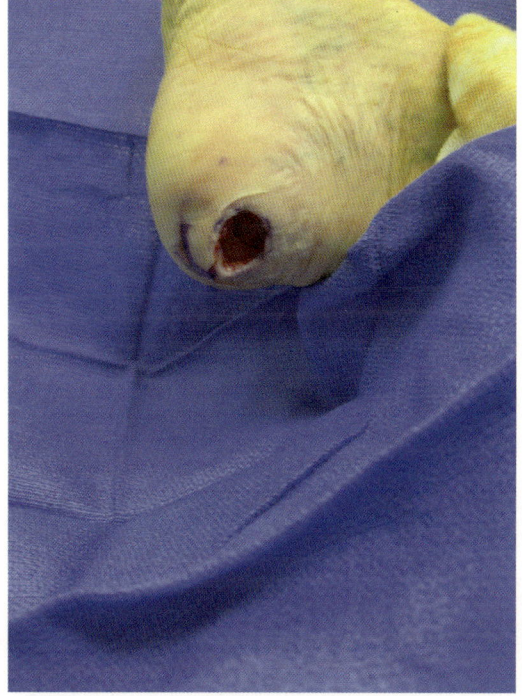

Fig. 6.5 Mal perforans ulcer at the heal immediately postdebridement ready to be closed

be falsely elevated and is not reliable to evaluate the level of ischemia. Toe brachial index, measured by placing small cuffs on toes, is a better indicator of foot perfusion due to the fact that toe vessels are relatively spared from the atherosclerotic disease process.

Neurologic Examination

The lower extremity neurologic examination is essential and should include testing for motor strength; deep-tendon reflexes; and vibratory, proprioceptive, and protective sensation [48]. Chronic ischemia can cause varying patterns of sensory loss that is usually within the affected arterial distribution. Neuropathy occurs in 42% of patients with diabetes within 20 years after diagnosis of the disease [21]. The neuropathy alters motor, sensory, and autonomic function, which directly affect the dynamic function of the foot during gait. The gait of the patient should be observed to detect any gross asymmetry or unsteadiness.

Motor neuropathy is associated with demyelinization and motor end-plate damage, which contribute to conduction defects. Atrophy of the small intrinsic muscles of the foot occurs secondary to the distal motor nerve damage. Wasting of the lumbric and interosseous muscles of the foot results in collapse of the arch and loss of stability of metatarsal–phalangeal joints during midstance of the gait. Overpowering by extrinsic muscles can lead to depression of the metatarsal heads, digital contractures, and cocked-up toes. These changes result in abnormal pressure points, increased shearing, and ulcer formation.

Diabetic sensory neuropathy is typically a glove-and-stocking distribution and is associated with a decrement in vibration and two-point

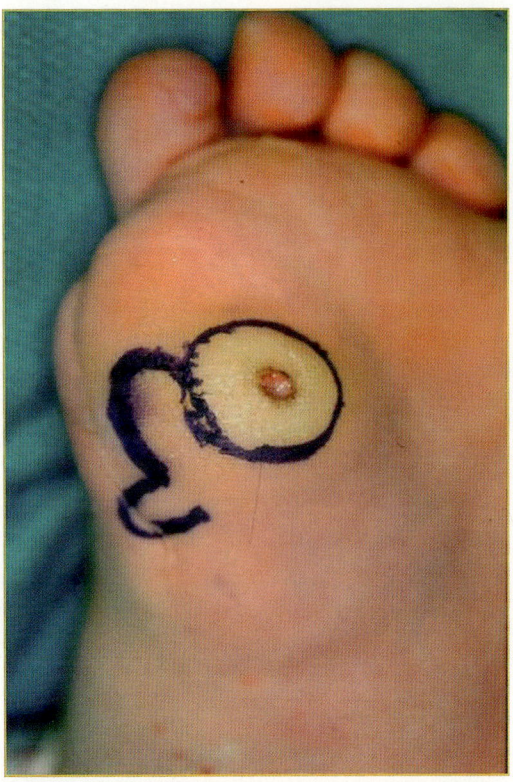

Fig. 6.6 Mal perforans ulcer over the first metatarsal head

discrimination. Loss of protective sensation due to peripheral neuropathy is the most common cause of ulceration in the diabetic population. The use of monofilament gauges (Semmes–Weinstein) is a good objective way of assessing diabetic neuropathy [48]. Patients with normal foot sensation usually can feel a 4.17 monofilament (equivalent to 1 g of linear pressure). Patients who cannot detect a 5.07 monofilament when it buckles (equivalent to 10 g of linear pressure) are considered to have lost protective sensation [49, 50]. Several cross-sectional studies have indicated that foot ulceration is strongly associated with elevated cutaneous pressure perception thresholds [48, 52]. Magnitudes of association, however, were provided in a case–control study, where an unadjusted sevenfold risk of ulceration was observed in those patients (97% male) with insensitivity to the 5.07 monofilament [51]. Screening is vital in identifying diabetic neuropathy early, thus enabling earlier intervention and management to reduce the risk of ulceration and lower extremity amputation. Although the nerve conduction test is the gold standard, its expense and limited availability prevent its widespread application as a screening tool for diabetic neuropathy. Semmes–Weinstein monofilament is a convenient, inexpensive, painless alternative to NCS that should be utilized in the initial evaluation of all patients with diabetes mellitus as a screen for peripheral neuropathy. A positive Semmes–Weinstein monofilament result is a significant predictor of future ulceration and likely lower extremity amputation as well in patients with diabetes mellitus [52]. If diabetic patients have positive monofilament results, their chances of ulceration increase with 10–20%, corresponding with a 2.5–5 times higher risk than patients with normal sensation as determined by monofilament. Additionally, the risks of leg amputation increase 5–15%, which corresponds with a 1.5–15 times higher risk for patients with diabetes mellitus with positive monofilament results compared with those with negative monofilament results. The Semmes–Weinstein monofilament is an important evidence-based tool for determining which patients are at increased risk of complications during follow-up, leading to improved patient selection for early intervention and management. Ultimately, screening with Semmes–Weinstein monofilament may lead to improved clinical outcomes for patients with diabetic foot [52].

The presence of neuropathy mandates attention to the biomechanics of the foot. The role of the podiatrist or podiatric foot and ankle surgeon in the evaluation of these patients cannot be underscored enough [18]. Use of a computerized gait analysis system to assess abnormally high pressure areas has led to greater use of orthotic devices in the prevention of skin breakdown. For example, an F scan system uses an ultrathin Tekscan sensor consisting of 960 sensor cells (5 mm^2 each). The sensor is used in a floor mat system designed to measure barefoot or stocking-foot dynamic plantar pressures, indicating those subjects with pressures greater than or equal to 6 kg/cm^2. Abnormal mechanical forces that can result in ulcerations should be addressed with the

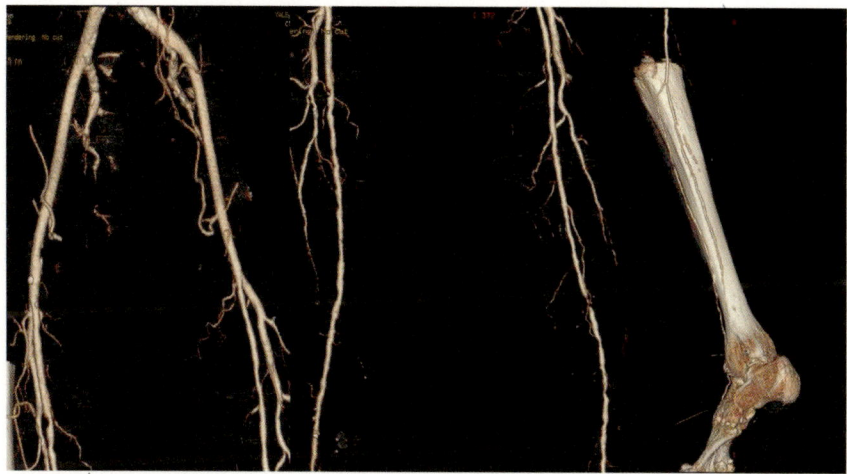

Fig. 6.7 CT angiogram of a patient with diabetic foot. Vascular disease in diabetics typically affects the tibial vessels as reflected by the third portion of this image

use of offloading devices or other modalities in order to assist in wound healing.

Particular attention should be paid to documenting a complete neurologic examination on patients who have suffered from a previous stroke, as much of the rationale for extremity salvage hinges on the potential for rehabilitation. The remainder of the physical examination should be undertaken with attention to the presence of comorbidities, which may influence the decision-making process.

Tests and Imaging Techniques

Duplex ultrasound is an integral component of diagnostic testing for the evaluation and management of arterial disease. This technology combines the acquisition of blood flow (pulsed Doppler spectral analysis) and anatomic (B-mode and color Doppler imaging) information. Contemporary duplex ultrasound systems provide high-resolution B-mode ultrasound imaging of tissue and vessel anatomy, including three-dimensional vessel reconstruction and evaluation of atherosclerotic plaque morphology. The duplex testing performed in the vascular laboratory is an extension of clinical assessment and is used to verify the presence and extent of disease, the involved arterial segment, and its severity. In selected patients, duplex testing can obviate the need for diagnostic arteriography for decisions regarding suitability for endovascular intervention or bypass grafting. For the diagnosis of stenosis or occlusion involving the femoropopliteal artery segment, diagnostic accuracy exceeds 95% [53]. Other noninvasive imaging methods useful in the assessment of patients with leg ulcers include plain radiography, MRI, MR angiography, and CT angiography (Fig. 6.7) [54]. Imaging techniques can be used to diagnose osteomyelitis and confirm the presence of bony deformities. Plain film radiography is used primarily to exclude bony lesions as a cause of a patient's pain complaints, assess the presence of osteomyelitis beneath a ulcerated foot lesion, and assess the degree of vascular wall calcification (usually in concert with standard IV contrast angiography). Plain films of the foot are relatively inexpensive and can show soft-tissue swelling, disruption of bone cortex, and periosteal elevation (Fig. 6.2). MRI can provide details of pathologic anatomic features and has a high sensitivity for assessment of deep space infection and the presence of osteomyelitis in the diabetic foot.

The assessment of a patient with foot ulcers stemming from peripheral vascular disease encompasses a thorough history and physical

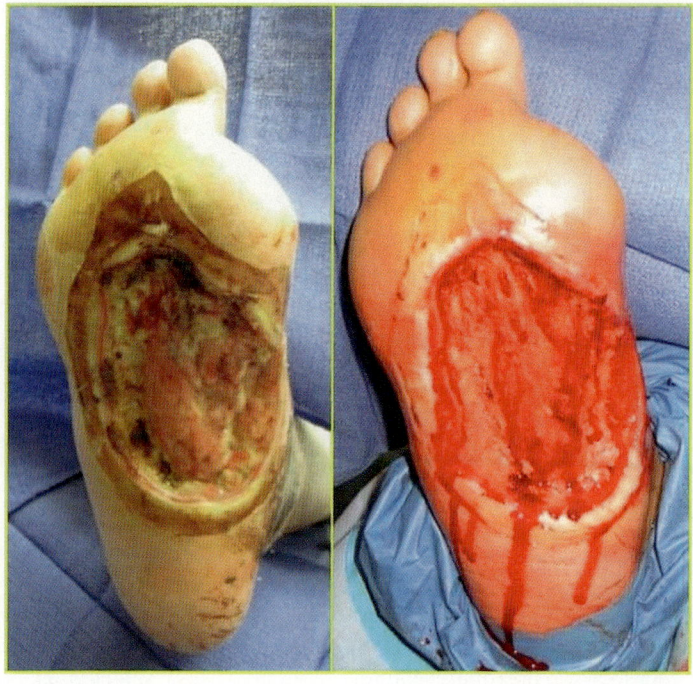

Fig. 6.8 Sharp debridement has removed all necrotic material down to healthy bleeding tissues in preparation of skin grafting

examination with the adjunctive use of the noninvasive vascular laboratory to confirm, localize, and grade lesions [47]. While multiple noninvasive and invasive methods are available to assess the peripheral vasculature, it should be obvious that not every patient requires an exhaustive battery of tests in order to evaluate his or her vascular status. In general, only those tests likely to provide information that alters the course of action should be performed. Differing clinical syndromes mandate the extent of peripheral vascular testing. It is imperative that flow-limiting arterial lesions are evaluated and reconstructed or bypassed if ischemic foot ulcers are to heal.

Management of Ulcers

General

Aggressive mechanical debridement, systemic antibiotic therapy, and strict nonweight bearing are the cornerstones for effective wound care [55]. The role of a multidisciplinary group of consultants in the management of diabetic ulcers cannot be overemphasized [56]. Successful management of foot ulcers involves recognition and correction of the underlying etiology, as well as appropriate wound care and prevention of recurrence. Sharp debridement in the operating room or at the bedside, when applicable, allows for thorough removal of all necrotic material and optimizes the wound environment (Fig. 6.8) [57]. Advanced debridement techniques like hydrosurgery (Versajet), ultrasonic debridement (Sonaca), and numerous recent modalities can be helpful in eliminating necrotic tissue in preparation for wound closure (Fig. 6.9). All necrotic bone and devascularized tissues, plus a small portion of the uninvolved bone and soft tissue should be excised to establish the degree of penetration of the infection (Fig. 6.4) [57]. Curettage of any exposed or remaining cartilage is important to prevent this avascular structure from becoming a nidus of infection. Foot soaks, whirlpool therapy, or enzymatic debridement have a use but are rarely effective and may lead to further skin maceration or wound breakdown. No prospective randomized studies have demonstrated the superiority of dressing products compared with standard saline wet to dry sterile gauze in establishing a granulation bed. Use of moist dressings in clean,

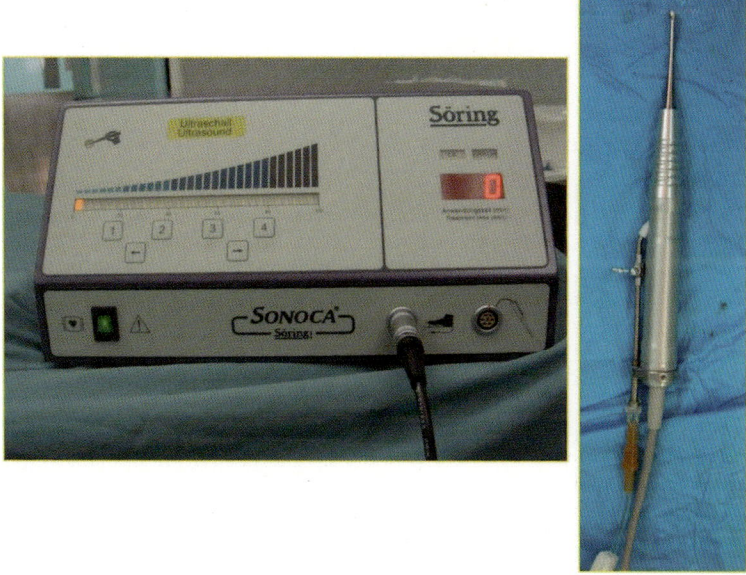

Fig. 6.9 Sonoca ultrasonic debridement apparatus

Table 6.3 Various types of dressings

Type of dressing	Characteristics
Hydrogels	Contain a large portion of water (70–90%). Cool the surface of the wound, with marked pain reduction. Maintain moist wound environment and are mostly suitable for use on dry or necrotic wounds or lightly exuding wounds. Not suitable for infected or heavily exuding wounds
Hydrocolloids	Slowly absorb fluids, leading to formation of gel covering the wound. Ensure the moist wound environment, promote the formation of granulation tissue, and provide pain relief by covering nerve endings. Are suitable for the dressing of both acute wounds and chronic wounds, for desloughing, and for different stages of light-to-heavily exuding wounds. These should not be used on infected wounds
Alginates	Are highly absorbable biodegradable dressings derived from seaweed. They control exudate by ion exchange, activate macrophages within the chronic wound bed to generate proinflammatory signals. Not the dressing of choice for infected wounds and should not be applied to dry or drying wounds. Most alginates require a secondary dressing

granulating wounds is recommended to enhance the wound environment [58, 59]. An "ideal" dressing not only provides protection against further bacterial contamination but also maintains moisture balance, optimizes the wound pH, absorbs fibrinous fluids, and reduces local pain. Many advanced moist wound therapies are available and each has its own distinct characteristics (Table 6.3). Hydrogels, hydrocolloids, alginates, and many silver compounds have been found to promote wound healing and reduce bacterial contamination (Fig. 6.10) [60]. Various dressings are currently available to target specific characteristics of the wound; however, moist normal-saline dressings are probably sufficient for most wounds [61]. These inexpensive dressings are highly absorptive of exudative drainage and maintain the moist environment.

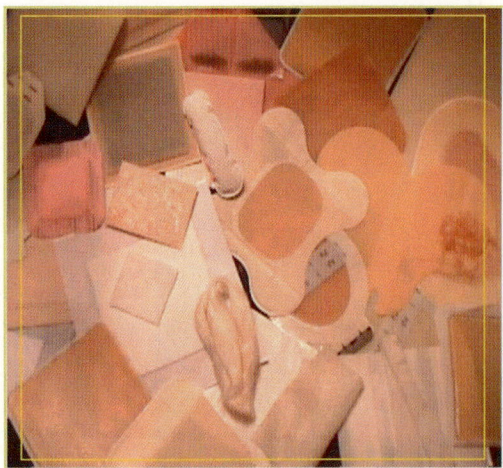

Fig. 6.10 Various types of specialized dressings available off the shelf

Advanced Surgical Debridement Techniques

While surgical debridement is swift and effective, it requires a skilled operator to carry it out safely and thoroughly. Debridement using a scalpel produces a very clean wound, but healthy collateral tissue around the wound is also removed. Nonsurgical methods of debridement include autolysis—often facilitated by dressings, larval therapy using sterile maggots, and chemical debridement using collagenases or papain–urea ointments. These are all effective in certain wounds but tend to be slow and sometimes unpredictable. Recent developments in hydrosurgery provide more control over the surgical debridement process. The VERSAJET system (Fig. 6.11) uses pressurized saline in a sterile circuit that is forced into a nozzle. The water executes a 180° turn and is forced out of a miniscule nozzle, less than 0.0005 in. diameter, where it emerges as a focused jet. The water jet passes parallel to the wound and is captured by an evacuator port creating a Venturi effect. Venturi effect associated with the flow carries the water jet, ablated tissue, and debris into the evacuator port without the need for separate suction. The debridement therapy of Versajet therapy is clearly visible without any accompanying thermal damage to the tissue. There is minimal bleeding with excellent preservation of the healthy collateral tissue.

Control of Infection

Infection control is paramount to the success of wound conversion. The absence of systemic manifestations such as fever, chills, or leukocytosis is an unreliable indicator of underlying infection, especially in the diabetic immune-compromised population. Systemic antibiotics must be given as early as possible in cases of clinically infected diabetic foot ulcers and the use of topical antibiotics and antiseptics is not recommended as the sole treatment of infection. In cases of gross wound infections and rampant cellulitis, use of a silver-containing medication such as Silvadene may be necessary in the initial setting to reduce the bacterial load. Oral antimicrobial therapy should be instituted on the basis of the suspected pathogen and clinical findings. IV antimicrobials should be administered for severe infections. Polymicrobial infections are common in the diabetic foot but the majority of pathogens remain gram positive [62, 63]. Severe infections, however, should be treated with broad-spectrum IV antibiotics with particular emphasis on the role of biofilms [64, 65]. Initial broad spectrum systemic therapy is continued until adequate cultures are available. A severity grading of the wound can assist in choice of antibiotics. The antibiotic regimen must always include an agent active against Gram-positive cocci, particularly *S. aureus*. Other factors to be considered when selecting an appropriate antibiotic combination and the route of administration include: severity of infection, previous allergy or intolerance, patient compliance, renal and/or hepatic dysfunction, peripheral arterial disease and any devitalization of the tissues surrounding the wound, recent exposure to antibiotic therapy or hospital admission, chronicity of the wound, knowledge of local potential pathogens, and antibiotic sensitivity patterns severity of infection. IDSA guidelines have been developed as a tool for determining appropriate antimicrobial therapies.

6 Diabetic Foot Ulceration and Management

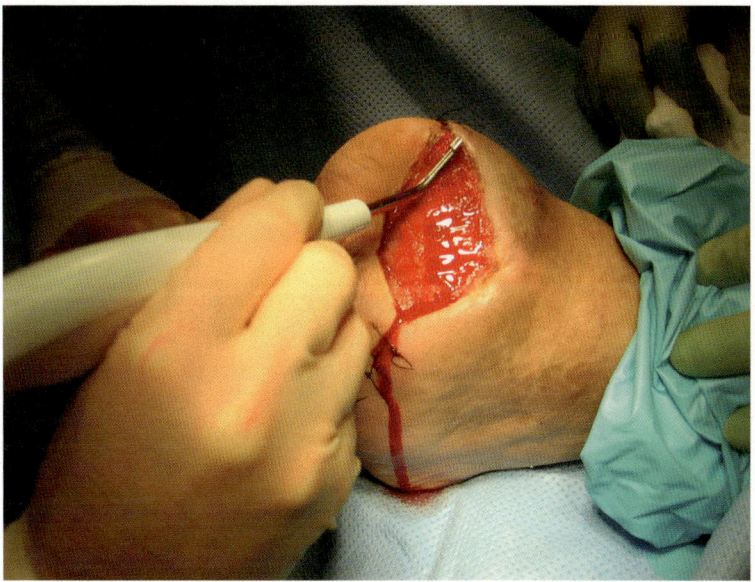

Fig. 6.11 Versajet system uses a venturing effect of a high pressure thin water stream to capture debris without the need of a separate suction. There is minimal bleeding with excellent preservation of healthy collateral tissue

The emergence of resistance poses many unique problems in reference to diabetic foot infections. MRSA, VRE, and gram negative resistance have created new challenges for those caring for the diabetic foot [66]. Development of newer antibiotic therapies for resistant pathogens is timely. Each drug has its own unique properties. Daptomycin (Cubist), Linezolid (Zyvox), Ceftaroline (Teflaro), and Tygicycline (Tygicil) represent some of the new antibiotic therapies [67]. However, as emphasized by Lipsky et al. and recently confirmed in a systematic review, no one particular antimicrobial agent or regimen has yet been shown to be superior to others in curing diabetic foot infection [68]. Once antibiotic treatment is initiated, the wound must be regularly and carefully inspected to assess the response to therapy. Once microbiological culture and sensitivity testing results are available the initial regimen should be adjusted to use the most effective narrow-spectrum regimen. The optimal duration of antibiotic treatment is not clearly defined and depends on severity of infection and response to treatment. Most authorities suggest that 1- to 2-week antibiotic therapy for mild infections whereas treatment must be extended for up to 1 month or more for more severe infections.

Wound Closure and Foot Reconstruction

After bacterial contamination has been controlled, small ulcers can usually be excised and closed immediately. Use of local rotation flap helps in primary closure of the excised wounds without any undue tension on the suture line (Fig. 6.12). This allows the use of local tissue, which is more suited for weight bearing, for wound closure (Fig. 6.13). Large open wounds, however, are treated with a staged approach, with frequent debridement and establishment of a granulation base. The clean wounds can then be closed with healthy tissue, with the use of local or free-flap coverage and soft-tissue repair (Fig. 6.14). Meticulous surgical reconstruction of these wounds can help avert the production of inelastic scar tissue over weight-bearing surfaces. Any remaining extrinsic or intrinsic pressures can be reduced with the postoperative use of orthoses.

The endpoint for chronic diabetic foot wounds should include reduction in the number of major amputations, prevention of infection, decreased probability of ulceration, maintenance of skin integrity, and improvement of

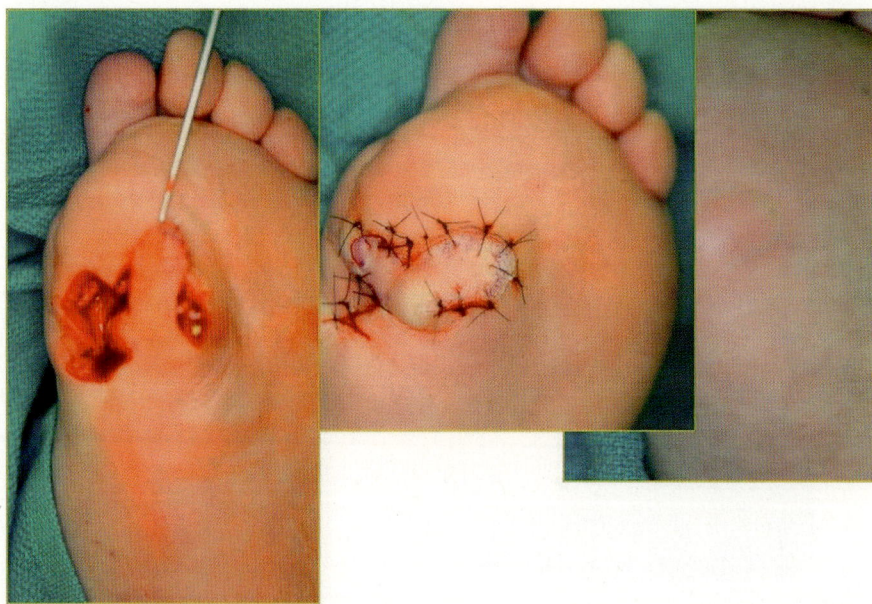

Fig. 6.12 Localized rotation flaps help in tension free primary closure of wounds

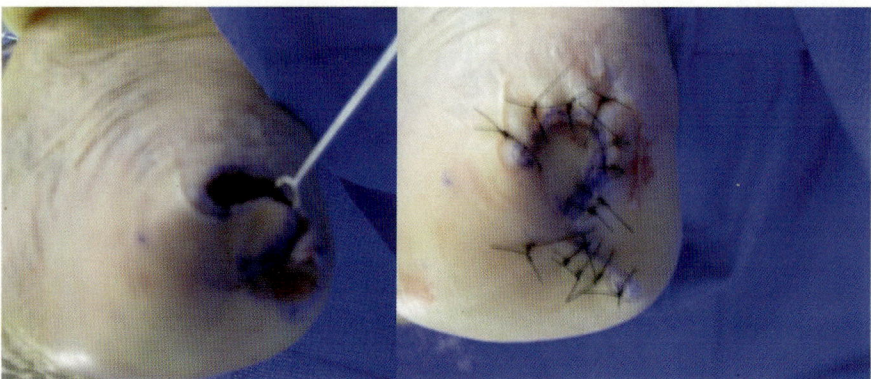

Fig. 6.13 Rotation flap allows the use of heel skin for wound closure

function. Reconstructive foot surgery plays a vital role in avoiding major amputations in these chronic neuropathic wounds. Successful outcomes for diabetic foot reconstruction should result in less intrinsic pressures via minor amputations, arthroplasties, osteotomies, condylectomies, exostosectomies, tendon procedures, and joint arthrodesis [56]. Open wounds can be treated in one stage and are primarily closed with premorbid tissue using local flap reconstruction and soft tissue repair [69]. Plastic surgical repair of these wounds can help avoid the production of inelastic scar tissue over weight-bearing surfaces [70]. Extrinsic and intrinsic pressures can be further neutralized with postoperative accommodative shoe gear [71, 72]. Prophylactic diabetic foot surgery is an increasingly used option to prevent recurrent ulceration and reduce the risk of major amputations [73, 74]. Surgical biomechanics, plastic and soft tissue reconstruction, and appropriate offloading are all essential to creating a stable platform from which to keep these difficult patients free from tissue breakdown and as functional as possible.

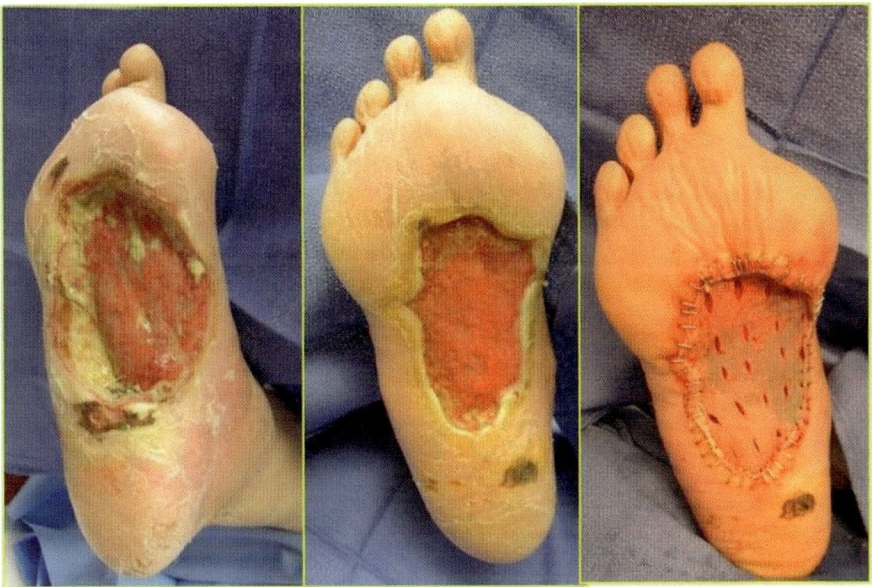

Fig. 6.14 Staged closure of large chronic wounds

Treatment of these pedal soft tissue deficits in the diabetic patient population continues to be a medical and surgical challenge, which extends the length of the patient's disability and significantly increases the cost of medical care. Simple closure of these wounds is often difficult because of preexisting bone deformity, tissue inelasticity, location of the defect, and superimposed osteomyelitis.

Negative Pressure Wound Therapy in Diabetic Foot

Management of even for the most superficial wounds in a diabetic foot is difficult with poor healing responses and high rates of complications. Although several advanced debridement and dressing techniques have been developed to improve wound healing, achieving adequate wound closure is a major problem. Negative pressure wound therapy (NPWT) has emerged as an effective treatment for these complex wounds [56]. This involves application of subatmospheric pressure to the wound through open celled foam dressing in a closed environment. The pump is connected to a canister, which collects the wound exudates. Besides the convenience of wound care, NPWT has been shown to stimulate angiogenesis, increase rate of granulation tissue, and decrease bacterial colonization while decreasing edema and increasing blood flow [75]. Multiple studies have indicated that NPWT is a safe and effective treatment for complex diabetic foot wounds and could lead to a higher proportion of healed wounds, faster healing rates, and potentially fewer re-amputations than standard care. When compared to advanced moist wound therapy in a multicenter randomized control trial, NPWT achieved wound closure in 43% patients as opposed to 29% patients being treated by conventional techniques ($P=0.007$). Patients with NPWT also experienced fewer secondary amputations and a significantly shorter healing time [76].

Once healthy granulation of deep complex wounds is achieved, restoration of intact skin barrier is of utmost importance following to prevent infection, minimize wound contraction to maintain function, minimize cosmetic disfigurement, and to avoid volume depletion. Traditionally, split-thickness skin grafts (STSGs) are used to cover large areas of skin loss, granulating tissue beds, tissue loss across joints in areas where contraction will cause deformity and where epithelialization alone will produce an unstable wound cover. STSGs currently represent the most rapid,

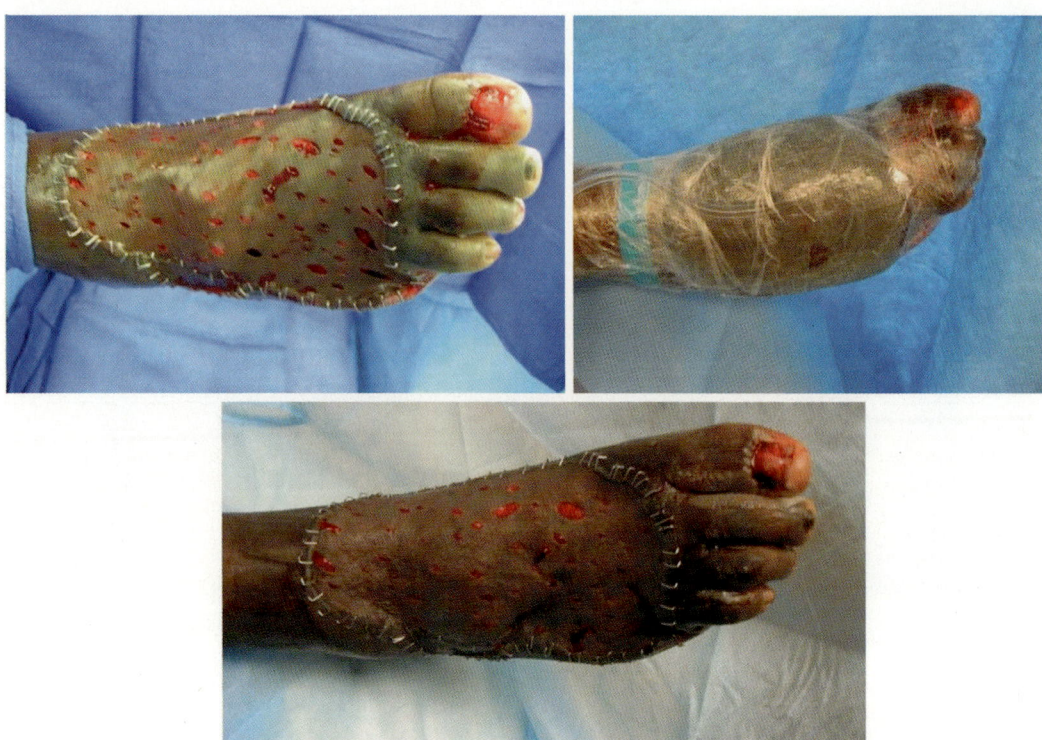

Fig. 6.15 Negative pressure wound therapy is very effective in stabilizing the fresh skin grafts on the wound bed and also aid in removal of seroma from under the graft

effective method of reconstructing large skin defects. The conventional therapy dressing of choice, to secure the graft while it is healing, is a cotton bolster or sterile compressive or stainless steel gauze dressing that is used for at least five days. NPWT has been increasingly used as an alternative dressing following STSG and has achieved improved graft survival while reducing the incidence of complications such as seroma, hematoma, and infection (Fig. 6.15). Mechanisms of action of NPWT include reducing edema from extracellular tissues, decreasing the bacterial load on the wound, and promoting tissue perfusion and healthy granulation tissue formation [77–79].

Off-Loading Techniques

Surgical correction of biomechanical defects, plastic and soft-tissue reconstruction, and appropriate measures to minimize foot pressure are all essential to enable the patient to walk effectively again. Likewise, the use of negative pressure wound therapy has been a big advance in the care of advanced wounds [76, 80, 81].

Off-loading strategies such as total contact casting or removable walkers has resulted in significant decreases in healing times [71, 72]. The stresses placed on the foot can be intrinsic, as was previously described with respect to digital contractures, or extrinsic in nature. These external forces can result from inappropriate footwear, traumatic injury, or foreign bodies. Shoes that are too tight or too shallow are a frequent yet preventable component to the development of neuropathic ulcers. Various shoe modifications such as the rocker-sole design and different types of insoles have made it possible to reduce plantar foot pressures, thus decreasing the risks of ulceration [82–84].

Revascularization

Management of ischemic ulcers follows some basic guiding principles. It is imperative that flow-limiting arterial lesions be evaluated and reconstructed or bypassed [85]. In general, the optimal strategy is to perform revascularization, if indicated, as soon as possible. Closure of the ulcer by primary healing or secondary reconstructive surgery will then be expedited. If revascularization of an ischemic ulcer is not possible for medical or technical reasons, amputation of the foot or limb will most likely result. Contraindications to revascularization include nonambulatory patients and a foot phlegmon with sepsis or excessive foot gangrene, precluding a functional foot despite adjunctive plastic surgical procedures such as skin grafts and free flaps.

Nonoperative management of patients with lower extremity ischemia consists of general wound care measures. As a rule, however, severe ischemia of the lower limb generally requires an interventional approach. The method of revascularization of the affected limb depends on several factors, among the most important being the indications for surgery, the patient's operative risk, arteriographic findings, and available graft material.

Bioengineered Alternative Tissues and Adjunctive Therapies for Diabetic Foot Wounds

Even when properly managed, the wounds may not heal in a timely fashion. Foot ulcers that do not heal in an expedient amount of time are expected to be more likely to become complicated by intervening infection, hospitalization, and amputation and, thus, to be more costly because of the increased utilization of healthcare resources. Therapists generally rely on good clinical judgment and personal experience in deciding when to use more aggressive or more expensive technologies and interventions. In a prospective randomized controlled trial in 203 patients, wound area reduction of greater than 52%, both absolute and relative, over a 4-week period was a strong predictor of complete wound healing over an extended 12-week period (58% healing rate vs 9% healing rate) [86].

Many agents have been suggested to be used as adjuvants, to aid healing, in the treatment of diabetic ulcers. These therapies include topical agents for application to the wound bed (e.g., Recombinant PDGF, Regranex), systemic therapies (hyperbaric oxygen) to treat the patient, and skin substitutes (e.g., Apligraf, Dermagraft) (Figs. 6.16 and 6.17). These agents have shown promising results and have proven useful under specific circumstances. There is level I evidence that platelet-derived growth factor (PDGF) is effective in treating diabetic neurotrophic foot ulcers. PDGF is a powerful chemoattractant and mitogen, exerting its action on fibroblasts, smooth muscle cells, and endothelial cells. It also induces production of fibronectin and hyaluronic acid. Margolis and colleagues examined the effectiveness of recombinant PDGF (becaplermin) in actual clinical practice in a study including 24,898 subjects with neuropathic foot ulceration between 1998 and 2004, of whom 2,394 (9.6%) received becaplermin. Healing rates were 33.5% and 25.8% in the becaplermin and control group, respectively ($P<0.0001$) consistent with increased likelihood of healing by 32%. Moreover, amputation rates were significantly ($P<0.0001$) lower in the becaplermin (4.9%) than in the control group (6.4%) [87]. Other cytokine growth factors do not yet have enough data on efficacy to recommend any of them for treatment of diabetic ulcers, although isolated reports suggest their potential usefulness [88].

Tissue-engineered skin (Apligraf, Organogenesis) comprises a cultured living dermis and sequentially cultured epidermis, the cellular components of which are derived from neonatal foreskin. In a randomized trial involving 208 patients, the rate of healing at 12 weeks was higher among those who used tissue-engineered skin (applied weekly for up to 5 weeks) and received good wound care (debridement and elimination of pressure) than among those who received good wound care alone (56% vs. 38%, $P=0.004$). Treatment with tissue-engineered skin was associated with

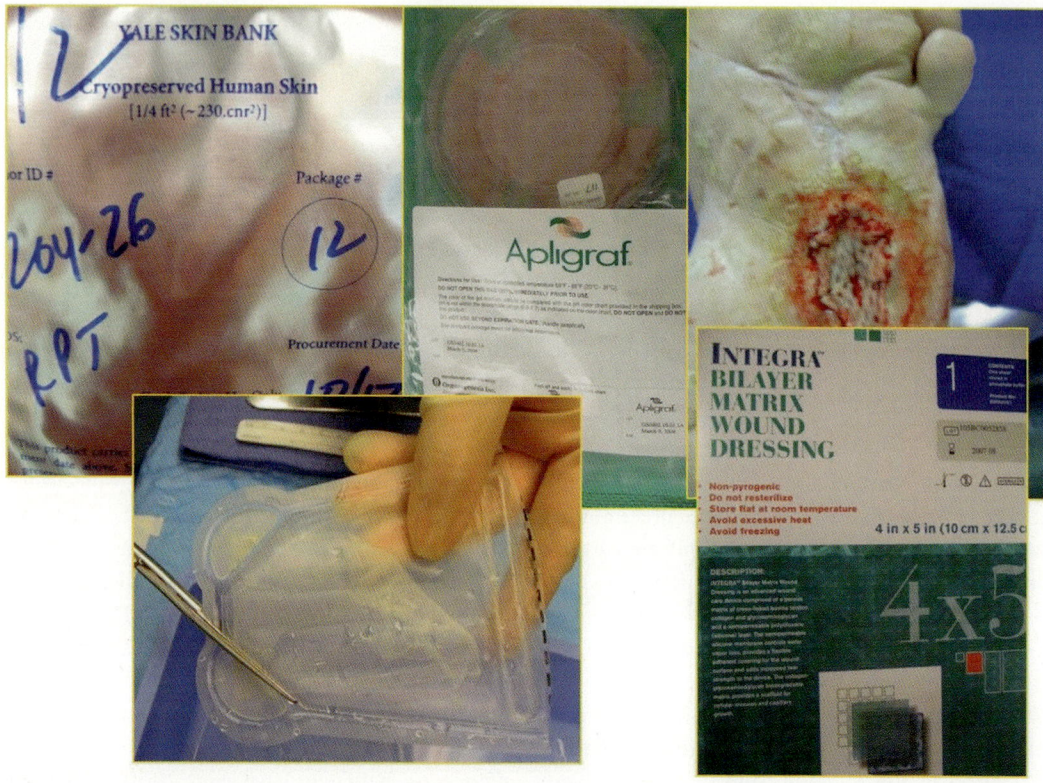

Fig. 6.16 Various adjuvant therapies available to aid in the healing of chronic wounds

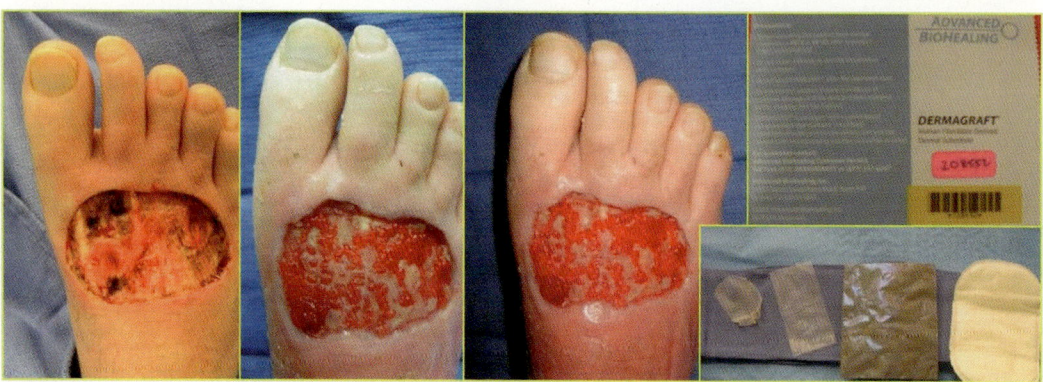

Fig. 6.17 Dermagraft®, a living dermal substitute, has been shown to increase the proportion of diabetic foot ulcers that heal at 12 weeks by 64% when compared to conventional therapy

faster healing and lower rates of osteomyelitis (3%, vs. 10% in the control group; $P=0.04$) and lower-limb amputation (6 percent vs. 16 percent, $P=0.03$) [89]. The failure to reduce the size of an ulcer after four weeks of treatment that includes appropriate debridement and pressure reduction should prompt consideration of adjuvant therapy (Fig. 6.18). Current adjunctive therapies are in general limited due to a combination of their substantial costs and poor reproduction of results of

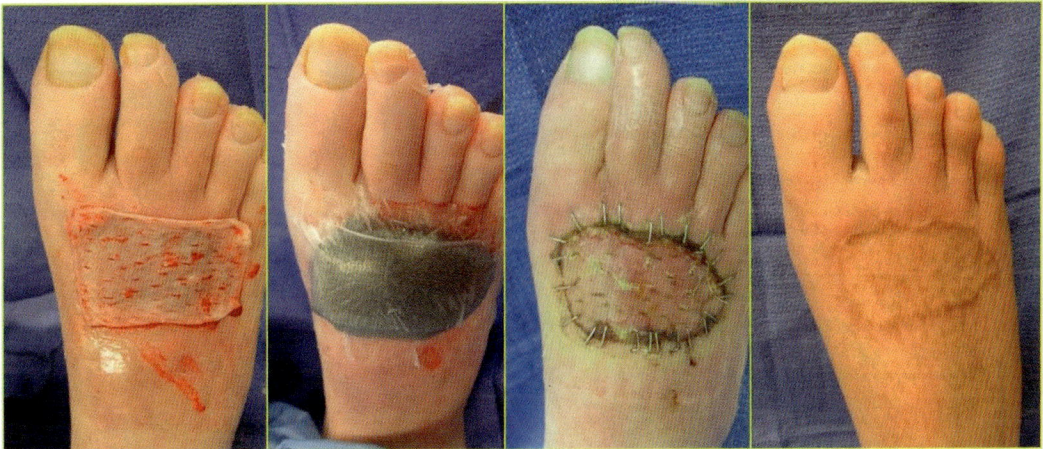

Fig. 6.18 Multiple adjunctive therapies may be required to achieve a good outcome from a chronic diabetic foot wound

controlled clinical trials in actual clinical practice [90]. Other investigational adjuvant therapies for diabetic foot include electrical stimulation of the ulcer bed, therapeutic ultrasound, application of electromagnetic fields, and therapeutic heat.

Metabolic Control in Diabetic Foot

People with diabetes should receive medical care from a physician-coordinated team. Such teams may include, but are not limited to, physicians, nurse practitioners, physician's assistants, nurses, dietitians, pharmacists, and mental health professionals with expertise and a special interest in diabetes. Two primary techniques are available for health providers and patients to assess the effectiveness of the management plan on glycemic control: patient self-monitoring of blood glucose (SMBG) and A1C. Since A1C is thought to reflect average glycemia over several months, and has strong predictive value for diabetes complications, A1C testing should be performed routinely in all patients with diabetes, at initial assessment and then as part of continuing care [91]. Lowering A1C to below or around 7% has been shown to reduce microvascular and neuropathic complications of diabetes and, if implemented soon after the diagnosis of diabetes, is associated with long-term reduction in macrovascular disease. Therefore, a reasonable $A1_C$ goal for many nonpregnant adults is <7% [92].

The Reconstructive Ladder

Reconstructive surgery can range from simple metatarsal head resections to subtotal calcanectomies. Local flaps that are often difficult to elevate and inset are more easily mobilized and incised when concomitant bone resection is achieved at the time of flap creation. In addition, a local flap results in greater exposure and direct visualization of the underlying osseous structures compared with a single linear or semielliptical incision. The implementation of local random flaps can eliminate the need for additional incisions often deemed necessary to gain access to a forefoot, midfoot, or rearfoot bony defect (Fig. 6.19). The use of negative pressure wound therapy has greatly enabled the salvage of these complex limb wounds [56].

Prevention of Recurrence of Diabetic Foot Ulcers

Diabetic ulcers of lower extremity are a chronic problem with recurrence rates of 8–59%. Therefore, long-term maintenance must be addressed even for healed ulcers. This includes identification of high-risk patients, education of the patient, and institution of measures to prevent ulceration. High-risk patients should be identified

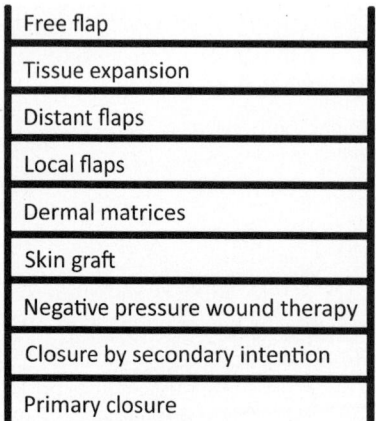

Fig. 6.19 The reconstructive ladder

during the routine foot examination performed on all patients with DM. Patient education should emphasize (1) careful selection of footwear, (2) daily inspection of the feet to detect early signs of poor-fitting footwear or minor trauma, (3) daily foot hygiene to keep the skin clean and moist, (4) avoidance of self-treatment of foot abnormalities and high-risk behavior (e.g., walking barefoot), and (5) prompt consultation with a health care provider if an abnormality arises. Any diabetic patient admitted to acute care setting should (1) have their feet examined on admission, (2) if it is judged that their feet are at risk of new ulceration, preventive steps should be taken immediately, which includes provision of a pressure mattress and suitable protective footwear, (3) those with new ulcers should be referred promptly to an expert multidisciplinary team for expert assessment and management [93]. There is strong evidence that introduction of a specialist podiatry service and a comprehensive diabetes education and care management program in the dialysis unit results in a prompt decline in the incidence of amputation. McMurray et al. demonstrated that introduction of such a program in dialysis unit results in significant stabilization of the diabetes-related peripheral vascular/neuropathic disease and the 12-month foot risk assessment score. While there was no difference in the mortality, the study group had a statistically significant lower hospitalization rate for diabetes, peripheral vascular, infection, and amputation-related admissions ($P<0.05$) [94].

Summary Diabetic Foot Ulcers and Management

Chronic diabetic foot ulcers are frequently encountered in clinical practice. The cost of chronic non-healing wounds is enormous and is accompanied with a considerable morbidity and mortality. The role of the primary care physician in the evaluation, diagnosis, and management of lower extremities wounds is critical. Careful assessment of vascular disease, evaluation and management of biomechanical and metabolic abnormalities, and aggressive treatment of any infections are required. The multidisciplinary approach provides a comprehensive treatment protocol and significantly increases the chances of successfully healing the ulcer and preventing recurrence.

Clinical pathways related to diabetic foot ulcers frequently involve persistent sharp debridement, expensive wound care products, long-term IV antibiotics, total contact casting, total contact casting with tendo-Achilles lengthening, use of skin equivalents, electrical stimulation, multiple offloading orthopedic devices, and even amputation.

References

1. Knox RC, Dutch W, Blume P, Sumpio BE. Diabetic foot disease. Int J Angiol. 2000;9(1):1–6.
2. Reiber GE, Lipsky BA, Gibbons GW. The burden of diabetic foot ulcers. Am J Surg. 1998;176(2A): 5S–10.
3. Boulton AJ. The diabetic foot: a global view. Diabetes Metab Res Rev. 2000;16 Suppl 1:S2–5.
4. Weiss JS, Sumpio BE. Review of prevalence and outcome of vascular disease in patients with diabetes mellitus. Eur J Vasc Endovasc Surg. 2006;31(2): 143–50.
5. Stockl K, Vanderplas A, Tafesse E, Chang E. Costs of lower extremity ulcers among patients with diabetes. Diabetes Care. 2004;27:2129–34.
6. Lavery LA, Armstrong DG, Wunderlich RP, Mohler MJ, Wendel CS, Lipsky BA. Risk factors for foot infections in individuals with diabetes. Diabetes Care. 2006;29:1288–93.
7. Ellison DA, Hayes L, Lane C, Tracey A, McCollum CN. Evaluating the cost and efficacy of leg ulcer care provided in two large UK health authorities. J Wound Care. 2002;11(2):47–51.
8. Lloyd A, Sawyer W, Hopkinson P. Impact of long-term complications on quality of life in patients with

type 2 diabetes not using insulin. Value Health. 2001;4: 392–400.
9. Ragnarson TG, Apelqvist J. Health-related quality of life in patients with diabetes mellitus and foot ulcers. J Diabetes Complications. 2000;14:235–41.
10. Goodridge D, Trepman E, Embil JM. Health-related quality of life in diabetic patients with foot ulcers. Literature review. J Wound Ostomy Continence Nurs. 2005;32:368–77.
11. Phillips TJ. Chronic cutaneous ulcers: etiology and epidemiology. J Invest Dermatol. 1994;102(6): 38S–41.
12. Ashford RL, McGee P, Kinmond K. Perception of quality of life by patients with diabetic foot ulcers. Diab Foot. 2000;3:150–5.
13. Browse NL. The etiology of venous ulceration. World J Surg. 1986;10(6):938–43.
14. Goldman M, Fronek A. The Alexander House Group: Consensus paper on venous leg ulcers. J Dermatol Surg Oncol. 1992;18:592.
15. Phillips T, Stanton B, Provan A. A study of the impact of leg ulcers on quality of life: financial, social, and psychological implications. J Am Acad Dermatol. 1994;31:49–53.
16. Hutton W, Stokes I. The mechanics of the foot. In: Klenerman L, editor. The foot and its disorders. Oxford: Blackwell; 1991. p. 11.
17. Murray H, Boulton A. The pathophysiology of diabetic foot ulceration. Clin Podiatr Med Surg. 1995;12:1.
18. Sumpio BE, Armstrong DG, Lavery LA, Andros G. The role of interdisciplinary team approach in the management of the diabetic foot: a joint statement from the Society for Vascular Surgery and the American Podiatric Medical Association. J Vasc Surg. 2010;51(6):1504–6.
19. Sumpio BE, Aruny J, Blume PA. The multidisciplinary approach to limb salvage. Acta Chir Belg. 2004;104(6):647–53.
20. American Diabetes Association. Preventive foot care in people with diabetes [position statement]. Diabetes Care. 2003;26 Suppl 1:78.
21. O'Brien IA, Corrall RJ. Epidemiology of diabetes and its complications. N Engl J Med. 1988;318(24): 1619–20.
22. Kamal K, Powell RJ, Sumpio BE. The pathobiology of diabetes mellitus: implications for surgeons. J Am Coll Surg. 1996;183(3):271–89.
23. Laing P. The development and complications of diabetic foot ulcers. Am J Surg. 1998;176(2A):11S–9.
24. Levin ME. Diabetes and peripheral neuropathy. Diabetes Care. 1998;21(1):1.
25. Boulton AJ, Hardisty CA, Betts RP, Franks CI, Worth RC, Ward JD, et al. Dynamic foot pressure and other studies as diagnostic and management aids in diabetic neuropathy. Diabetes Care. 1983;6(1):26–33.
26. Fernando DJ, Masson EA, Veves A, Boulton AJ. Relationship of limited joint mobility to abnormal foot pressures and diabetic foot ulceration. Diabetes Care. 1991;14(1):8–11.
27. Lee L, Blume PA, Sumpio B. Charcot joint disease in diabetes mellitus. Ann Vasc Surg. 2003;17(5): 571–80.
28. Veves A, Fernando D, Walewski P, et al. A study of plantar pressures in a diabetic clinic population. Foot. 1991;2:89.
29. Boulton AJ, Armstrong DG, Albert SF, Frykberg RG, Hellman R, Kirkman MS, et al. Comprehensive foot examination and risk assessment: a report of the task force of the foot care interest group of the American Diabetes Association, with endorsement by the American Association of Clinical Endocrinologists. Diabetes Care. 2008;31(8):1679–85.
30. Masson E, Hay E, Stockley I, Veves A, Betts R, Boulton A. Abnormal foot pressures alone may not cause ulceration. Diabet Med. 1989;6:426–8.
31. Morag E, Pammer S, Boulton A, Young M, Deffner K, Cavanagh P. Structural and functional aspects of the diabetic foot. Clin Biomech (Bristol, Avon). 1997;12(3):S9–10.
32. Saltzman C, Pedowitz W. Diabetic foot infection. AAOS Instr Course Lect. 1999;48:317–23.
33. Habershaw G, Chzran J. Management of diabetic foot problems. In: Kozak GP, Campbell DR, Frykberg RG, Habershaw GM, editors. Biomechanical considerations of the diabetic foot. Philadelphia, PA: W.B. Saunders; 1995. p. 53–65.
34. Sumpio BE. Foot ulcers. N Engl J Med. 2000;343(11): 787–93.
35. Bullock G, Stavosky J. Surgical wound management of the diabetic foot. Surg Technol Int. 2001;6:301–10.
36. Bild DE, Selby JV, Sinnock P, Browner WS, Braveman P, Showstack JA. Lower-extremity amputation in people with diabetes. Epidemiology and prevention. Diabetes Care. 1989;12(1):24–31.
37. Kannel WB, McGee DL. Diabetes and cardiovascular disease. The Framingham study. JAMA. 1979;241(19):2035–8.
38. Melton 3rd LJ, Macken KM, Palumbo PJ, Elveback LR. Incidence and prevalence of clinical peripheral vascular disease in a population-based cohort of diabetic patients. Diabetes Care. 1980;3(6):650–4.
39. Eggers PW, Gohdes D, Pugh J. Nontraumatic lower extremity amputations in the Medicare end-stage renal disease population. Kidney Int. 1999;56: 1524–33.
40. Lavery LA, Hunt NA, Ndip A, Lavery DC, Van Houtum W, Boulton AJ. Impact of chronic kidney disease on survival after amputation in individuals with diabetes. Diabetes Care. 2010;33(11):2365–9.
41. Johnson BL, Glickman MH, Bandyk DF, Esses GE. Failure of foot salvage in patients end-stage renal disease after surgical revascularization. J Vasc Surg. 1995;22:280–6.
42. Adam DJ, Naik J, Hartshorne T, Bello M, London NJ. The diagnosis and management of 689 chronic leg ulcers in a single-visit assessment clinic. Eur J Vasc Endovasc Surg. 2003;25(5):462–8.
43. Weitz JI, Byrne J, Clagett GP, Farkouh ME, Porter JM, Sackett DL, et al. Diagnosis and treatment of

chronic arterial insufficiency of the lower extremities: a critical review. Circulation. 1996;94(11):3026–49.
44. Pressley Z, Foster J, Kolm P, Zhao L, Warren F, Weintraub W, et al. Digital image analysis: a reliable tool in the quantitative evaluation of cutaneous lesions and beyond. Arch Dermatol. 2007;143(10):1331–3.
45. Grayson ML, Gibbons GW, Balogh K, Levin E, Karchmer AW. Probing to bone in infected pedal ulcers. A clinical sign of underlying osteomyelitis in diabetic patients. JAMA. 1995;273(9):721–3.
46. Lozano RM, Fernández LG, Hernández DM, Montesinos JVB, Jiménez SG, Jurado MAG. Validating the probe-to-bone test and other tests for diagnosing chronic osteomyelitis in the diabetic foot. Diabetes Care. 2010;33:2140–5.
47. Collins KA, Sumpio BE. Vascular assessment. Clin Podiatr Med Surg. 2000;17(2):171–91.
48. Feng Y, Schlosser FJ, Sumpio BE. The Semmes Weinstein monofilament examination as a screening tool for diabetic peripheral neuropathy. J Vasc Surg. 2009;50(3):675–82, 682.e1.
49. Armstrong DG, Lavery LA. Diabetic foot ulcers: prevention, diagnosis and classification. Am Fam Physician. 1998;57(6):1325–32, 1337-8.
50. Birke J, Sims D. Plantar sensory threshold in the ulcerative foot. Lepr Rev. 1986;57:261.
51. McNeely M, Boyko E, Ahroni J, Stensel V, Reiber G, Smith D. The independent contributions of diabetic neuropathy and vasculopathy in foot ulceration: how great are the risks? Diabetes Care. 1995;18:216–9.
52. Feng Y, Schlosser FJ, Sumpio BE. The Semmes Weinstein monofilament examination is a significant predictor of the risk of foot ulceration and amputation in patients with diabetes mellitus. J Vasc Surg. 2011;53(1):220–226.e1–5.
53. Cossman DV, Ellison JE, Wagner WH, Carroll RM, Treiman RL, Foran RF, et al. Comparison of contrast arteriography to arterial mapping with color-flow duplex imaging in the lower extremities. J Vasc Surg. 1989;10:522–9.
54. Sumpio BE, Lee T, Blume PA. Vascular evaluation and arterial reconstruction of the diabetic foot. Clin Podiatr Med Surg. 2003;20(4):689–708.
55. Steed DL, Donohoe D, Webster MW, Lindsley L. Effect of extensive debridement and treatment on the healing of diabetic foot ulcers. Diabetic Ulcer Study Group. J Am Coll Surg. 1996;183(1):61–4.
56. Sumpio BE, Driver V, Gibbons G, Holloway G, Joseph W, McGuigan F, et al. A Multidisciplinary approach to limb preservation – the role of VAC therapy. Wounds. 2009;21(9 Suppl 2):1–19.
57. Granick M, Boykin J, Gamelli R, Schultz G, Tenenhaus M. Toward a common language: surgical wound bed preparation and debridement. Wound Repair Regen. 2006;14 Suppl 1:S1–10.
58. Bergstrom N, Bennett M, Carlson C. Treatment of pressure ulcers. Clinical practice guidelines, no. 15 (AHCPR publication no. 95-0652). Rockville, MD: Agency for Health Care Policy and Research; 1994. p. 1–102.
59. Singer AJ, Clark RA. Cutaneous wound healing. N Engl J Med. 1999;341(10):738–46.
60. Blume P, Driver VR, Tallis AJ, Kirsner RS, Kroeker R, Payne WG, et al. Formulated collagen gel accelerates healing rate immediately after application in patients with diabetic neuropathic foot ulcers. Wound Repair Regen. 2011;19:302–8.
61. Bello YM, Phillips TJ. Recent advances in wound healing. JAMA. 2000;283(6):716–8.
62. Lipsky BA, Armstrong DG, Citron DM, Tice AD, Morgenstern DE, Abramson MA. Ertapenem versus piperacillin/tazobactam for diabetic foot infections (SIDESTEP): prospective, randomised, controlled, double-blinded, multicentre trial. Lancet. 2005;366(9498):1695–703.
63. Lipsky BA, Berendt AR, Deery HG, Embil JM, Joseph WS, Karchmer AW, et al. Diagnosis and treatment of diabetic foot infections. Clin Infect Dis. 2004;39:885–910.
64. Joshi N, Caputo GM, Weitekamp MR, Karchmer AW. Infections in patients with diabetes mellitus. N Engl J Med. 1999;341(25):1906–12.
65. Davis SC, Martinez L, Kirsner R. The diabetic foot: the importance of biofilms and wound bed preparation. Curr Diab Rep. 2006;6(6):439–45.
66. Lipsky BA, Tabak YP, Johannes RS, Vo L, Hyde L, Weigelt JA. Skin and soft tissue infections in hospitalised patients with diabetes: culture isolates and risk factors associated with mortality, length of stay and cost. Diabetologia. 2010;53:914–23.
67. Citron DM, Goldstein EJ, Merriam CV, Lipsky BA, Abramson MA. Bacteriology of moderate-to-severe diabetic foot infections and in vitro activity of antimicrobial agents. J Clin Microbiol. 2007;45(9):2819–28.
68. Nelson EA, O'Meara S, Golder S, Dalton J, Craig D, Iglesias C. Systematic review of antimicrobial treatments for diabetic foot ulcers. Diabet Med. 2006;23:348–59.
69. Blume P, Partagas L, Attinger C, Sumpio B. Single stage surgical treatment of noninfected diabetic foot ulcers. J Plast Reconstr Surg. 2002;109:601–9.
70. Blume P, Salonga C, Garbalosa J, Pierre-Paul D, Key J, Gahtan V, et al. Predictors for the healing of transmetatarsal amputations: retrospective study of 91 amputations. Vascular. 2007;15(3):126–33.
71. Bus SA, Valk GD, van Deursen RW, Armstrong DG, Caravaggi C, Hlavacek P, et al. The effectiveness of footwear and offloading interventions to prevent and heal foot ulcers and reduce plantar pressure in diabetes: a systematic review. Diabetes Metab Res Rev. 2008;24 Suppl 1:S162–80.
72. Bus SA, Valk GD, van Deursen RW, Armstrong DG, Caravaggi C, Hlavacek P, et al. Specific guidelines on footwear and offloading. Diabetes Metab Res Rev. 2008;24 Suppl 1:S192–3.
73. Armstrong D, Lavery L, Stern S, Harkless L. Is prophylactic diabetic foot surgery dangerous? J Foot Ankle Surg. 1996;35(6):585–9.
74. Catanzariti A, Blitch E, Karlock L. Elective foot and ankle surgery in the diabetic patient. J Foot Ankle Surg. 1995;34(1):23–41.

75. Orgill DP, Manders EK, Sumpio BE, Lee RC, Attinger CE, Gurtner GC, et al. The mechanisms of action of vacuum assisted closure: more to learn. Surgery. 2009;146(1):40–51.
76. Blume PA, Walters J, Payne W, Ayala J, Lantis J. Comparison of negative pressure wound therapy using vacuum-assisted closure with advanced moist wound therapy in the treatment of diabetic foot ulcers: a multicenter randomized controlled trial. Diabetes Care. 2008;31(4):631–6.
77. Vig S, Dowsett C, Berg L, Caravaggi C, Rome P, Birke-Sorensen H, et al. International Expert Panel on Negative Pressure Wound Therapy. Evidence-based recommendations for the use of negative pressure wound therapy in chronic wounds: steps towards an international consensus. J Tissue Viability. 2011;20 Suppl 1:S1–18.
78. Blume PA, Key JJ, Thakor P, Thakor S, Sumpio B. Retrospective evaluation of clinical outcomes in subjects with split-thickness skin graft: comparing V.A.C.® therapy and conventional therapy in foot and ankle reconstructive surgeries. Int Wound J. 2010;7(6):480–7.
79. Sumpio BE, Thakor P, Mahler D, Blume PA. Negative pressure wound therapy as postoperative dressing in below knee amputation stump closure of patients with chronic venous insufficiency. Wounds. 2011;23(10):301–8.
80. Orgill DP, Manders EK, Sumpio BE, Lee RC, Attinger CE, Gurtner GC, et al. The mechanisms of action of vacuum assisted closure: more to learn. Surgery. 2009;146(1):40–51.
81. Sumpio BE, Allie DE, Horvath KA, Marston WA, Meites HL, Mills JL, et al. Role of negative pressure wound therapy in treating peripheral vascular graft infections. Vascular. 2008;16(4):194–200.
82. Barrow J, Hughes J, Clark P. A study of the effect of wear on the pressure-relieving properties of foot orthosis. Foot. 1992;1:195–9.
83. Nawoczenski D, Birke J, Coleman W. Effect of rocker sole design on plantar forefoot pressures. J Am Podiatr Med Assoc. 1988;78:455–60.
84. Tang PC, Ravji K, Key JJ, Mahler DB, Blume PA, Sumpio B. Let them walk! Current prosthesis options for leg and foot amputees. J Am Coll Surg. 2008;206(3):548–60.
85. Sarage A, Yui W, Blume P, Aruny J, Sumpio B. Aggressive revascularization options using cryoplasty in patients with lower extremity vascular disease. In: Geroulakos G, editor. Re-do vascular surgery. London: Springer; 2009. p. 79–84.
86. Sheehan P, Jones P, Caselli A, Giurini JM, Veves A. Percent change in wound area of diabetic foot ulcers over a 4-week period is a robust predictor of complete healing in a 12-week prospective trial. Diabetes Care. 2003;26(6):1879–82.
87. Margolis DJ, Bartus C, Hoffstad O, Malay S, Berlin JA. Effectiveness of recombinant human platelet-derived growth factor for the treatment of diabetic neuropathic foot ulcers. Wound Repair Regen. 2005;13:531–6.
88. Steed DL, Attinger C, Colaizzi T, Crossland M, Franz M, Harkless L, et al. Guidelines for the treatment of diabetic ulcers. Wound Repair Regen. 2006;14(6):680–92.
89. Veves A, Falanga V, Armstrong DG, Sabolinski ML. Graftskin, a human skin equivalent, is effective in the management of noninfected neuropathic diabetic foot ulcers: a prospective randomized multicenter clinical trial. Diabetes Care. 2001;24:290–5.
90. Boulton AJ, Kirsner RS, Vileikyte L. Clinical practice. Neuropathic diabetic foot ulcers. N Engl J Med. 2004;351(1):48–55.
91. DCCT: The effect of intensive treatment of diabetes on the development and progression of long-term complications in insulin-dependent diabetes mellitus. The Diabetes Control and Complications Trial Research Group. N Engl J Med. 1993;329:977–86.
92. American Diabetes Association. Executive summary: standards of medical care in diabetes – 2011. Diabetes Care. 2011;34 Suppl 1:S4–10.
93. Tan T, Shaw EJ, Siddiqui F, Kandaswamy P, Barry PW, Baker M, Guideline Development Group. Inpatient management of diabetic foot problems: summary of NICE guidance. BMJ. 2011;342:d1280.
94. McMurray SD, Johnson G, Davis S, McDougall K. Diabetes education and care management significantly improve patient outcomes in the dialysis unit. Am J Kidney Dis. 2003;40:566–75.

Diabetic Foot Infections: Microbiology and Antibiotic Therapy

Brian Scully

Keywords

Diabetic foot • Ulceration • Bone biopsy • Osteomyelitis • Cellulitis • Antibiotic

Introduction

Infection of the feet in patients with diabetes is a common and potentially devastating complication of the disease. It is a frequent reason for the hospitalization of patients with diabetes. It is also the most important proximate reason for nontraumatic amputations [1]. Many patients have serious comorbid conditions such as chronic renal failure, congestive heart failure, or immunosuppression by virtue of solid organ transplantation. Effective management thus requires a sharp clinical acumen and judgment on the part of the primary physician aided by the frequent recourse to Vascular and Infectious Disease consultations.

B. Scully, M.B., B.Ch. (✉)
Department of Medicine & Infectious Disease,
New York Presbyterian Hospital, 161 Ft. Washington Avenue, New York, NY 10032, USA
e-mail: bs4@columbia.edu; scullyfam@yahoo.com

Pathogenesis

Table 7.1 lists the main factors contributing to the pathogenesis of infection of the feet in patients with diabetes. Peripheral neuropathy plays a central role [2]. The resultant reduced sensation and deformities allow minor pressure or trauma to go unnoticed and eventually cause the painless skin ulcers. This breach in the barrier defenses allows bacteria to first colonize and then to actively infect the ulcer and surrounding tissues. This process can be aided by tissue hypoxia from poor circulation and by poor glycemic control with its deleterious effects on immune function. Hyperglycemia adversely affects intracellular killing of bacteria and also impairs leukocyte chemotaxis [3, 4]. Chronic renal failure, if present, will further impair immune function. Neglect of the ulcer, related to poor vision, reduced sensation, and sometimes social issues, are other factors. Finally, the inherent virulence of the infecting pathogen will determine the clinical presentation—for example, acute if Group B

Table 7.1 Risk factors for diabetic foot infection

Risk factor	Impairments
Neuropathy	Protective sensation, reduced sweating, abnormal anatomy, and mechanics
Arterial insufficiency	Tissue hypoxia, impaired healing, and tissue viability
Hyperglycemia/metabolic derangements, e.g., chronic renal failure	Neutrophil function, healing

Streptococcus or *Staphylococcus aureus*, and indolent if *Staphylococcus epidermidis* or *Streptococcus* Group D.

Clinical Syndromes and Microbiology

A variety of clinical syndromes may occur. These include simple cellulitis, the infected ulcer with or without adjacent cellulitis, necrotizing fasciitis, deep space infections and abscesses, osteomyelitis and septic arthritis. Table 7.2 lists some of these syndromes with their main associated pathogens. Generally, Gram-positive pathogens such as *Staphylococcus aureus* and the beta-hemolytic Streptococci are most common especially in patients who are less antibiotic experienced and have at least a fair blood supply [5, 6]. Gram-negatives and anaerobes become more important in patients with longer standing problems and in those with severe ischemia [7–9]. Low virulence pathogens such as coagulase-negative staphylococci, enterococci, and various diphtheroid species can colonize chronic ulcerations and may become pathogenic. Infections in patients with chronic ulcers or severe ischemia are frequently polymicrobial. Previous antibiotic therapy and prior hospitalizations will influence the flora of these infections, favoring the selection of methicillin-resistant *Staphylococcus aureus* (MRSA) and multiple antibiotic-resistant Gram-negative pathogens and fungi such as *Candida* species [10, 11]. Soaking favors the colonization of ulcers and the skin with nonfermenting Gram-negatives such as *Pseudomonas aeruginosa*, *Stenotrophomonas maltophilia*, and *Serratia marcescens*.

Table 7.2 Clinical syndromes and microbiology

Syndrome	Microbiology
Cellulitis	Beta-hemolytic streptococci especially Group B *Staphylococcus aureus*
Infected ulcer with cellulitis	As above
Chronic or previously treated ulcer	*S. aureus*, beta Strep, Enterobacteriaceae[a], *Pseudomonas aeruginosa*, fungi
Ulcer with maceration	*Pseudomonas aeruginosa* other Gram-negatives
Extensive necrosis/gangrene	Polymicrobial, Gram-negatives—enterobacteriaceae, *Pseudomonas* and other nonfermenters[b], obligate anaerobes[c]

[a]*Escherichia coli*, *Proteus* sp., *Citrobacter* sp., *Klebsiella*
[b]*Stenotrophomonas maltophilia*, *Acinetobacter* sp.
[c]*Bacteroides* sp.

Patient Evaluation

For each patient, one has to accurately assess (1) the extent and systemic consequences of the infection, (2) the contributing factors, particularly circulatory, and (3) the microbiology of the infection (Table 7.3). The clinical examination requires particular attention to the pulses, capillary blood flow, extent of inflammatory changes, the depth of the ulcer, if present, and the presence of any fluctuance. The latter can be very subtle and is easily missed. The presence of neuropathy is best assessed by testing light touch. Noninvasive arterial and venous flow studies should be done in selected cases. CT scanning or ultrasound can be used to detect collections.

The microbiology of the infection is determined by cultures. Blood cultures are only occasionally positive but should be obtained in all serious infections. Traditional teaching states that superficial wound swab cultures are of limited value [5, 12]. Certainly, if *Staphylococcus aureus* or beta-hemolytic Streptococci are recovered they are likely to be true pathogens but for Gram-negatives the result is much less reliable. Ideally, any callus should first be debrided, then the ulcer or wound surface should be vigorously cleansed

Table 7.3 Assessment of the patient

Systemic consequences	History, physical examination, labs
Local limb/wound	Depth of wound—does it probe to bone?; tendon/joint involvement; extent of erythema, presence of crepitus, bullae
	Deformities, e.g., Charcot foot
	Imaging as needed
Contributing factors	Assess the circulation
	Presence of neuropathy—light touch
	Psychosocial issues
Microbiology	Blood cultures in selected cases; local cultures

and a deep specimen obtained with a curette or scalpel [13]. The specimen should then be rapidly transported to the lab and processed for aerobes and anaerobes. Swabs should be sent in transport media capable of supporting anaerobic as well as aerobic growth. Recent studies show a good correlation between superficial and deep cultures for diabetics with deep soft tissue infection but not for osteomyelitis [14]. Culture of a needle aspirate of a collection is useful. Bone biopsy obtained either by a needle through uninfected skin or at operative debridement should be obtained when possible in patients with suspected osteomyelitis. Unfortunately, many patients will already have been placed on antibiotics by the time a biopsy can be arranged. For these patients if clinically stable, it is worth suspending antibiotic therapy for 48 h to obtain a bone biopsy to more accurately determine the infecting bacteria and to confirm the diagnosis histologically.

Management

Antibiotics: General Remarks

There are a veritable multitude of effective antibiotic regimens, which can be used to treat diabetic foot infections. No one regimen has been shown to be superior [15, 16]. Table 7.4 lists most of the commonly used antibiotics by class and highlights their antimicrobial spectra. It also has a column containing remarks about unique properties or risks of treatment.

The beta-lactams are well tolerated as a group and have good tissue penetration. Effective bone levels are obtained with intravenous administration but are borderline with oral administration of even high doses [17]. They have no activity against MRSA except for the recently introduced Ceftaroline. None of the cephalosporins are effective against Enterococci. Toxicities are generally forgiving. Most serious is a profound but reversible neutropenia that can occur with prolonged intravenous use. This typically occurs 3–4 weeks into a course. I have seen it with penicillins, cephalosporins, and carbapenems. It is therefore important that the blood count be monitored in patients on extended intravenous courses of these drugs. Drug-induced hepatitis and thrombocytopenia may also occur.

The quinolones are well absorbed from the intestine and can achieve levels in bone by this route, which are adequate to treat osteomyelitis due to susceptible organisms [17]. When treating staphylococcal infections levofloxacin or moxifloxacin are preferred over ciprofloxacin because of their superior activity against Gram-positive organisms. Resistance developing on therapy is seen most frequently in pathogens with higher MICs such as *Pseudomonas aeruginosa* and *Staphylococcus aureus*. To minimize this risk, necrotic poorly vascularized tissue should be debrided prior to starting the quinolone and dosage should be on the higher side, for example Ciprofloxacin at 750 mg PO bid to treat *Pseudomonas* or Levofloxacin at 750 mg PO daily to treat *S. aureus*. Tendinitis, tendon rupture, and QT interval prolongation and arrhythmias are potential serious toxicities. The last is sometimes an issue in patients with renal failure or those already on drugs which can affect the QT interval such as amiodarone and macrolides.

Clindamycin is an effective drug against susceptible staphylococci and streptococci, but resistance has been on the rise in some areas. It has good oral bioavailability and achieves levels of up to 70% of serum in bone [17]. It is also effective in infections where the organisms may be in a stationary growth phase due to a high density of organisms—the Eagle effect [18]. For this reason, it is often added to a beta-lactam in severe

Table 7.4 Antibiotics

Drug	Spectrum of activity	Comments
Penicillin G [IV or PO]; Amoxicillin [PO]	Mainly streptococci	Narrow spectrum; good oral absorption of Amoxicillin
Amoxicillin/Clavulanate [PO]; Ampicillin/Sulbactam [IV]	Strep, *S. aureus*, many anaerobes, selected Gram-negatives, e.g., many *E. coli* and *Proteus* sp.	Twice daily dosing of Amox/Clavulanate but frequent diarrhea; sensitivity of Gram-negatives is variable
Ticarcillin/Clavulanate [IV]; Piperacillin/Tazobactam [IV]	Expanded Gram-negative spectrum to include many strains of *Pseudomonas*, *Serratia* and other Gram-negatives; excellent anaerobic activity; P covers Enterococci well, T does not	Ideal spectrum for many infections where Gram-negatives are a consideration especially if the patient is not heavily antibiotic experienced
1st generation Cephalosporins—Cefazolin [iV]/Cephalexin [pO]	*S. aureus* but not MRSA or many coag negative staph; Strep but not Enterococci; some Gram-negatives; poor anaerobic activity	Good oral tolerance of Cephalexin in doses of up to 1 g
2nd—Cefoxitin [IV]	Fair anaerobic activity when dosed at 2 g; weak staph activity; no activity against *Pseudomonas* or *Enterobacter*	Strong beta-lactamase inducer
3rd—Ceftriaxone [IV]; Cefotaxime [IV] Ceftazidime [IV]; Cefpodoxime [PO] Cefixime [PO]	Good *S. aureus*, beta-strep and Gram-negatives; Ceftazidime covers *Pseudomonas* well; poor anaerobic coverage	Increasing Gram-negative resistance; once daily dosing of Ceftriaxone; the oral third generation are weak Staph drugs
4th—Cefepime [IV]	MSSA, beta-strep, Gram-negatives including *Pseudomonas* and *Enterobacter*. Weak anaerobic activity	
5th—Ceftaroline [IV]	MSSA and MRSA; poor *Pseudomonas* activity	New agent; once daily dosing
Monobactam—Aztreonam	Only Gram-negative activity including *Pseudomonas*	Safe in most patients with Penicillin or Cephalosporin allergy
Carbapenems—Imipenem [iV], Meropenem [IV] and Ertapenem [IV]	Very broad spectrum including anaerobes; Ertapenem does not have activity against *Pseudomonas*; *E. fecium* and *S. maltophilia* are always resistant	Increasing resistance in *Klebsiella* and other Gram-negatives due to Carbapenamases; Ertapenem is given once daily
Quinolones—Ciprofloxacin, Levofloxacin, Moxifloxacin [IV] or [PO]	Gram-negatives; some Staph and Strep; resistance an issue	Good oral bioavailability
Aminoglycosides—Gentamicin, Tobramycin, Amikacin all [IV] or [IM]	Predominately facultative Gram-negatives including *Pseudomonas*	Effective tissue penetration and issue and the need for precise dosing; toxicities
Vancomycin [IV]	*S. aureus*; coag negative Staph and Enterococci	Vancomycin resistance in Enterococci an issue in nosocomial infections intermediate sensitivity in Staph
Clindamycin [IV] or [PO]	*S. aureus*; Strep but not Enterococci; occasional resistance in Strep; good anaerobic activity though some resistance	Excellent oral bioavailability and bone penetration
Linezolid [IV] or [PO]	Gram-positives including MRSA, MRSE, and VRE	Excellent oral bioavailability; potential serious toxicities with prolonged courses
Daptomycin [IV]	Gram-positives including MRSA, MRSE and VRE	Well tolerated; some Enterococci are only borderline susceptible

(continued)

Table 7.4 (continued)

Drug	Spectrum of activity	Comments
Tigecycline [IV]	Gram-positives including MRSA, VRE, many Anaerobes and Enterobacteriaceae but not *Pseudomonas*	Blood levels are low
Doxycycline [IV] or [PO]; Minocycline [IV] or [PO]	Mostly Gram-positives often MRSA and selected Gram-negatives such as *S. maltophilia*	GI tolerance may be problematic; inexpensive oral treatment of some MRSA infections
Trimethoprim/Sulfamethoxazole [PO] or [IV]	Many Staph; selected Gram-negatives	Excellent oral absorption
Metronidazole [PO] or [IV]	Obligate anaerobes	Excellent oral bioavailability; potential toxicities with extended courses
Rifampin	Staphylococci and beta-hemolytic Streptococci	Should always be used in combination with another agent; good efficacy in osteomyelitis

cellulitis or necrotizing fasciitis. Toxicities and side effects tend to be minor but Clindamycin has been notorious for predisposing to Clostridium difficile colitis. Allergy is common as is nausea with the oral administration of higher doses.

Metronidazole is a very effective bacteriocidal anaerobic antibiotic. It is highly active against *Bacteroides* sp., *Prevotella* sp., *Fusobacteria*, and *Clostridia* sp. Actinomyces and Propionebacteria are intrinsically resistant. As with the quinolones, oral bioavailability is excellent allowing for oral therapy of serious infections. Bone levels are similar to serum levels [17]. Thus far, the development of resistance has been uncommon. Frequent side effects are abdominal pain and a profound nausea. A painful peripheral neuropathy which is irreversible in most cases becomes a risk with courses lasting more than 1 month. Caution is therefore warranted in treating patients with osteomyelitis.

Linezolid has excellent activity against MRSA and vancomycin-resistant enterococci (VRE). It has excellent tissue penetration and oral bioavailability. Bone levels are about 50% of those in serum [17]. It is at least as effective as vancomycin in treating soft tissue infections. There are several potentially serious toxicities that can occur when treatment is prolonged beyond 10–14 days—bone marrow suppression, especially affecting the platelets and peripheral or optic neuritis. Close monitoring is therefore advised. Potential drug reactions, especially with the selective serotonin reuptake inhibitors (SSRI) and monoamine oxidase (MAO) inhibitor antidepressants, should be considered when prescribing Linezolid.

Tigecycline is a recently introduced tetracycline active against many tetracycline-resistant Gram-negatives, VRE and MRSA. Its volume of distribution is very high but blood levels are low making it an unsuitable choice to treat bacteremia. Significant toxicities include hepatitis and nausea and vomiting.

Daptomycin is a cell wall antibiotic active against staphylococci and streptococci including methicillin and vancomycin-resistant strains. Limited data show good efficacy in soft tissue and bone infections despite poor bone penetration [19, 20]. It is highly protein bound and is administered once daily in patients with creatinine clearances greater than 35 ml/min. The main toxicity is myositis, which occurs in about 15% of treatment courses. It can only be administered intravenously.

Trimethoprim/sulfamethoxazole (T/S) traditionally has been used to treat UTIs and exacerbations of chronic bronchitis. Its spectrum includes Gram-negative bacilli such as *E. coli*, *Proteus* and *Hemophilus* sp., Gram-positive cocci such as *Staphylococcus aureus*, and to a lesser extent streptococci and some uncommonly encountered bacteria such as *Nocardia*. Resistance has been increasing among the Gram-negatives but many strains of staphylocooci remain susceptible. Oral bioavailability and penetration into bone and soft tissues are excellent. T/S has shown good efficacy when given in combination with Rifampin in staphylococcal osteomyelitis [21]. Dosage should be higher than that used for UTIs when given for these indications, e.g., 7–8 mg/kg/day in divided doses.

Aminoglycosides such as gentamicin are active against many aerobic and facultative Gram-negatives. As a group they have the potential to cause severe renal, auditory and vestibular toxicities and have narrow therapeutic/toxic ratio. Dosing has thus to be precise. The aminoglycosides require oxygen for transport into the bacterial cell and so they are not effective in an anaerobic environment. For these reasons, they are not often used in the treatment of diabetic foot infections.

The polymyxins, colistin, and polymyxin B have a predominately Gram-negative spectrum. Like the aminoglycosides they may cause serious toxicities, especially renal. They are sometimes, however, the only agents active against the carbapenem-resistant Gram-negatives and so have a role under consultation with specialists in Infectious Disease.

Rifampin, besides its well-known activity against *Mycobacterium tuberculosis* has substantial antistaphylococcal activity and excellent absorption and penetration into bone. Resistance can develop rapidly on therapy and so it should always be given in combination with another active antibiotic. Favorable results when combined with T/S or Linezolid have been seen in patients with chronic osteomyelitis [22]. My own practice is to add rifampin to the other agent after a week or so of therapy, when hopefully the microbial burden has been reduced, so as to minimize the potential for selecting rifampin-resistant strains. Finally, rifampin is a potent inducer of the hepatic cytochrome p450 enzyme system. As many diabetic patients will be on drugs metabolized by this system, a careful review of concomitant drug therapy should be done prior to starting rifampin.

Cellulitis, Without an Open Wound

Most cases are due to infection with a beta-hemolytic Strep or *Staphylococcus aureus*. They are well managed with cefazolin or Ampicillin/Sulbactam. Patients with a severe beta-lactam allergy can be treated with Vancomycin or Daptomycin. Clindamycin is sometimes added to the regimen in patients with severe cellulitis or necrotizing fasciitis because of its efficacy against stationary growth phase bacteria. If, for epidemiologic or historical reasons MRSA is suspected, then Vancomycin, Linezolid or Daptomycin should be included in the initial regimen. If a deep space infection or necrotizing fasciitis is present, prompt surgical intervention is critical to a successful outcome as pus under pressure in a foot abscess can be very destructive within a short period of time. For patients with less severe infections in whom systemic toxicity is mild and in whom co-morbid illnesses such as renal failure, vascular disease or heart failure are not critical, an oral antibiotic regimen can be given with provision for follow-up within 4 or 5 days. Cephalexin, Cefadroxil, and Amoxicillin/Clavulanate are all effective. Doxycycline is also effective and treats many MRSA strains.

Diabetic Foot Ulcer

Lipsky et al. have proposed a classification system for diabetic ulcers in the IDSA guidelines in the management of DFI and the International Consensus on the Diabetic Foot—Table 7.5 [23].

Uninfected ulcers are classified as Grade 1. Superficial infections, extending less than 2 cm from the ulcer, are classified as mild or Grade 2. More extensive infections or those with lymphangitic streaking, spread beneath superficial tissue or into bone but without systemic toxicity or metabolic instability are classified as Grade 3. Patients with systemic inflammatory response syndrome are classified as severe—Grade 4.

Many ulcers are not infected (Grade 1) and do not require antibiotic therapy even though the ulcers may be heavily colonized. In some, the distinction may be difficult and a short course of culture-directed therapy or perhaps a topical agent such as mupirocin may be beneficial.

Table 7.5 Clinical classification of diabetic foot infection

Clinical signs	IWDGF classification-grade, IDSA
Wound without purulence/inflammation	Grade 1-uninfected
Two or more signs of infection[a], <2 cm of surrounding erythema/induration, superficial, no systemic illness or local complications	Grade 2-infected, mild
As above but also cellulitis>2 cm beyond the wound *or* lymphangitic streaking *or* evidence of any spread beneath the superficial fascia	Grade 3-infected, moderate
Infection with evidence for systemic toxicity or metabolic instability	Grade 4-infected, severe

Adapted from Lipsky BA, Berendt AR, Deery HG, et al. Diagnosis and treatment of diabetic foot infections. Clin Infect Dis. 2004;39:885–910. With permission from Oxford University Press
[a]Local swelling or induration, erythema, tenderness or pain, warmth, purulent discharge

Most patients with Grade 2 and some patients with Grade 3 infection can be well treated with an oral antibiotic regimen with close follow-up. The predominant pathogens are *Staphylococcus aureus* and beta-hemolytic Streptococci. Potential regimens are listed in Table 7.6. Cephalexin and Amoxicillin/Clavulanate are effective and well tolerated. Doxycycline has the advantage of covering many MRSA strains, though nausea and abdominal pain are frequent side effects. Gram-positive quinolones, such as Levofloxacin or Moxifloxacin are effective also but, my own opinion is that these drugs should not be used as a first-line therapy due to their expense, some potential toxicities, e.g., tendon rupture, and the risk of jeopardizing their effectiveness in Gram-negative infections.

Patients with more extensive infections or where there is a critical ischemia should be treated with intravenous antibiotics. The program chosen should cover Staph, Strep, a wide variety of Gram-negatives and in most cases anaerobic organisms. MRSA coverage should be included in the initial regimen in limb or life-threatening infections and in patients with recent hospitalizations. There are many effective regimens.

Follow-up

Hospitalized patients will be followed closely for signs of clinical improvement particularly in temperature, pain, redness, and swelling. Failure to respond should suggest the presence of a resistant organism or the need for a surgical intervention such as drainage, debridement, or amputation. Culture results are usually available by day 4 and should be used to broaden or narrow the coverage. With some frequency, multiple organisms are cultured. In general, the more virulent, such as *Staphylococcus aureus*, beta Strep and *Pseudomonas* should be treated. Coagulase negative Staph and enterococci need not always be treated, especially if isolated in combination with more virulent species. In the patient who is not responding well to antibiotics, it is best to treat all of the cultured isolates. In some who are responding poorly, consideration might be given to adjunctive treatment, such as hyperbaric oxygen or neutrophil growth factors. Strong data to support their use are lacking, however [24, 25].

Osteomyelitis

Osteomyelitis should be suspected whenever the ulceration is over a bony prominence or has been chronic or when the ulcer probes to the bone. Elevated inflammatory markers or a leukocytosis may be present. Plain radiography is useful in more chronic cases but X-ray changes take at least 2–3 weeks to appear. Radionuclide studies are sensitive but often falsely positive. MRI is the most sensitive imaging study [23]. Specificity is high except in the situation of the Charcot foot where false-positives are common. Bone biopsy can be very helpful [see above]. Initial antibiotics should be chosen according to the stage of the ulceration and then adjusted according to the culture results. The sensitivities of the organisms cultured will determine whether an oral regimen can be given. It is preferable that the local tissue

Table 7.6 Suggested antibiotic regimens

Cellulitis, Stage 2 ulcerations	Cefazolin 1 g IV q8 h[a] or Ampicillin/Sulbactam 3 g q6 h
	Vancomycin 15 mg/kg q12 h if severe penicillin allergy or if MRSA is suspected
	Alternatives—Daptomycin at 6 mg/kg/day or Linezolid at 600 mg IV q12 h
	In severe cases, especially if Group A Strep necrotizing fasciitis is suspected, Clindamycin 600 mg IV q8 h may be added
	Oral regimens for less severe cases or as follow-up to the IV regimens
	Cephalexin 500 mg qid
	Cefadroxil 1,000 mg daily
	Amoxicillin/Clavulanate 875 mg bid
	Doxycycline 100 mg bid
	Levofloxacin 500–750 mg daily
	Moxifloxacin 400 mg daily
Stage 3 or 4 ulcerations Chronic ulcers	Piperacillin/Tazobactam 4.5 g q6–8 h ± agent for MRSA
	Cefepime 2 g q12 h ± MRSA agent ± metronidazole 500 mg IV Q8 h or Clindamycin
	Meropenem 500 mg q6 h or Imipenem 500 mg q6 h
	For patients with beta-lactam allergies consider substituting Aztreonam 1–2 g q8 h for Cefepime

[a]Dosages suggested are those for patients with normal renal function

conditions be optimized prior to starting quinolone therapy due to the easy selection of resistant strains. Consider T/S ± rifampin for staphylococcal osteomyelitis dosed at 7–8 mg/kg of the trimethoprim component.

Duration of Therapy

The duration of therapy will vary according to the severity and extent of the infection and whether there is osteomyelitis. Mild soft tissue infections should be treated for 7–14 days, generally for about 4 days following clinical resolution. More severe soft tissue infections require longer, up to 4 weeks, depending on the depth and severity of the infection and the pace of the response to therapy. The latter part of the course can usually be completed with an oral antibiotic program, assuming the culture data are supportive. Antibiotics should usually be discontinued when the infection has resolved clinically even if the ulcer has not completely healed. For patients with osteomyelitis, much depends on the extent of the bone and adjacent soft tissue infection and on whether a complete debridement of infected bone or an amputation has been performed. For example, where there has been a transmetatarsal amputation in a patient with osteomyelitis of a phalanx who does not have proximal soft tissue infection, several days of antibiotics may be sufficient. If in addition, there was a significant cellulitis or plantar space infection, several weeks, at least 2 and perhaps 4–6 weeks of antibiotics should be given. The same thought process applies to the patient who has residual infected, but viable bone. For the patient with osteomyelitis who has nonviable bone that has not been debrided, a more extended course of 3 or even 6 months should be given. Frequently, antibiotics can be switched to an oral regimen after an initial period of intravenous treatment, depending on the infecting organism and the ability to achieve adequate tissue levels with an oral antibiotic agent. Inflammatory markers such as the C-reactive protein and erythrocyte sedimentation rate (ESR) can be helpful in guiding therapy but many patients will have confounding illnesses which can affect their measurement. Healing of the overlying soft tissue and reconstitution of the bone on plain radiographs are favorable signs. Unfortunately, recurrences at the same or a new site occur in 20–30% of patients [26].

References

1. Pecoraro RE, Reiber GE, Burgess EM. Pathways to diabetic limb amputation: basis for prevention. Diabetes Care. 1990;13:513–21.
2. Frykberg RG. Diabetic foot ulcers: current concepts. J Foot Ankle Sur. 1998;37:440–6.
3. Marhoffer W, Stein M, Maeser E, Federlin K. Impairment of polymorphonuclear leukocyte function and metabolic control of diabetes. Diabetes Care. 1992;15:256–60.
4. Geerlings SE, Hoepelman AI. Immune dysfunction in patients with diabetes mellitus (DM). FEMS Immunol Med Microbiol. 1999;26:259–65.
5. Wheat IJ, Allen SD, Henry M, et al. Diabetic foot infections. Bacteriologic analysis. Arch Intern Med. 1986;146(10):1935–40.
6. Lipsky BA, Pecoraro RE, Wheat LJ. The diabetic foot: soft tissue and bone infection. Infect Dis Clin North Am. 1990;7:467–81.
7. Jones EW, Edwards R, Finch R, Jeffcoate WJ. A microbiological study of diabetic foot lesions. Diabet Med. 1985;2:213–5.
8. Gerding DN. Foot infections in diabetics: the role of anaerobes. Clin Infect Dis. 1995;20 Suppl 2:S283–8.
9. Pathare NA, Bal A, Talvalkar GV, Antani DU. Diabetic foot infections: a study of microorganisms associated with different Wagner grades. Indian J Pathol Microbiol. 1998;41:437–41.
10. Bansal E, Garg A, Bhatia S, Attri AK, Chander J. Spectrum of microbial flora in diabetic foot ulcers. Indian J Pathol Microbiol. 2008;51(2):204–8.
11. Eleftheriadou I, Tentolouris N, Argiana V, Jude E, Boulton AJ. Methicillin-resistant Staphylococcus aureus in diabetic foot infections. Drugs. 2010;70(14):1784–97.
12. Pellizzer G, Strazzabosco M, Presi S, et al. Deep tissue biopsy vs superficial swab culture monitoring in the microbiological assessment of limb-threatening diabetic foot infection. Diabet Med. 2001;18(10):822–7.
13. Lipsky BA, Pecoraro RE, Larson SA, Hanley ME, Ahroni JH. Outpatient management of uncomplicated lower extremity infections in diabetic patients. Arch Int Med. 1990;150(4):790–7.
14. Senneville E, Meliez H, Beltrand E, et al. Culture of percutaneous bone biopsy specimens for diagnosis of diabetic foot osteomyelitis: concordance with ulcer swab cultures. Clin Infect Dis. 2006;42:57–62.
15. Crouzet J, Lavigne JP, Richard JC, Sotto A. Diabetic foot infection; a critical review of recent randomized clinical trials on antibiotic therapy. Int J Infect Dis. 2011;15(9):e601–10.
16. Lipsky BA, Peters EJ, Senneville E, Berendt AR, et al. Expert opinion on the management of infections in the diabetic foot. Diabetes Metab Res Rev. 2012;28 Suppl 1:163–78.
17. Spellberg B, Lipsky BA. Systemic antibiotic therapy for chronic osteomyelitis in adults. Clin Infect Dis. 2012;54(3):393–407.
18. Stevens DL, Gibbons AE, Bergstrom R, Winn V. The Eagle effect revisited; efficacy of clindamycin, erythromycin and penicillin in streptococcal osteomyelitis. J Infect Dis. 1988;158(1):22–8.
19. Holtom PD, Zalavras CG, Lamp KC, Park N, Friedrich LV. Clinical experience with daptomycin treatment of foot and ankle osteomyelitis: a preliminary study. Clin Orthop Relat Res. 2007;461:35–9.
20. Traunmuller F, Schintler MV, Metzler J, et al. Soft tissue and bone penetration abilities of daptomycin in diabetic patients with bacterial foot infections. J Antimicrob Chemother. 2010;65:1252–7.
21. Nguyen S, Pasquet A, Legout L, et al. Efficacy and tolerance of rifampicin-linezolid compared with rifampicin-cotrimoxazole combinations in prolonged oral therapy for bone and joint infections. Clin Microbiol Infect. 2009;15:1163–9.
22. Norden CW, Bryant R, Palmer D, Montgomerie JZ, Wheat J. Chronic osteomyelitis caused by Staphylococcus aureus: controlled clinical trial of nafcillin therapy and nafcillin-rifampin therapy. South Med J. 1986;79:947–51.
23. Lipsky BA, Berendt AR, Deery HG, et al. Diagnosis and treatment of diabetic foot infections. Clin Infect Dis. 2004;39:885–910.
24. Lipsky BA, Holroyd KJ, Zasloff M. Topical versus systemic antimicrobial therapy for treating mildly infected diabetic foot ulcers: a randomized, controlled, double-blinded multicenter trial of pexiganan cream. Clin Infect Dis. 2008;47(12):1537–45.
25. Londahl M, Katzman P, Nilsson A, Hammarlund C. Hyperbaric oxygen therapy facilitates healing of chronic foot ulcers in patients with diabetes. Diabetes Care. 2010;33(5):998–1003.
26. Gottrup F. Management of the diabetic foot: surgical and organisational aspects. Horm Metab Res. 2005;37 Suppl 1:69–75.

Arterial Imaging

Rodney P. Bensley and Marc L. Schermerhorn

Keywords

Noninvasive arterial imaging • Arterial duplex scanning • Computed tomographic angiography • Magnetic resonance angiography • Digital subtraction arteriography

Various arterial imaging modalities are available to image the arterial tree in diabetic patients. These include noninvasive arterial studies (NIAS), arterial duplex scanning, noninvasive angiography, such as computed tomographic angiography (CTA) or magnetic resonance angiography (MRA), and invasive digital subtraction arteriography (DSA), which is the current gold standard.

NIAS and arterial duplex scanning provide a wealth of information regarding peripheral arterial occlusive disease (PAOD). They can confirm the presence of PAOD, its location and severity, its physiologic consequences, the potential for primary healing of a wound, surgical incision, or amputation, as well as determine what type of intervention is most appropriate for the patient.

DSA has superior image resolution and is the gold standard for arterial imaging. It is also the only imaging modality that can be used for both diagnosis and treatment. With improvements in technology and image quality, MRA and CTA have become reasonable alternatives to DSA, but the image resolution with DSA remains superior.

Precise arterial imaging is crucial in patients with diabetes as these patients often have multisegmental disease most commonly involving the tibial and peroneal arteries, calcifications of both the atherosclerotic lesions and the arterial wall, and the presence of renal insufficiency.

Noninvasive Arterial Studies

NIAS are useful in screening patients with diabetes for PAOD. In patients with clinical signs and symptoms of PAOD, NIAS provide critical information on the location and severity of PAOD as well as an assessment of the potential for healing of a wound, surgical incision, or amputation. NIAS include pressure measurements, pulse volume recordings (PVRs), stress testing, and Doppler waveforms.

R.P. Bensley, M.D. (✉) • M.L. Schermerhorn, M.D.
Division of Vascular and Endovascular Surgery,
Department of Surgery, Beth Israel Deaconess
Medical Center, 110 Francis St., Suite 5 B,
Boston, MA 02115, USA
e-mail: rbensley@bidmc.harvard.edu

Pressure Measurements

Ankle–Brachial Index

Measurement of the ankle–brachial index (ABI) is the simplest noninvasive method for determining the presence of lower extremity arterial occlusive disease. The American Diabetes Association consensus statement on PAOD recommends screening of diabetic patients over 50 years of age for PAOD utilizing the ABI [1]. The brachial pressure is used to estimate the central pressure and is accurate except in cases of occlusive disease of arteries supplying the upper extremity. For this reason, the brachial pressure is measured in both upper extremities and the highest value is used. The ankle pressures are measured in each ankle at both the dorsalis pedis and posterior tibial artery, and the greater of these in each ankle is divided by the higher of the two brachial pressures giving the ABI for each ankle. The goal of the ABI is to detect occlusive disease by identifying pressure drops between the proximal aorta and ankle. The normal ankle pressure is approximately 10% higher than the brachial pressure (ABI of 1.1). Table 8.1 lists the ranges of ABI measurements and their interpretation. ABIs in the range of 0.9–1.29 are considered normal. ABIs decrease as the severity of the occlusive disease increases. ABIs between 0.5 and 0.9 reveal mild to moderate PAOD and these patients usually have intermittent claudication of varying severity. Patients with critical limb ischemia (rest pain and gangrene) generally have ABIs less than 0.4. The sensitivity of the ABI in detecting PAOD ranges from 80 to 95% and the specificity from 95 to 100% with positive and negative predictive values above 90%. Patients with diabetes often have medial calcification of their tibial vessels (medial calcinosis) and the presence of this calcium in the arterial wall makes the artery noncompressible giving a falsely elevated ABI greater than 1.3 [2]. Diabetic patients with severe PAOD can have a normal ABI of 1.0 due to medial calcification. This can be deceptive and misleading as the falsely elevated ABI underestimates the prevalence of arterial disease in the diabetic population [3].

Table 8.1 Ankle–brachial index measurements and their interpretation

>1.30	Noncompressible
0.91–1.29	Normal
0.71–0.90	Mild peripheral arterial disease
0.41–0.70	Moderate peripheral arterial disease
0.00–0.40	Severe peripheral arterial disease

Digital Pressures

The digital vessels are usually spared from calcification in diabetic patients. Therefore, a measurement of the toe pressures is more accurate in quantifying PAOD in the diabetic patient. Toe pressures of 30 mmHg are associated with ischemic symptoms and pressures greater than 40 mmHg are associated with the ability to heal a lesion. The toe to brachial index (TBI) is calculated similar to the ABI. A TBI > 0.75 is considered normal. A TBI < 0.25 is consistent with severe PAOD.

Segmental Pressures

Segmental pressures can be used to indirectly localize PAOD. They are obtained by placing blood pressure cuffs at the upper thigh, lower thigh, below the knee, and at the ankle. The upper thigh pressure is usually higher than the brachial pressure. Pressure gradients are measured between successive cuffs. A pressure gradient of 20 mmHg or more from one cuff to the cuff directly above it indicates significant disease. Multilevel disease can be difficult to identify as a proximal stenosis can limit distal blood flow and pressure. Well-developed collateral vessels can mask PAOD as well.

Pulse Volume Recordings

Another useful NIAS in patients with diabetes is the PVR. Pulse contours are obtained by air plethysmography and their waveforms can be interpreted to infer the presence and location of PAOD. Pressure cuffs are placed around the thigh, calf, and metatarsal heads and the PVR is measured as changes in volume of blood flow across the cuff. The PVR is not affected by arterial calcification making it a very useful test in diabetic patients. A normal pulse waveform contains a rapid upstroke, a sharp systolic peak, a prominent dicrotic notch, and a downslope that returns toward the baseline (Fig. 8.1). However, in patients with PAOD the dicrotic notch is lost and the pulse waveform becomes more dampened, and this decrease in amplitude and/or upstroke of the waveform indicates the presence of a stenosis upstream (Fig. 8.2). Comparisons can be made between the PVR of different segments in the same leg or at a single level between the right and left legs. Interpretation of the PVR can be altered by the blood pressure, peripheral resistance, and cardiac output, as well as by proximal stenoses that may limit distal blood flow.

Stress Testing

Most patients with claudication and ischemic symptoms usually have decreased resting pressures detected by ABI, so exercise testing is rarely required to diagnose PAOD. Exercise testing is most useful in patients with normal resting ABIs in whom claudication is harder to diagnose. Exercise testing will help distinguish between cardiopulmonary, orthopedic, and vascular disease as the etiology of the patient's difficulty in walking. In patients with claudication and a normal resting ABI, 31% were found to have a drop in their ABI after exercise testing [4]. The patient's ABI is measured at rest and after standard exercise. Various protocols such as the Skinner–Gardner protocol consist of a graded workload. The patient walks on a treadmill at a constant speed of 2 mph and an increase in grade of 2% every 2 min [5]. Patients are instructed to walk for 5 min or until forced to stop due to symptoms. The severity of the PAOD is reflected by the post-exercise drop in ABI and length of time required to return to baseline levels. Patients with mild PAOD may have normal resting pressures, a mild drop in ABI post-exercise, with return of normal pressures within minutes. Patients with severe PAOD have abnormal ABIs at rest with further decreases after exercise that may not return to pre-exercise levels in the allotted observation period. A normal individual is generally able to walk for 5 min with little or no fall in ankle pressure post-exercise. The exercise test tends to be more positive for proximal rather than distal PAOD.

Doppler Waveform Analysis

Doppler waveform analysis is the interpretation of velocity frequency shifts both aurally and visually. A handheld Doppler probe that couples an ultrasound transducer and receiver analyzes blood flow and creates velocity waveforms. These velocity waveforms are based on the Doppler principle and are more sensitive in detecting subclinical PAOD than the ABI. The ultrasound waveform undergoes a frequency shift proportional to the velocity of a moving object, in this case, red blood cells. Velocities are measurements of these frequency shifts and are displayed on the vertical axis with time on the horizontal axis.

A normal peripheral artery has a triphasic (Fig. 8.3) or biphasic (Fig. 8.4) quality at rest. In a triphasic waveform, there is a brisk upstroke of forward flow in systole followed by a brief reversal of flow in diastole, and lastly, a small forward flow component in late diastole. The reversal of flow and second wave of forward flow are due to the elasticity of the peripheral arteries. A normal triphasic waveform usually rules out clinically significant PAOD at or proximal to the interrogated level of the arterial tree. PAOD and areas of stenosis alter the normal triphasic velocity waveform. The normal reversal of blood flow in early diastole is progressively lost and results in spectral broadening of the waveform. As with pressure measurements, Doppler waveforms can change after exercise stress testing.

In low-resistance vascular beds such as the splenic, renal, mesenteric, and internal carotid arteries, there is no reverse flow component and the normal velocity waveform is monophasic. This occurs as there is continued forward flow through the artery even in diastole.

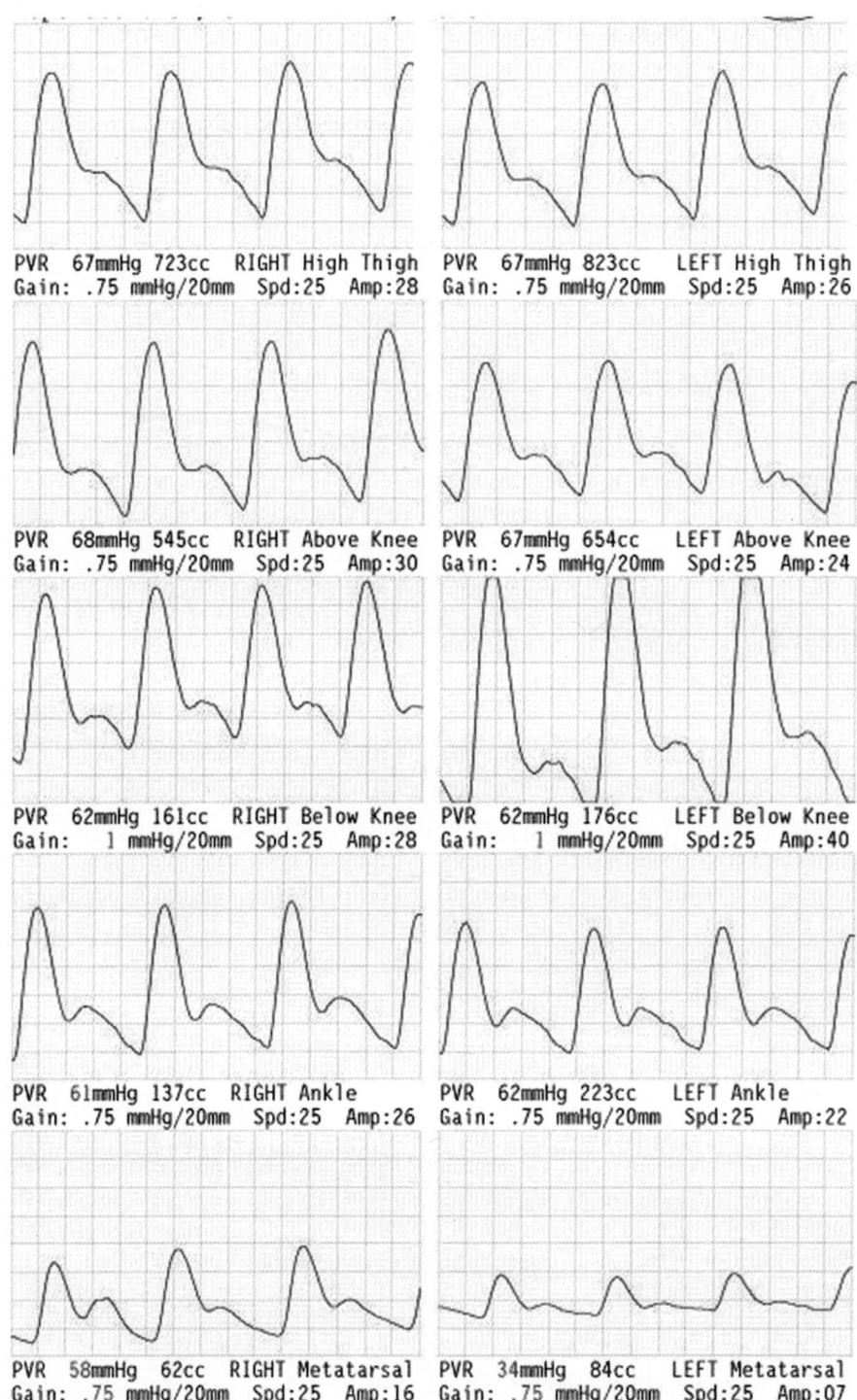

Fig. 8.1 Normal pulse volume recording

8 Arterial Imaging

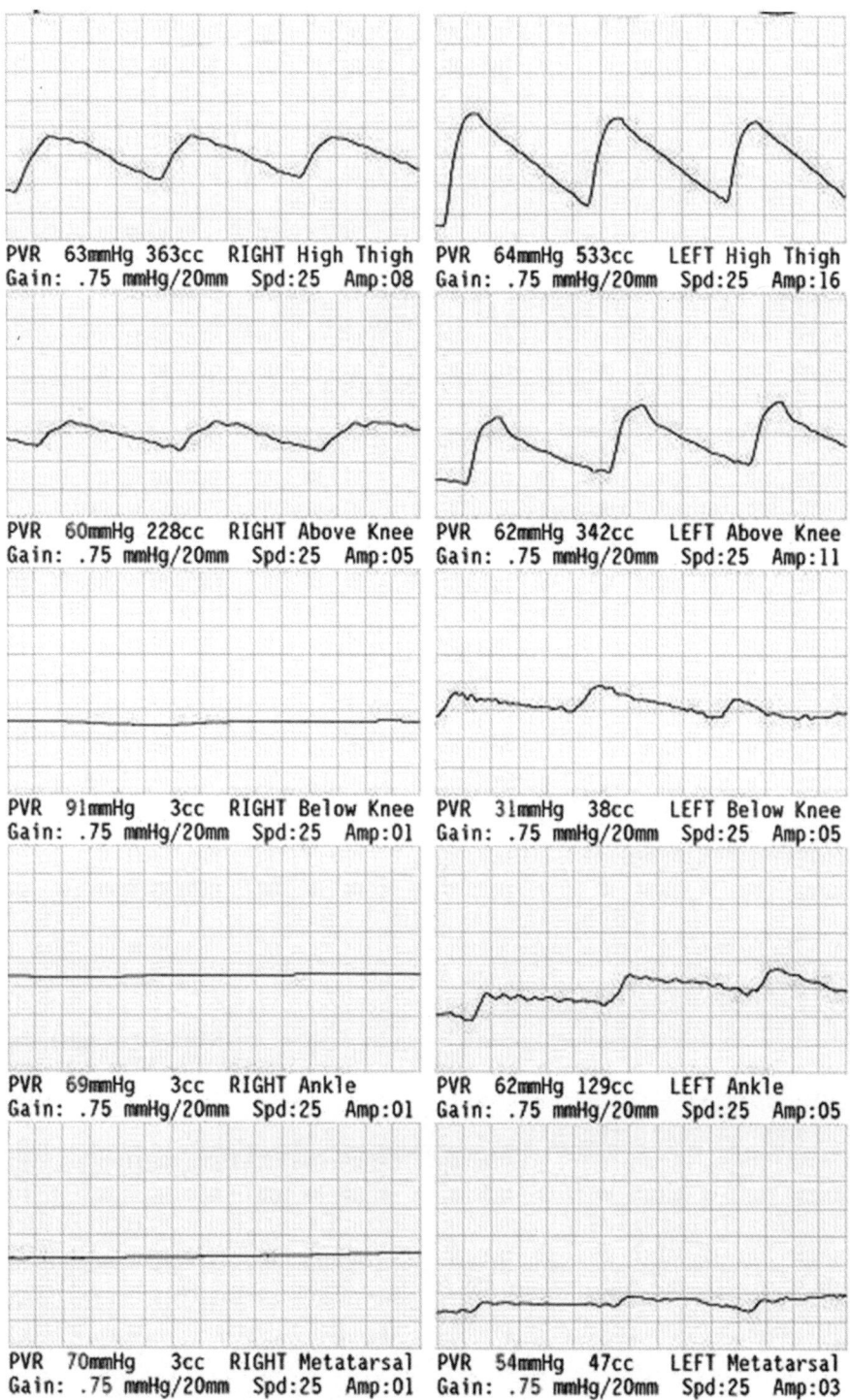

Fig. 8.2 Abnormal pulse volume recording showing bilateral peripheral arterial occlusive disease

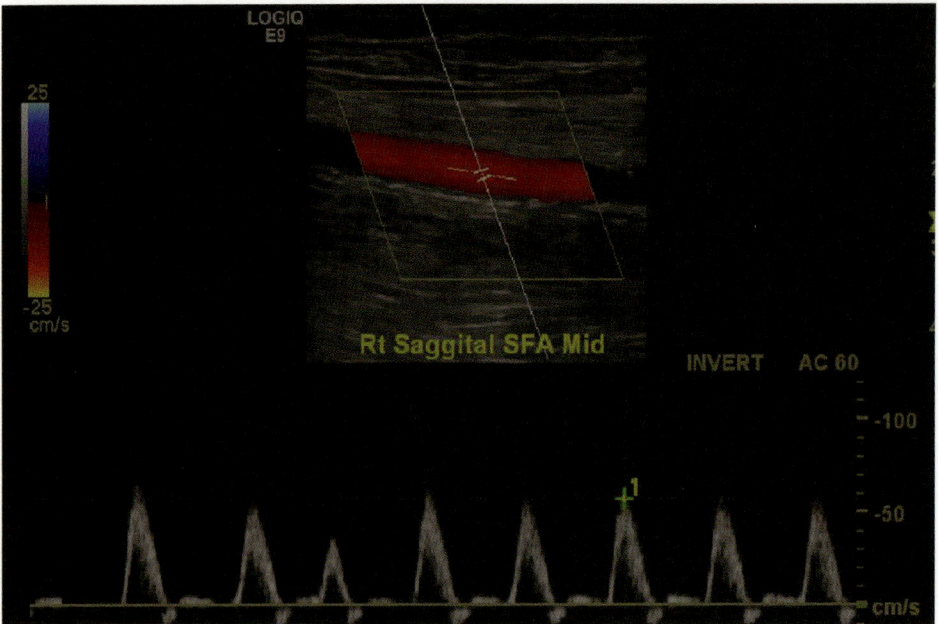

Fig. 8.3 Triphasic velocity waveform of a peripheral artery

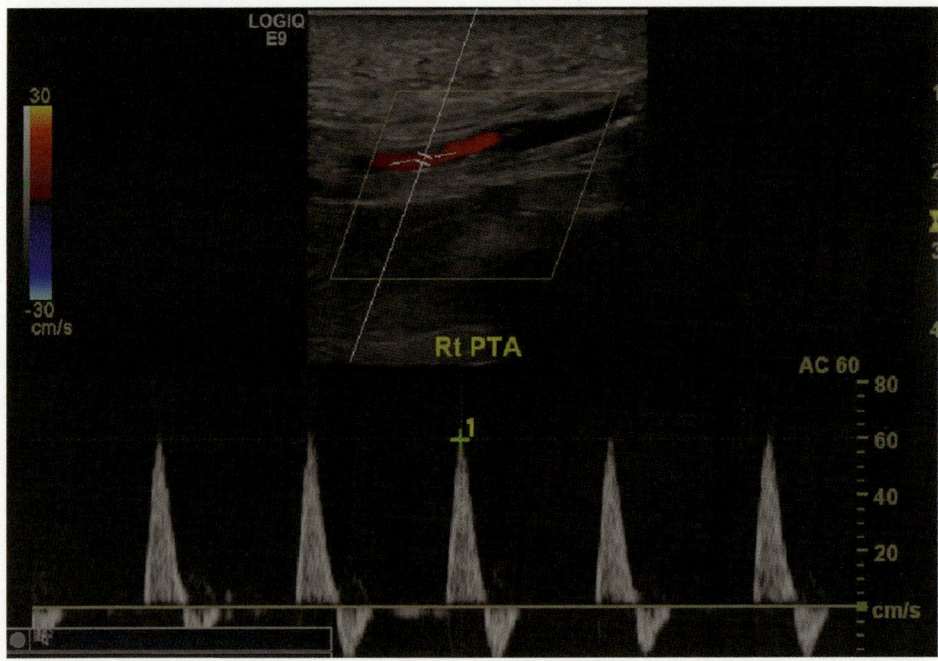

Fig. 8.4 Biphasic velocity waveform of a peripheral artery

Arterial Duplex Scanning

Arterial duplex scanning allows for the direct visualization of the artery and identification of the anatomic site of arterial lesions. It can also evaluate the hemodynamic consequences of lesions by measuring the velocity of blood flow across them. As with Doppler waveform analysis, arterial duplex scanning employs the Doppler principle.

The benefit of arterial duplex for Doppler waveform analysis is the availability to visualize the acoustic window. A triphasic signal with brisk flow results in a "clear" acoustic window beneath the velocity waveform. Spectral broadening (widening of the waveform) or dampening is the earliest visible change in the waveform at the site of stenosis and is manifested as a blunted monophasic waveform with "filling in" of the normally clear acoustic window (Fig. 8.5). This occurs as there is a wide range of flow velocities within the area of turbulent flow. Spectral broadening can be seen in triphasic waveforms as well.

In addition to being able to analyze the Doppler waveform (as discussed in the previous section), with arterial duplex scanning one is able to quantify the hemodynamic consequences of a site of stenosis. Specifically, the peak systolic velocity (PSV) proximal to and across an area of stenosis can be measured. The ratio of these velocities can be used to quantify the amount of stenosis within the artery. An area of severe stenosis can cause a marked increase in PSV, as well as spectral broadening. The PSV can be doubled at these sites compared to adjacent segments, and generally, a twofold step up in PSV across an area of stenosis equates to greater than 50% stenosis of the artery at that segment (Fig. 8.6). The velocity waveforms downstream from a site of stenosis are dampened. Arterial duplex scanning combined with B-mode imaging allows the velocity spectra of any location along the artery to be recorded and analyzed.

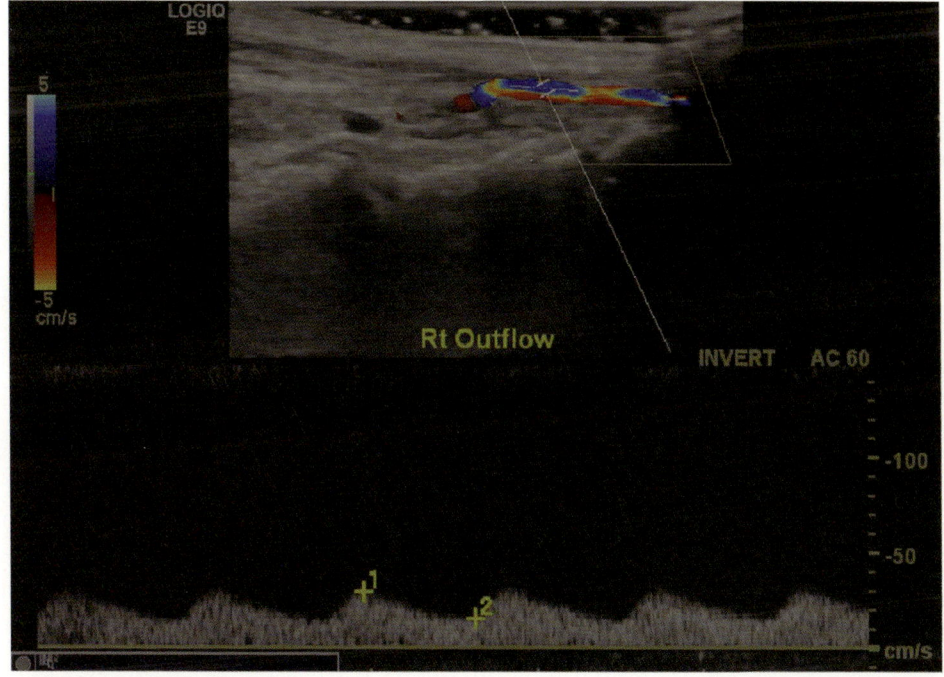

Fig. 8.5 Monophasic velocity waveform of a peripheral artery showing spectral broadening of "filling in" of the acoustic window

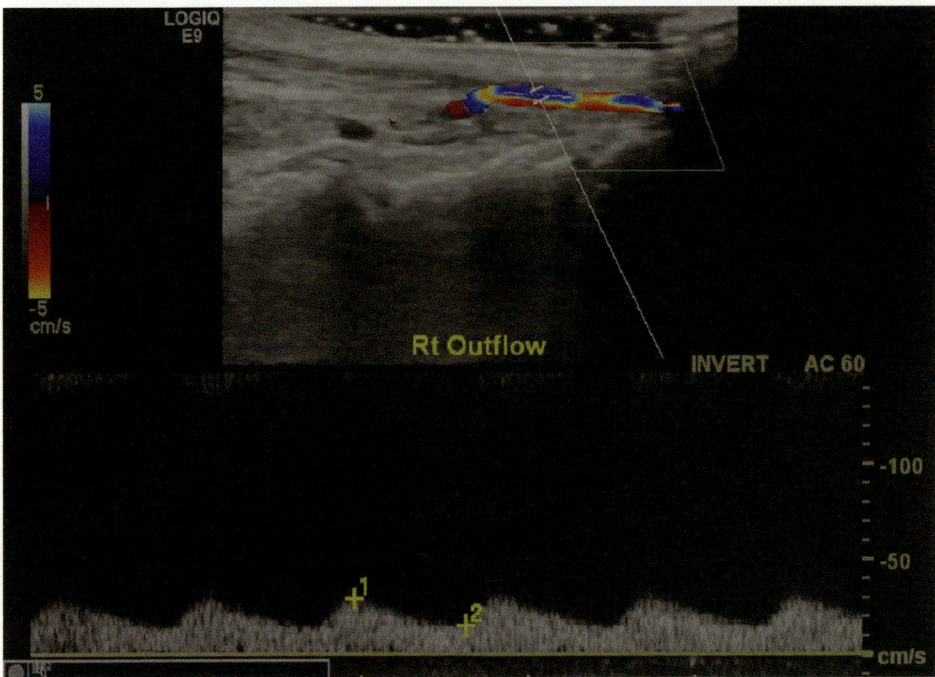

Fig. 8.6 Arterial duplex scan of a peripheral artery showing a peak systolic velocity of 55 cm/s pre-stenosis (*left*) and a peak systolic velocity of 125 cm/s post-stenosis (*right*) resulting in a 2.3-fold step up in velocity

Arteriography

Contrast arteriography is the gold standard arterial imaging modality due to its superior image resolution coupled with the ability to be both diagnostic and therapeutic. However, it is an invasive procedure with certain well-documented complications, especially in diabetic patients with renal insufficiency. With improvements in technology and image quality, an alternative to invasive contrast arteriography has become available in the form of CTA and MRA. Each of these three modalities has advantages and disadvantages that will be discussed below.

Computed Tomographic Angiography

With the development of spiral computed tomography (CT) scanning and multi-detector CT scanners, data are acquired rapidly over a continuous volume and CT scanners are able to capture multiple separate slices per 360° rotations. Continuous slices can be acquired at submillimeter thickness, and complete imaging of the lower extremity vasculature can be accomplished in a matter of seconds. Current CT scanners display images in a 512×512 or greater matrix with a resolution of 0.2–1 mm^2 for each pixel, which is twice that of typical magnetic resonance imaging (MRI).

CTA has been made possible with the development of multi-detector spiral CT scanners. Imaging of the vasculature requires the administration of intravenous contrast and "chasing" of the bolus of contrast over a long distance. CT image acquisition must occur rapidly as contrast flows rapidly through the blood stream. The timing of the initiation of image acquisition is determined by computer algorithms and contrast protocols that have been developed by CT scanner manufacturers. These algorithms allow for image acquisition of the maximum opacification of the vessels over the scanned volume. Image acquisition may out run the contrast bolus in patients with multisegment disease or slow transit times. When this occurs, a second acquisition sequence is acquired in reverse. As large distances must often be covered when scanning a patient's lower extremity, CTA requires a larger volume of contrast material. Up to 150 to 180 cc of full-strength nonionic contrast may be required [6].

As data are acquired over an entire volume, rather than in discontinuous slices, multiplanar reconstruction into coronal, sagittal, and other nonaxial planes is possible [7]. New software and computer technology has made three-dimensional (3D) reconstruction of the vasculature possible. As conventional CT slices often do not cut perpendicular to the vessel, this results in an elliptical cross section of the vessel. 3D reconstruction and CT reformats perpendicular to the vessel make diameter measurements more accurate [8–10]. 3D reconstructions are portrayed as shaded surface displays and allow the vasculature to be rotated and viewed from any perspective. While other structures such as bone can be cut away and "erased" when formatting 3D reconstructions, calcium within the vessel wall cannot be erased and is generally included in the reconstruction of the vasculature. Figure 8.7 is a 3D CTA reconstruction revealing occluded anterior tibial and peroneal arteries with a narrowed tibioperoneal trunk due to calcified atherosclerotic disease.

CTA images are artificial reconstructions and subject to potential reconstruction-based artifacts. Partial-volume effects occur when objects are only partially included in the scan plane. This may give the appearance of a lesion where none exists. Beam hardening artifacts occur when dense material is within the scan plane, such as prosthetic hips or metallic stents. Motion artifacts occur with patient movement and respiratory efforts or vessel movement as is often seen at the aortic root. Image quality depends on a compliant patient as they are instructed to hold their breath during scanning.

One of the most important concepts to understand when evaluating occlusive lesions on CTA is the window and level settings. Small changes in the brightness of the window-level setting may obscure small differences in contrast. This can occur in diabetic patients with heavily calcified small vessels (e.g. tibial arteries) where it may be

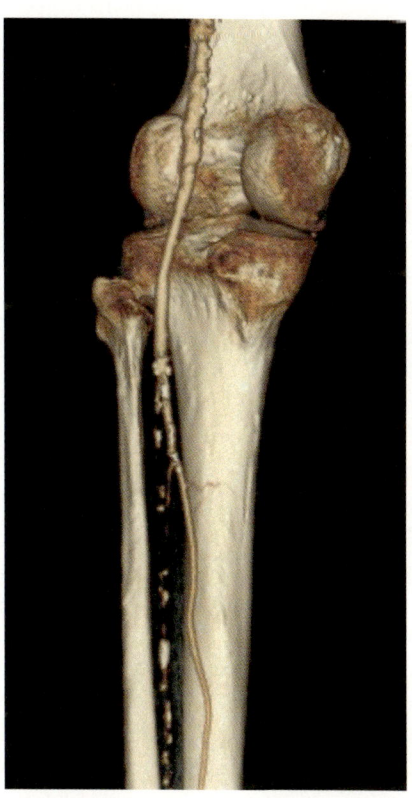

Fig. 8.7 Three-dimensionsal computed tomography reconstruction of tibial vessels revealing occluded anterior tibial and peroneal arteries with a narrowed tibioperoneal trunk due to calcified atherosclerotic disease

difficult to determine what a total occlusion versus a calcified stenosis is. Adjustments can usually be made to distinguish calcium from contrast but this can be difficult.

Although CTA is a good imaging modality for the lower extremity vasculature, it is not without its complications. It is estimated that 1.5–2% of all cancers in the United States are attributable to CT scans [11]. The high radiation dose coupled with the increased utilization of CT scans has prompted more radiation awareness among physicians, particularly with clinical decision making on whether or not a CTA is required.

Nephrotoxicity is especially important in patients with diabetes and underlying renal insufficiency. Contrast induced nephropathy (CIN) is the third leading cause of acute renal failure in hospitalized patients [12, 13]. CIN can range from a reversible rise in serum creatinine to end-stage renal failure requiring permanent hemodialysis or death. Preexisting renal insufficiency remains the most important factor in developing CIN. The risk of CIN in patients with normal renal function is only 1–2% [14]. The risk increases to 10% in patients with serum creatinine levels of 1.3–1.9 mg/dl and up to 62% in patients with serum creatinine levels greater than 2 mg/dl [15]. Diabetes itself is not an independent risk factor for the development of CIN, but the incidence of CIN is higher in patients with diabetes presumably due to subclinical renal insufficiency. CIN is particularly worrisome with CTA as up to 180 cc of contrast may be required to accurately image lower extremity vessels [6].

Many studies have been performed analyzing the prevention of CIN. Intravenous hydration with normal saline or sodium bicarbonate solution before exposure to contrast material appears to be the most effective preventive tool [16, 17]. The antioxidant N-acetylcysteine has been shown in some studies to help with prevention of CIN [18–21]. Other more recent studies show no benefit [22, 23]. Other agents studied include fenoldopam, theophylline, prostaglandin E1, calcium channel blockers, dopamine, and diuretics, but none of these can be recommended for the prevention of CIN [24–32].

Magnetic Resonance Angiography

Magnetic resonance angiography has become a common method for the evaluation of PAOD. When compared to DSA, its sensitivity for detecting a hemodynamically significant stenosis is as high as 99.5% with a specificity of 98.8% [33].

Magnetic resonance imaging uses a large external magnetic field, magnetic field gradients, and a radiofrequency field to produce images. These three magnetic fields manipulate the protons inside a patient's body and produce signals that can be used to generate images. MR pulse sequences are specific combinations of radiofrequency and magnetic field gradients used to create the image. The contrast in MR images depends on the characteristics of the object being imaged and on the specifics of the MR pulse sequence chosen. Images are T1-weighted or T2-weighted images. In T2-weighted images, simple fluids are bright and other tissues are black. Magnetic resonance angiography is performed with T1-weighted image sequences. Objects bright on T1-weighted images include fat, methemoglobin, flow effects, and MRI contrast.

MRA can be performed with or without contrast, but MRA with contrast has superior image resolution; so contrast-enhanced MRA has generally replaced non-contrast techniques [34, 35]. The most common non-contrast MRA technique is time of flight (TOF) angiography. TOF images are gathered as fully magnetized protons in a vessel flow into the slice of interest and produce much greater signals than the surrounding tissue resulting in a white image.

MRA with contrast uses the rare element gadolinium as its contrast agent. The gadolinium is chelated to another substance to prevent its release into the body, as it is a toxic substance. The gadolinium itself is not imaged, but rather its effect on the protons in T1-weighted imaging is captured. Similar to CTA, image acquisition involves imaging a large volume over a long distance. The gadolinium flows into the studied volume in a time-dependent fashion and as such the images can be obtained before contrast reaches the area of interest, or if images are obtained too late, there can be venous contamination by adjacent veins filled with contrast. As with CTA, the data gathered with MRA can undergo 3D reconstruction as well.

A rare condition called nephrogenic systemic fibrosis (NSF) was first associated with gadolinium contrast in 2006 in a cohort of patients on dialysis undergoing MRA [36]. All reported cases of NSF to date have occurred in patients with renal insufficiency. Predisposing factors to NSF include a larger dose of gadolinium contrast agents or patients undergoing repeated contrast studies. The use of gadolinium contrast agents is now contraindicated in patients with glomerular filtration rates of less than 30 ml/min or acute renal insufficiency. There have been no reported cases of NSF in patients with normal renal function. This potential complication has limited the utility of MRA with contrast in patients with diabetes and renal insufficiency. Some formations of gadolinium may be less likely to produce NSF.

Contrast Arteriography

Digital subtraction arteriography is the "gold standard" and most accurate method available to evaluate the circulation of the lower extremity. The lower extremity arterial tree can be completely visualized easily and rapidly. In patients with diabetic arterial occlusive disease, DSA provides superior imaging of distal small caliber vessels. Selective catheterizations of the superficial femoral or popliteal arteries allow excellent imaging of the foot vessels with a much reduced contrast load. DSA is an invasive technique that can be performed in an operating room or imaging suite. It is the only imaging modality in which the diagnosis and treatment of arterial disease can be performed simultaneously. When endovascular techniques were first developed, these minimally invasive procedures were performed in operating rooms with mobile C-arms or imaging suites with fixed mount imaging, such as interventional radiology suites or the cardiac catheterization laboratory. Recently, many hospitals have built hybrid operating rooms to allow vascular surgeons to perform complex and sophisticated procedures involving both open surgery and endovascular techniques. The advantage of fixed mount imaging units is their more powerful generators that allow for detailed imaging with superior resolution. They also have large high-resolution flat panel detectors that provide a larger field of view. This allows the surgeon to cover a larger imaging area with less radiation exposure and contrast volume. The advantage of portable C-arms is that they are mobile and can be taken from room to room or even to the patient if the patient is too unstable to be transported. This portability is at the expense of reduced image quality and resolution. DSA requires an injection of contrast that can be performed manually or with a power injector. A power injector allows for the precise control of the pressure setting, amount of contrast injected, timing of the injection, and the rate of rise of the injection.

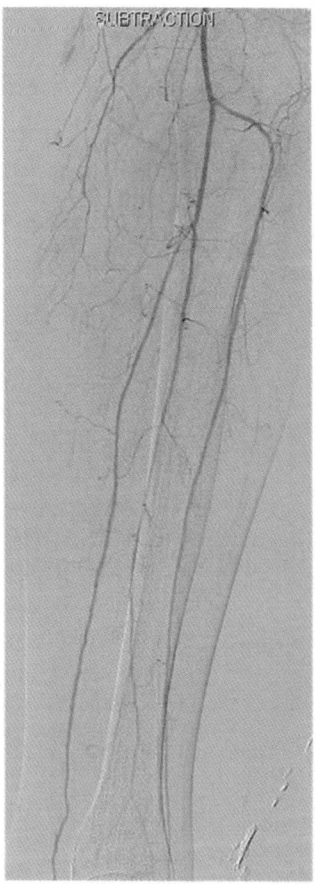

Fig. 8.8 Arteriogram of normal tibial vessels

Use of a power injector also allows the surgeon to leave the room during the acquisition of high-dose DSA images. Improvements in computers and image processors allow the surgeon to utilize subtraction, masking, view tracing, stacking, roadmapping, and unsubstracted image referencing when performing contrast arteriography and when viewing angiographic images. Figure 8.8 is an arteriogram of normal, but diminutive tibial arteries and Fig. 8.9 is an arteriogram of diseased tibial arteries.

Angiographic imaging requires a contrast agent that has a radiodensity that is higher or lower than the surrounding tissues. Typical contrast agents have a radiodensity that is greater than the surrounding tissue; however, carbon dioxide (CO_2) has a lower radiodensity but still provides adequate contrast to image anatomic details of the vascular tree [37, 38]. Conventional

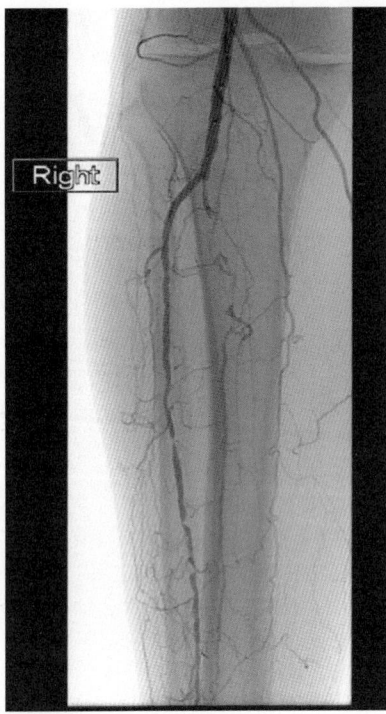

Fig. 8.9 Arteriogram of diseased tibial vessels

contrast agents are iodine-containing compounds that are either ionic or nonionic. Ionic agents dissociate into anions and cations thus doubling their osmolality making them hyperosmolar agents (1,500–1,700 mosm). Nonionic agents do not dissolve and have less osmolality (320–880 mosm). For comparison, plasma has an osmolality of 285. Table 8.2 lists the pros and cons of CTA, MRA, and contrast arteriography.

The toxic side effects of iodinated contrast agents are due to their hyperosmolality [39]. Common side effects include nausea, vomiting, pain in the arterial bed being studied, and allergic reactions. Adverse reactions can be minor, such as urticaria, or severe, such as anaphylactic shock and cardiopulmonary arrest. One study revealed the overall incidence of adverse reactions to be as high as 12% with ionic contrast and 3% with nonionic contrast. The incidence of severe adverse reactions was 0.2% with ionic contrast and 0.04% with nonionic contrast [40]. A history of a prior reaction is the best predictor of a future adverse event and the incidence of recurrent reactions ranges from 8 to 25% [41]. Premedication with oral corticosteroids has been shown to significantly reduce the incidence of adverse reactions [42]. At our institution we have both an intravenous and an oral regimen. The intravenous regimen entails the administration of solumedrol (120 mg), famotidine (20 mg), and diphenhydramine (25–50 mg) all given intravenously 1 h prior to the contrast study. The oral regimen entails prednisone (50 mg) administered at 16, 8, and 1 h before the contrast study as well as diphenhydramine (25–50 mg) and ranitidine (300 mg) both administered 1 h before the contrast study. In the event of adverse reactions, contrast administration should be stopped immediately. Mild adverse reactions are usually self-limiting and require no treatment. Anaphylactic reactions can be much more severe. If a patient develops bronchospasm or upper airway edema, inhalers and epinephrine should be administered promptly. Antihistamines and H2 blockers can be administered as well. Hypotension can be treated with intravenous iso-osmolar fluid such as normal saline or Ringer's lactate.

As stated earlier, nephrotoxicity is a side effect of contrast injection that can adversely affect diabetic patients with renal insufficiency. This is particularly important with contrast arteriography as studies have shown a higher rate of CIN with intra-arterial contrast injections as compared to intravenous contrast injections [43]. As diabetic patients have clinical and subclinical renal insufficiency, they are at a greater risk of developing CIN as compared to patients with normal renal function. As such, protective measures should be employed to try to prevent CIN such as the use of a low-volume nonionic isosmolar contrast agent and prehydration with either normal saline or bicarbonate solution.

Special consideration should be taken when performing angiography on diabetic patients taking Metformin (dimethylbiguanide) as the use of metformin in a patient with renal dysfunction can result in lactic acidosis. It is recommended that patients refrain from taking Metformin for 2 days after contrast arteriography.

CO_2 has been used in place of iodinated contrast agents in patients with renal insufficiency or severe allergic reactions, although image quality remains inferior to that of conventional contrast

Table 8.2 Pros and cons of CTA, MRA, and contrast arteriography

	Pros	Cons
CTA	Noninvasive	Radiation exposure
	Fast scanning time	Contrast volume
	Good image resolution	Reactions to contrast
	Multiplanar and 3D reconstructions	
MRA	Noninvasive	Lowest image resolution
	No radiation exposure	Slow scanning time
	3D reconstructions	Nephrogenic systemic fibrosis
Contrast arteriography	Gold standard	Invasive
	Best image resolution	Radiation exposure
	Allows for diagnosis and treatment	Access site complications
		Reactions to contrast

agents. CO_2 has a radiodensity that is lower than surrounding tissues. It is nontoxic when injected, rapidly displaces blood, and then dissolves quickly. Due to the rapidity with which the CO_2 dissolves, image acquisition settings must be changed compared to those used for image acquisition during iodinated contrast studies. If the CO_2 dissolves too quickly and is unable to completely fill the lumen of the artery, an overestimation of the stenosis can occur [44]. CO_2 is lighter than water and blood and tends to rise, so performing arteriography with the legs elevated on top of pillows or with the patient in Trendelenburg, if possible, may allow for more accurate imaging of the distal lower extremity arteries. One can also rotate the table laterally or place a pillow under the patient's flank to aid in evaluation of the renal arteries. CO_2 can be combined with iodinated contrast agents where CO_2 is used for most of the image acquisition and limited use of iodinated contrast is employed for areas where CO_2 cannot accurately define the anatomy. Complications with CO_2 injection are uncommon, although mesenteric ischemia has been reported due to gas trapping within the mesenteric vessels [45, 46].

References

1. American Diabetes Association. Peripheral arterial disease in people with diabetes (consensus statement). Diabetes Care. 2003;26:3333–41.
2. Smith FB, Lee AJ, Price JF, et al. Changes in ankle brachial index in symptomatic and asymptomatic subjects in the general population. J Vasc Surg. 2003;38:1323–30.
3. Potier L, Halbron M, Bouilloud F, et al. Ankle-to-brachial ration index underestimates the prevalence of peripheral occlusive disease in diabetic patients at high risk for arterial disease. Diabetes Care. 2009;32:c44.
4. Stein R, Hriljac I, Halperin JL, et al. Limitation of the resting ankle-brachial index in symptomatic patients with peripheral arterial disease. Vasc Med. 2006;11:29–33.
5. Hiatt WR, Hirsch AT, Regensteiner JG, et al. Clinical trials for claudication. Assessment of exercise performance, functional status, and clinical end points. Vascular Clinical Trialists. Circulation. 1995;92:614–21.
6. Prokop M. CT angiography of the abdominal arteries. Abdom Imaging. 1998;23:462–8.
7. Ibukuro K, Charnsangavej C, Chasen MH, et al. Helical CT angiography with multiplanar reformation: techniques and clinical applications. Radiographics. 1995;15:671–82.
8. Broeders IA, Blankensteijn JD, Olree M, et al. Preoperative sizing of grafts for transfemoral endovascular aneurysm management: a prospective comparative study of spiral CT angiography, arteriography, and conventional CT imaging. J Endovasc Surg. 1997;4:252–61.
9. Sprouse LR, Meier III GH, Parent FN, et al. Is three-dimensional computed tomography reconstruction justified before endovascular aortic aneurysm repair? J Vasc Surg. 2004;40:443–7.
10. Parker MV, O'Donnell SD, Chang AS, et al. What imaging studies are necessary for abdominal aortic endograft sizing? A prospective blinded study using conventional computed tomography, aortography, and three-dimensional computed tomography. J Vasc Surg. 2005;41:199–205.
11. Brenner DJ, Hall DJ. Computed tomography – an increasing source of radiation exposure. N Engl J Med. 2007;357:2277–84.
12. Waybill MM, Waybill PN. Contrast media-induced nephrotoxicity: identification of patients at risk and

algorithms for prevention. J Vasc Interv Radiol. 2001;12:3–9.
13. Agrawal M, Stouffer GA. Cardiology grand rounds from the University of North Caroline at Chapel Hill: contrast induced nephropathy after angiography. Am J Med Sci. 2002;323:252–8.
14. Parfrey PS, Griffiths SM, Barrett BJ, et al. Contrast material-induced renal failure in patients with diabetes mellitus, renal insufficiency, or both: a prospective controlled study. N Engl J Med. 1989;320:143–9.
15. Hall KA, Wong RW, Hunter GC, et al. Contrast-induced nephrotoxicity: the effects of vasodilator therapy. J Surg Res. 1992;53:317–20.
16. Trivedi HS, Moore H, Nasr S, et al. A randomized prospective trial to assess the role of saline hydration on the development of contrast nephrotoxicity. Nephron Clin Pract. 2003;93:C29–34.
17. Mueller C, Buerkle G, Buettner HJ, et al. Prevention of contrast media-associated nephropathy: randomized comparison of 2 hydration regimens in 1620 patients undergoing coronary angioplasty. Arch Intern Med. 2002;162:329–36.
18. Tepel M, van der Giet M, Schwarzfeld C, et al. Prevention of radiographic-contrast-agent-induced reductions in renal function by acetylcysteine. N Engl J Med. 2000;343:180–4.
19. Kay J, Chow WH, Chan TM, et al. Acetylcysteine for prevention of acute deterioration of renal function following elective coronary angiography and intervention: a randomized controlled trial. JAMA. 2003;289:553–8.
20. Diaz-Sandoval LJ, Kosowsky BD, Losordo DW. Acetylcysteine to prevent angiography-related renal tissue injury (the APART trial). Am J Cardiol. 2002;89:356–8.
21. Shyu KG, Cheng JJ, Kuan P. Acetylcysteine protects against acute renal damage in patients with abnormal renal function undergoing a coronary procedure. J Am Coll Cardiol. 2002;40:1383–8.
22. Durham JD, Caputo C, Dokko J, et al. A randomized controlled trial of N-acetylcysteine to prevent contrast nephropathy in cardiac angiography. Kidney Int. 2002;62:2202–7.
23. Hoffmann U, Fischereder M, Kruger B, et al. The value of N-acetylcysteine in the prevention of radio-contrast agent-induced nephropathy seems questionable. J Am Soc Nephrol. 2004;15:407–10.
24. Stevens MA, McCullough PA, Tobin KJ, et al. A prospective randomized trial of prevention measures in patients at high risk for contrast nephropathy: results of the P.R.I.N.C.E. Study. Prevention of Radiocontrast Induced Nephropathy Clinical Evaluation. J Am Coll Cardiol. 1999;33:403–11.
25. Weisberg LS, Kurnik PB, Kurnik BR. Risk of radio-contrast nephropathy in patients with and without diabetes mellitus. Kidney Int. 1994;45:259–65.
26. Solomon R, Werner C, Mann D, et al. Effects of saline, mannitol, and furosemide to prevent acute decreases in renal function induced by radiocontrast agents. N Engl J Med. 1994;331:1416–20.
27. Weinstein JM, Heyman S, Brezis M. Potential deleterious effect of furosemide in radiocontrast nephropathy. Nephron. 1992;62:413–5.
28. Sketch Jr MH, Whelton A, Schollmayer E, et al. Prevention of contrast media-induced renal dysfunction with prostaglandin E1: a randomized, double-blind, placebo-controlled study. Am J Ther. 2001;8:155–62.
29. Huber W, Schipek C, Ilgmann K, et al. Effectiveness of theophylline prophylaxis of renal impairment after coronary angiography in patients with chronic renal insufficiency. Am J Cardiol. 2003;91:1157–62.
30. Allaqaband S, Tumuluri R, Malik AM, et al. Prospective randomized study of N-acetylcysteine, fenoldopam, and saline for prevention of radiocontrast-induced nephropathy. Catheter Cardiovasc Interv. 2002;57:279–83.
31. Stone GW, McCullough PA, Tumlin JA, et al. Fenoldopam mesylate for the prevention of contrast-induced nephropathy: a randomized controlled trial. JAMA. 2003;290:2284–91.
32. Neumayer HH, Junge W, Kufner A, et al. Prevention of radiocontrast-media-induced nephrotoxicity by the calcium channel blocker nitrendipine: a prospective randomized clinical trial. Nephrol Dial Transplant. 1989;4:1030–6.
33. Steffens JC, Schafer FK, Oberscheid B, et al. Bolus-chasing contrast-enhanced 3D MRA of the lower extremity. Comparison with intraarterial DSA. Acta Radiol. 2003;44:185–92.
34. Meaney JF. Magnetic resonance angiography of the peripheral arteries: current status. Eur Radiol. 2003;13:836–52.
35. Sharafuddin MJ, Stolpen AH, Sun S, et al. High-resolution multiphase contrast-enhanced three-dimensional MR angiography compared with two-dimensional time-of-flight MR angiography for the identification of pedal vessels. J Vasc Interv Radiol. 2002;13:695–702.
36. Grobner T. Gadolinium – a specific trigger for the development of nephrogenic fibrosing dermopathy and nephrogenic systemic fibrosis? Nephrol Dial Transplant. 2006;4:1104–8.
37. Weaver FA, Pentecost MJ, Yellin AE, et al. Clinical applications of carbon dioxide/digital subtraction angiography. J Vasc Surg. 1991;13:266–73.
38. Seeger JM, Self S, Harward TR, et al. Carbon dioxide gas as an arterial contrast agent. Ann Surg. 1993;217:688–97.
39. Smith D, Yahiku PY, Maloney MD, et al. Three new low-osmolality contrast agents: a comparative study of patient discomfort. Am J Neuroradiol. 1988;9:137–9.
40. Katayama H, Yamaguchi K, Kozuka T, et al. Adverse reactions to ionic and nonionic contrast media. A report from the Japanese Committee on the Safety of Contrast Media. Radiology. 1990;175(3):621–8.
41. Bettmann MA, Heeren T, Greenfield A, et al. Adverse events with radiographic contrast agents: results of the SCVIR Contrast Agent Registry. Radiology. 1997;203(3):611–20.

42. Lasser EC, Berry CC, Talner LB, et al. Pretreatment with corticosteroids to alleviate reactions to intravenous contrast material. N Engl J Med. 1987;14:845–9.
43. Katzberg RW, Barrett BJ. Risk of iodinated contrast material-induced nephropathy with intravenous administration. Radiology. 2007;243:622–8.
44. Lang EV, Gossler AA, Fick LJ, et al. Carbon dioxide angiography: effect of injection parameters on bolus configurations. J Vasc Interv Radiol. 1999;10:41–9.
45. Rundback JH, Shah PM, Wong J, et al. Livedo reticularis, rhabdomyolysis, massive intestinal infarction, and death after carbon dioxide angiography. J Vasc Surg. 1997;26:337–40.
46. Caridi JG, Hawkins Jr IF, Klioze SD, et al. Carbon dioxide digital subtraction angiography: the practical approach. Tech Vasc Interv Radiol. 2001;4:57–65.

The Role of Endovascular Therapy in Peripheral Arterial Disease

9

Andrew J. Meltzer and James F. McKinsey

Keywords
Endovascular • Angioplasty • Atherectomy • Outcomes

Introduction

The prevalence of peripheral arterial disease (PAD) among American adults is estimated at 4% [1]. Among the elderly, the prevalence exceeds 20%, affecting over four million individuals, and accounting for over $20 billion in annual healthcare costs [1, 2]. Its most advanced form, critical limb ischemia (CLI), is a highly morbid condition with 1-year mortality and major amputation rates estimated at 20% and 35%, respectively [3]. Treatment options to avoid amputation (limb salvage therapy) include surgical bypass and minimally invasive, endovascular interventions. Although the durability of peripheral bypass surgery is proven, it is associated with significant perioperative morbidity and mortality [4]. Conversely, endovascular interventions are associated with reduced durability and may require serial interventions to achieve limb salvage [5–7].

However, due to the minimally invasive nature of these procedures, they are associated with reduced perioperative risk. Although patients with severe CLI associated with extensive gangrene that require prompt revascularization may be best served with primary surgical bypass; for many patients endovascular therapy is a reasonable option.

Given the high prevalence of medical comorbidities among patients with PAD, many vascular specialists advocate aggressive use of endovascular therapy as first-line treatment for PAD. Therefore, it is imperative that practitioners involved in the care of patients with PAD and diabetes are familiar with endovascular techniques, expected outcomes (including risk factors for failure), and potential complications.

Endovascular Techniques

Arterial Access and Diagnostic Angiography

The first step in an endovascular intervention is access to the arterial circulation. For the treatment of infrainguinal disease, this may be obtained by an antegrade approach with puncture

A.J. Meltzer, M.D. (✉) • J.F. McKinsey, M.D., F.A.C.S.
Division of Vascular Surgery and Endovascular
Interventions Columbia University
College of Physicians and Surgeons
New York Presbyterian Hospitall,
526 East 68th Street, P706, New York, NY 10021, USA
e-mail: andrewjmeltzer@gmail.com

of the ipsilateral common femoral artery, or by arterial access via the contralateral common femoral artery followed by access to the target extremity after intraluminal catheter crossing the aortic bifurcation. In unusual circumstances (i.e., following endovascular aneurysm repair or extra-anatomic reconstruction) it may be necessary to perform lower extremity endovascular interventions via the upper extremity or direct puncture of an extra-anatomic bypass graft.

The approximate location of the common femoral artery (CFA) can be determined with fluoroscopy (generally in the medial middle third of the femoral head in the majority of patients), and punctured with an 18-gauge needle using this radiographic landmark in the presence of a palpable pulse. Alternatively, ultrasound guidance, with or without the routine use of a small bore micropuncture needle and access sheath, may be used to visualize the CFA during arterial access. The authors have found this technique to be particularly beneficial in the setting of an absent femoral pulse, significant arterial calcification, or in the vicinity of prior surgical bypass grafts. This technique has also been advocated for the percutaneous access of a large-diameter catheter with planned use suture-mediated closure devices to avoid a surgical cut down. With the ultrasonic guidance, the user can identify the femoral bifurcation as well as significant femoral plaque and precisely access the CFA and give the best opportunity to safely seal the CFA with the closure devices.

Following placement of the guidewire via the access needle, an in-dwelling arterial sheath is placed. The peripheral arteries of interest are accessed using hydrophilic wires and selective catheters under fluoroscopic guidance. Digital subtraction or cine angiography is performed with intravascular administration of contrast to confirm anatomic location and acquire diagnostic information. During this diagnostic stage of the procedure, the catheter may be advanced distally to permit better imaging of the infrapopliteal and pedal vessels (Fig. 9.1). It is imperative to perform angiography from orthogonal projections, as the two-dimensional nature of the resulting image may lead to underestimation of the true burden of disease.

Review of the diagnostic angiography is performed and the vascular specialist determines if the patient's clinical presentation and pattern of disease are consistent with candidacy for endovascular therapy.

Crossing Lesions

Systemic heparin is administered, and an arterial sheath (of sufficient caliber to subsequently permit introduction of devices for treatment) is introduced over a stiff wire. Once therapeutic levels of anticoagulation are achieved, using selective catheter and wire combinations, wire access is obtained across the diseased arterial segment. Although a number of wire and selective catheter combinations may be used, the authors routinely use a hydrophilic 0.035″ angled wire and 5 French angled catheter during the initial attempt to cross lesions. Based on the interventionalist's preference and experience, different combinations of wire diameter (0.014″, 0.018″, 0.035″), stiffness, and angulation may be combined with differently shaped selective catheters to traverse lesions intraluminally.

When lesions cannot be crossed via the true lumen, due to inability to cross through a complete occlusion, a subintimal (technically subadventitial) route may be chosen. By initiating a purposeful dissection in this plane, access around a lesion may be attained. This is usually accomplished by purposefully creating a "J" with the floppy tip of the wire and propagating the looped wire in a dissection flap distal to the area of significant disease. This is followed by true lumen reentry at a more distal site. The lumen may be reentered with the wire alone, angled catheter, or occasionally a commercially available device to facilitate true lumen reentry are sometimes required. These devices include the Outback Re-entry System (Cordis Corporation, Bridgewater, NJ) and the Pioneer catheter (Medtronic, Inc, Minneapolis, MN). Likewise, as an alternative to crossing lesions in the subintimal plane, commercially available devices may be used to facilitate crossing lesions. The role of these commercially available devices remains a

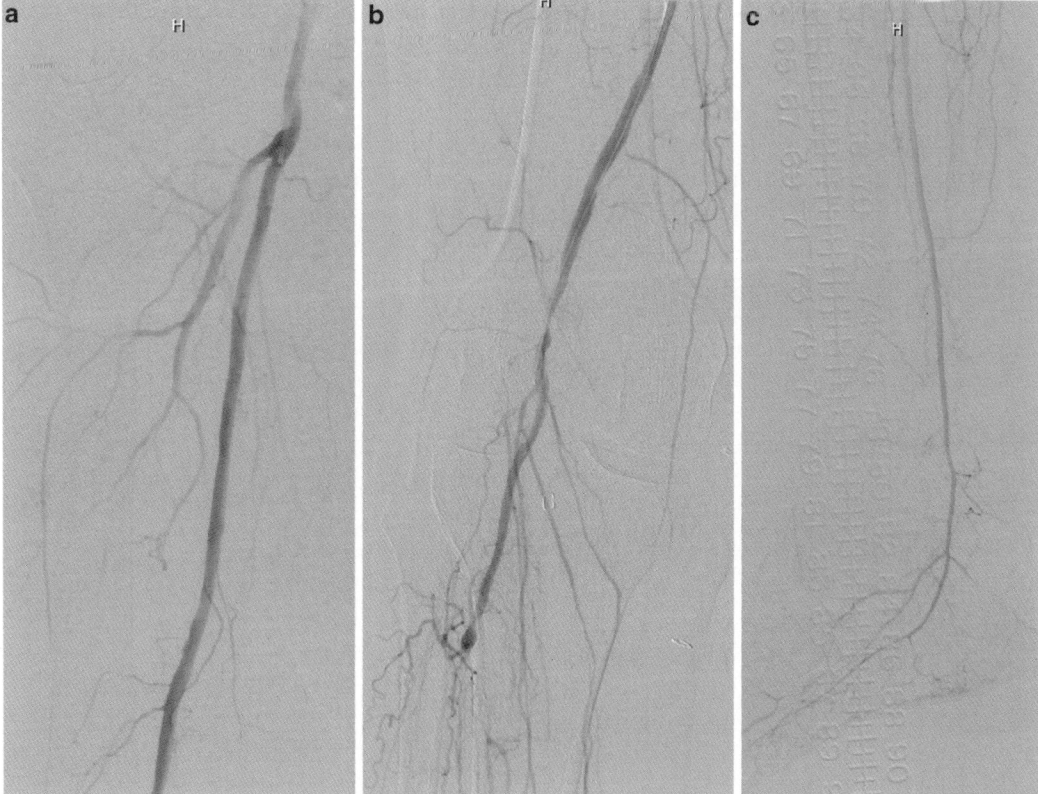

Fig. 9.1 Diagnostic angiography reveals (**a**) patent SFA; (**b**) chronic total occlusion of the retrogeniculate popliteal artery; (**c**) intact pedal runoff via the posterior tibial artery

matter of operator preference. The more recent technology utilizes specialized catheter devices including the Wildcat (Avinger, Redwood City, CA), Crosser (Bard Peripheral Vascular, Inc, Tempe, AZ), and Frontrunner (Cordis Corporation, Bridgewater, NJ) devices to theoretically cross the total occlusion in a central luminal position rather than a subadventitial plane.

Treatment

Angioplasty

After arterial lesions have been traversed, either intraluminally or in the subadventitial plane, the vascular specialist selects an appropriate treatment modality. The most commonly applied endovascular technique is percutaneous transluminal angioplasty (PTA). In instances in which lesions are traversed in the subintimal plane, as described above, the term subintimal angioplasty (SIA) may be used. With wire access across a lesion, an angioplasty balloon of appropriate length and diameter is inflated to create a focal dissection in the artery, restoring a lumen. There should be a 10–15% oversizing of the balloon relative to the reference lumen diameter of treated vessel. Whenever possible, the length of the balloon should span the entire length of the lesion so that the shoulders of the balloon have a lower probability of creating a dissection within the plaque. There are additional balloon devices that incorporate additional wires along the axis of the balloon which act as a focal point of cleavage. These focal point balloons theoretically decrease the incidence of dissections as well as prevent migration of the balloon during its inflation. Differing from the standard PTA balloon, the focal point balloons should be chosen to be the diameter of the reference vessel with minimal to no oversizing.

Prior to the introduction of endovascular stents and peripheral atherectomy devices, isolated PTA was the only treatment modality for endovascular interventions. The rapid evolution of endovascular techniques is evident in that this therapeutic mainstay is now often referred to as "POBA" (or "plain old balloon angioplasty"), a nickname that denotes the relative technological simplicity of the technique.

Much of the literature regarding outcomes after endovascular therapy remains fundamentally PTA-based; therefore, one must interpret results of early trials and treatment guidelines with caution. The introduction of novel devices and improved angioplasty balloons with smaller crossing profiles has fundamentally revolutionized endovascular interventions.

Bare Metal Stents

For disease in the relatively large-caliber vessels above the knee (particularly in the superficial femoral artery), PTA is often followed by the placement of intravascular stents. Bare metal stents (usually nitinol-based) and covered stents are both options in vessels of sufficient caliber. While numerous studies, and subsequent meta-analyses, have failed to demonstrate improved patency with stent placement, it is important to consider the burden of arterial disease [8, 9]. In general, the anatomic pattern of disease encountered in the setting of randomized trials included in meta-analyses is less severe than the "real-world" disease routinely encountered by the vascular specialist. Therefore, most interventionalists have adopted a liberal approach to adjunctive stenting, particularly in the setting of long-segment disease and chronic total occlusions. Results of a meta-analysis comparing PTA to stents in the SFA are shown in Fig. 9.2.

Covered Stents

In an effort to avoid the problems of in-stent restenosis seen following angioplasty and bare-metal stent placement in the SFA, some vascular specialists have adopted the use of covered stents in the SFA, both for treatment of primary atherosclerotic disease or for the treatment of in-stent restenosis after prior bare-metal stent placement. The primary rationale for the use of covered stents in the SFA is that this approach provides a direct mechanical barrier to prevent the ingrowth of neointimal hyperplasia through the interstices of the stent. Furthermore, some surgeons accustomed to performing femoropopliteal bypass grafts to the above knee popliteal artery with PTFE have embraced the "percutaneous fem-pop" as an endovascular alternative to the open procedure, with comparable short-term results [10].

The potential advantages of covered stent usage include the combination of radial force supplied by the metal stent component as well as the ePTFE mechanical barrier to intimal hyperplasia. A characteristic feature of covered stent failure, however, is "edge stenosis" at the proximal

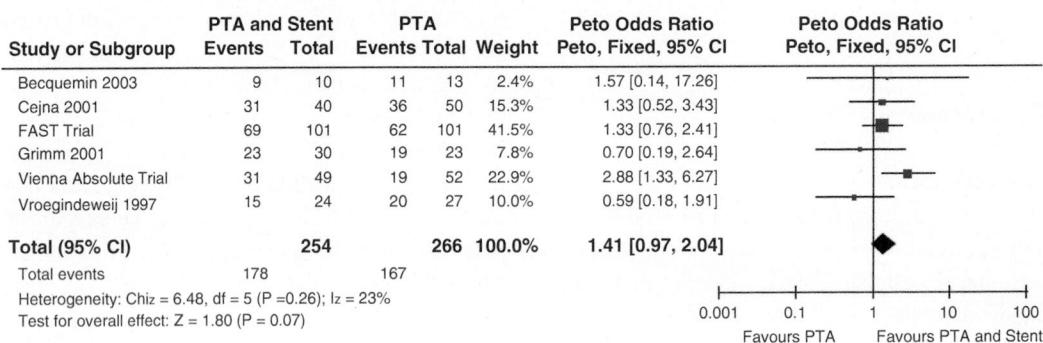

Fig. 9.2 Meta-analysis of PTA vs. PTA + S for SFA disease

and distal margins of the treated segment, where intimal hyperplasia may occur in the absence of the physical barrier provided by the ePTFE covered stent. This phenomenon may predispose stent grafts to acute thrombosis as a primary mode of failure. Because both inflow and outflow obstructions can occur, edge stenosis can lead to a challenging presentation of an acutely thrombosed graft that may require thrombolysis or thrombectomy to treat, as opposed to the diffuse pattern of in-stent restenosis observed after self-expanding nitinol stent placement. With the acute occlusion of the stent graft there can also be an associated distal embolization of thrombotic material resulting in distal ischemia and in some cases acute CLI.

Cryoplasty

Cryoplasty combines a standard dilation force and inflation time of balloon angioplasty with the delivery of cold thermal energy to the vessel wall. Theoretically, cryoplasty is believed to induce arterial smooth muscle cell apoptosis (rather than necrosis), therefore providing the theoretical advantage of reduced myointimal hyperplasia and improved long-term patency. Despite this novel mechanism, however, clinical results have yet to demonstrate any advantage in comparison to angioplasty alone, as summarized in a recent meta-analysis [11]. Much like covered stent placement, cryoplasty has been touted as a potential solution to in-stent restenosis. Unfortunately, it has not proven superior to other techniques in this setting [12]. Moreover, while randomized controlled trials are uncommon, specific efforts to evaluate the role of cryoplasty in diabetics have suggested that this technology is inferior compared to angioplasty alone, with respect to primary patency and need for re-intervention [13].

Atherectomy

Atherectomy is the only therapeutic modality that actually permits removal of the atherosclerotic burden from the peripheral vasculature. Potential benefits of this technique include avoidance of stents and the inherent problem of in-stent restenosis. Given the limited durability of all peripheral endovascular interventions, atherectomy does not require the placement of permanent implant that may negate subsequent interventions to maintain assisted and/or secondary patency by a new therapeutic modality that has not been FDA approved.

A number of devices are currently available including the directional Silverhawk (EV3, Minneapolis, MN) device, orbital atherectomy devices, including the CSI DiamondBack 360 (CSI, Minneapolis, MN) rotational atherectomy devices, such as the Pathway Jetstream (Pathway Medical Technologies, Inc., Kirkland, WA) and Rotablator device (Boston Scientific, Natick, MA), and laser atherectomy devices, including the Spectranetics Excimer Laser (Spectranetics, Colorado Springs, CO). The Silverhawk device is perhaps the best studied [14–19]. In fact, the Definitive LE study, which evaluated outcomes in a real-world patient population, is the largest peripheral device study to date, enrolling 800 patients at 50 centers. Interim analysis showed that from 87.4% primary patency at 6 months. Notably, there was no significant difference in short-term outcome among diabetic patients. Long-term follow-up will further address results with this device, and assess the potential efficacy in the diabetic population. Our group has reported the largest single-center experience with the device [19]. In this retrospectively reviewed series, 275 patients (62.5% male, 46.2% smokers, 67.6% diabetic) underwent Silverhawk atherectomy to treat 579 lesions (199 superficial femoral arteries, 110 popliteal, 218 tibials, and 52 multilevel). Eighteen-month primary and secondary patency for all lesions was 52.7%±2.8 and 75.0%±2.4. Eighteen-month primary and secondary patency for claudicants was 58.0%±4.3 and 82.5%±3.5 ($P<0.0001$) and for CLI was 49.4%±3.7 and 69.9%±3.2 ($P<0.0001$), respectively. The reintervention rate was 25.3% in claudicants and 30.1% for CLI. Limb salvage was 100% in claudicants and overall limb salvage was 92.4% at 18 months; only 4.4% required bypass during follow-up. Further prospective studies will better elucidate the role of the Silverhawk device and the other FDA-approved atherectomy devices in the treatment of PAD.

Drug-Eluting Technology

Chapter 16 includes an in-depth discussion of emerging technologies to treat peripheral vascular disease. A brief mention of some of the newer modalities is made here.

Success with drug-eluting stents (DES) technology in the coronary circulation has led to its application in the periphery. Small series have suggested that drug-eluting coronary stents may lead to improved patency in the infrapopliteal vessels, particularly in the setting of an adjunctive "bail-out" procedure after failed angioplasty [20]. The first study to address the role of DES in the SFA were the SIROCCO (SIROlimus Coated Cordis SMART Nitinol Self expandable Stent for the Treatment of Obstructive Superficial Femoral Artery Disease) studies [21–23]. The SIROCCO stent (Cordis, Miami Lakes, FL) was based on the SMART stent platform, loaded with sirolimus and delivered its drug over 7–8 days. While there was initially a distinct advantage for the SFA DES compared to bare metal stents, the 18–24 months data demonstrated no difference in patency compared to bare metal stents alone, a finding that has been attributed to inadequate drug delivery as well as stent fracture [24]. Recently, results from the STRIDES trial (Superficial Femoral Artery Treatment with Drug-Eluting Stents), using an everolimus-eluting platform, were reported. In STRIDES, technical success was achieved in 98% of cases. Clinical improvement was achieved in 80% of patients. Primary patency was 94±2.3% and 68±4.6% at 6 and 12 months, respectively [24]. Long-term outcomes remain unclear.

The Zilver-PTX platform (Cook Medical, Bloomington, IN), which consists of a polymer-free, paclitaxel-coated nitinol stent, was compared to PTA and provisional bare-metal stent placement in patients with femoropopliteal peripheral artery disease. Differing from the prior two studies discussed above, Zilver PTX results were favorable with this device: primary DES placement resulted in superior 12-month event-free survival (90.4% versus 82.6%; $P=0.004$) and primary patency (83.1% versus 32.8%; $P<0.001$) [25].

In addition to these reports and ongoing studies evaluating the efficacy of DES, drug-coated and drug-eluting balloons are a promising alternative. Early reports are favorable [26]. The potential benefits of drug-eluting balloons are most pronounced when one considers their applicability to the treatment of infrapopliteal disease, where results are generally poor and stent placement is generally avoided. Ongoing and future studies will hopefully clarify the role of drug-eluting technology in the treatment of PAD. However, new drug and delivery formulations, as well as improved balloon and stent platforms, may lead to improved outcomes with these techniques.

Peri-procedural Management

Although the role of dual antiplatelet therapy after peripheral endovascular intervention has not been evaluated in randomized, controlled trials, we routinely prescribe dual antiplatelet therapy including clopidogrel in the form of a 300 mg loading dose immediately following procedures. Patients that can tolerate antiplatelet therapy are prescribed a 1-month course of clopidogrel (75 mg daily) in addition to aspirin therapy (81 mg daily). This is an extrapolation of coronary intervention data showing that the use of clopidogrel can decrease the incidence of acute thrombosis after coronary stent intervention. The comprehensive medical management of patients with PAD is discussed in Chap. 3; nonetheless, it warrants reiteration that the procedural encounter affords an excellent opportunity for the vascular specialist to ensure that patients are following an appropriate regimen of medical management and risk factor modification. For the diabetic patient, specific attention should be made to peri-procedural glucose monitoring, particularly as perturbation in the normal diet and insulin regimen associated with preoperative NPO status and the stress of hospitalization requires careful attention to point-of-care blood glucose monitoring and potentially consultation with an endocrinologist.

Following procedures, patients require bed rest for 2–6 h after removal of the angiographic sheath. The use of arterial closure devices does allow more rapid ambulation at 2–3 h rather than the usual 6 h after manual compression. Routine post-intervention care includes frequent vascular examinations as well as frequent inspection of the access site to detect early signs of hemorrhage, pseudoaneurysm, and hematoma.

Follow-up and Surveillance

Outside of randomized, controlled trials in which follow-up is excellent and funding permits a regimented post-intervention surveillance protocol, there is significant variation with respect to follow-up surveillance schedules. Generally, reports include a combination of clinical follow-up and noninvasive imaging studies. For example, we routinely perform clinical examination, measure the ankle brachial index (ABI), and obtain pulse volume recording and duplex studies immediately after intervention, then at 1, 3, 6, and 12 months, and then yearly thereafter. Clinical recurrence of symptoms or duplex evidence of restenosis prompts consideration of re-intervention.

Guidelines, Outcomes, and Reporting Standards

The numerous treatment options, as well as variation in reported outcomes, have resulted in a confusing landscape for the vascular specialist in search of the appropriate treatment modality for any given patient. Although treatment guidelines and outcome definitions remain somewhat of a moving target, it is imperative that vascular specialists treating PAD are familiar with treatment guidelines, reporting standards, and outcome definitions.

Data from numerous randomized controlled clinical trials and the aggregate clinical experience with infrainguinal endovascular therapy have contributed to the evolution of treatment guidelines. The American Heart Association (AHA) Task Force compiled a list of recommendations for the use of endovascular therapy in the infrainguinal vascular tree in 1994. Recommendations included the application of endovascular therapy to mild disease, whereas more complex disease was deemed best treated with surgical revascularization. The revised Trans-Atlantic Inter-Society Consensus (TASC) guidelines are the commonly used both for clinical management as well as outcomes reporting. In the revised TASC criteria, surgery is recommended for TASC type D lesions due to the high failure rate with endovascular interventions [27]. The TASC guidelines do not delineate specific anatomic criteria for infrapopliteal endovascular therapy, nor is it recommended with the exception of a patient with CLI and significant medical comorbidities to allow in-line flow to the foot.

Commonly reported outcome measurements include technical success, clinical response, primary patency, assisted primary patency, secondary patency, target lesion (or limb) revascularization, and limb salvage. Additional measures include freedom from bypass surgery, and composite endpoints (such as amputation-free survival). In an effort to minimize variation in reported outcomes, the Society for Vascular Surgery has established reporting standards, including the Rutherford Reporting Guidelines as well as objective performance goals for endovascular therapy in CLI [28, 29]. The following definitions of accepted outcome measures represent a summary of pertinent points from these documents.

Technical and Hemodynamic Success

Technical success may be claimed after an endovascular intervention in the presence of: (1) antegrade flow through the treated lesion; (2) <30% residual stenosis; and (3) in-line flow to the pedal arch. Post-intervention vascular laboratory studies should reveal a peak systolic velocity ratio of 2.5 or less at the treatment site compared to adjacent segments and/or an ABI improvement of 0.15 or greater for patients with claudication. A more predictable indicator of success of SFA intervention in a patient with claudication is maintenance of ABI associated with pre- and post-exercise. Ongoing hemodynamic success relies on vascular laboratory evaluation, with a maintained ABI increase greater than 0.15 from the early postprocedural level biphasic or triphasic waveforms with a peak systolic velocity less than 200 cm/s or a treatment site peak systolic velocity ratio less than 2.5.

For clinical success to be claimed, these hemodynamic and technical measures must be attained in the setting of clinical improvement [28].

Clinical Success

Assessment of clinical success is perhaps the most ambiguous outcome metric, yet at the same time the most important from a patient-centered standpoint. Clinical improvement requires improvement by at least one Rutherford–Becker clinical category, with the exception of patients with tissue loss (Rutherford–Becker 5/6) who must advance two categories, to claudication or rest pain, respectively. In practical terms, the most important outcome measures in CLI are wound healing and limb salvage. In each case, wound healing must occur. Moreover, improvement must be clearly attributable to the intervention, and requires hemodynamic confirmation of success: a minimum change in ABI of 0.1 is recommended [28].

Primary Patency

Primary patency implies freedom from thrombosis and restenosis. It is generally reported using life-table analysis or Kaplan–Meier survival function. Generally, some degree of restenosis is allowable (0–50%), which correlates with noninvasive vascular studies indicating a systolic velocity ratio less than 2–2.5 or ABI decrease greater than 0.15 results in loss of primary patency (Fig. 9.3).

Assisted Patency and Secondary Patency

Assisted patency, also referred to as primary-assisted patency or assisted primary patency, refers to interventions necessitating a subsequent interventional procedure to maintain patency. Secondary patency refers to restoration of patency after re-occlusion. As duplex ultrasound surveillance is generally recommended after peripheral endovascular interventions, these outcome measures are generally comparable, with secondary patency calculations including those in which patency is maintained in the setting of restenosis detected by ultrasound (assisted patency) as well as re-interventions for occlusion.

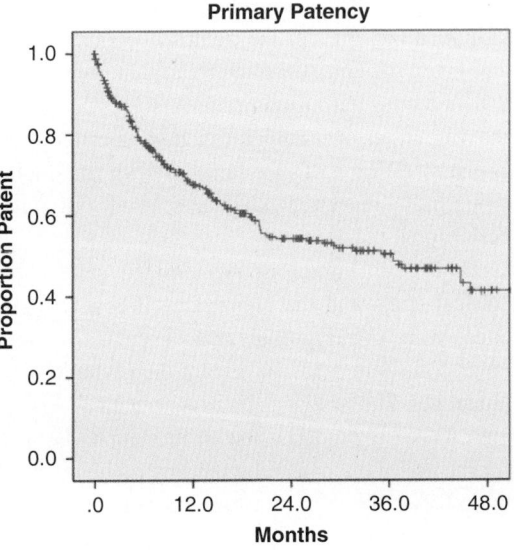

Fig. 9.3 Representative Kaplan–Meier curve of primary patency versus time after endovascular therapy for symptomatic PAD in over 400 patients treated at the New York-Presbyterian Hospital. Note that most instances of patency loss occur early due to re-stenosis

Assisted patency and secondary patency are reported with Kaplan–Meier function estimation or life-table analysis.

Target Lesion Revascularization

Target lesion revascularization (TLR) is a term derived from the cardiology literature, referring to re-intervention in a previously treated lesion. As applied to the periphery, TLR refers to re-intervention within 5 mm of the lesion treated during the index procedure. The terms target vessel revascularization and target limb revascularization refer to re-interventions elsewhere in the treated vessel or limb, respectively. The utility of TLR as an outcome measure is poor in the peripheral vasculature when compared to the coronary circulation. TLR overestimates the success of interventions, as re-interventions in the periphery are not mandated and patients do not necessarily undergo repeat intervention in the absence of symptoms or may opt to not undergo re-intervention despite the return of their original symptoms as is the case for claudication. Some patients can in fact have complete occlusion of their original intervention but still remain symptom-free and not require re-intervention. It would be erroneous to report these interventions as a success by TLR. For this reason, the authors prefer not to use TLR as an outcome measure after peripheral endovascular intervention.

Limb Salvage

For patients with CLI, limb salvage is generally accepted as the most significant outcome measure. Minor amputations (at the toe or trans-metatarsal level) are not considered limb loss. Though it should be noted when reporting outcomes if the toe or foot amputation was a planned procedure prior to the intervention or if it became necessary only after the intervention. The latter instance would represent the potential for embolization during the intervention and should be reported. When evaluating long-term limb salvage data, it is important to note that due to the high prevalence of significant comorbidities especially cardiac among these patients, survival is generally poor and therefore many patients are censored due to death throughout follow-up. This fact, combined with an unclear yet significant success rate with medical therapy and wound care alone, may artificially inflate limb salvage estimates after any revascularization procedure.

Outcome Determinants

Selection of appropriate candidates for endovascular intervention (versus surgical bypass) requires a knowledge of therapeutic options, technical facility with endovascular interventions, understanding of outcome measures, and a familiarity with the factors associated with success and failure. A separate factor, as we also see with carotid artery stenting, is the skill set and equipment availability for the interventionist. Many of the endovascular procedures do require added expertise to successfully complete the procedures. Numerous studies have demonstrated that results vary widely based on treatment details, patient demographics and comorbidities, and characteristics of treated lesions. This section reviews data regarding the contribution of various factors to the success or failure of endovascular therapy, with a specific focus on the role of diabetes mellitus on outcome.

Many factors associated with reduced patency after peripheral endovascular intervention are well known. Numerous reports have identified that diabetes, renal insufficiency, and CLI are associated with poor patency after endovascular therapy [7, 27, 30–36]. Moreover, clinical experience suggests that long lesions and chronic occlusions are predisposed to restenosis; these findings have also been demonstrated in prior published series [27]. In addition to these established factors that negatively impact patency, numerous other patient- and lesion-specific characteristics have been implicated in patency loss, with several recent series even suggesting differences in outcomes based on gender [37, 38].

The location of disease appears to affect outcome, at least in the current era in which endovascular stents suitable for the iliac and femoropopliteal distribution allow for a more durable solution when compared to the limited options (angioplasty alone or atherectomy) that may be applied to the smaller infrapopliteal vessels. This is reflected in the TASC guidelines, which support application of endovascular therapy to all but the most severe disease in the femoropopliteal distribution but remain restrictive with respect to infrapopliteal endovascular interventions. Also reflected in the TASC recommendations are the impact of lesion length and the presence of occlusion (versus stenosis) on outcome. Long-segment disease and the presence of chronic total occlusions are associated with reduced success across outcome measures [7, 35, 37, 39–41].

The status of runoff vessels, a factor clearly associated with reduced outcomes after surgical bypass, appears to impact the success of endovascular interventions as well [41, 42]. As previously discussed, female gender is associated with reduced patency and poor outcome in several studies [37, 38]. However, it is unclear if gender is truly an independent predictor of adverse outcome or if women have smaller vessels necessitating the use of smaller stents more prone to failure, and reduced caliber of outflow vessels.

The factors that affect outcome most profoundly are indications for intervention and comorbidities. Outcomes are clearly worse when interventions are undertaken for CLI (versus claudication), or in the setting of diabetes and chronic renal insufficiency. However, the independent contribution of CLI and these comorbidities is conflicting. Whether diabetes is an independent predictor of adverse outcome, or the infrapopliteal disease and CLI associated with diabetes predispose interventions to failure remains unclear. We recently reported a series of 1,220 patients undergoing intervention for claudication (22.5%) or CLI (77.5%). By multivariate analysis, predictors of primary patency loss included TASC C/D disease (Hazard Ratio: 1.375 (95% Confidence Interval: 1.164–1.624); P-value<0.001, presence of a CTO (1.225 [1.041–1.443]; 0.015); diabetes (1.243 [1.056–1.463]; 0.009), congestive heart failure (1.204 [1.011–1.434]; 0.038), and current smoking (1.529 [1.223–1.913]; 0.001) (Table 9.1). Factors associated with reduced secondary patency included TASC C/D disease (1.400 [1.111–1.764]; 0.004), diabetes (1.279 [1.017–1.608]; 0.036), congestive heart failure (1.463 [1.168–1.833]; 0.001), current smoking (1.789 [1.338–2.392]; <0.001), and CLI (4.007 [3.106–5.169]; 0.001) (Table 9.2). By multivariate analysis, the only independent risk factors for limb loss were current smoking (2.3 [1.24–4.01]; 0.007), end-stage renal disease, (1.9 [1.018–3.587]; 0.044), and diabetes (2.13 [1.21–3.76]; 0.008) [5].

The significance of diabetes as an independent predictor of poor outcome in this series is supported by prior reports. Abularrage and colleagues at the Massachusetts General Hospital (MGH) performed a retrospective analysis of over 1,000 limbs to assess the importance of diabetes on outcome after endovascular intervention. In this series, which compared 533 diabetic to 542 nondiabetic limbs, actuarial primary patency at 5 years was 42%±2.4%, assisted patency was 81%±2.0%, and limb salvage was 89%±1.6%. By univariate analysis, diabetes was associated with inferior 5-year primary patency (37%±3.4% vs. 46%±3.3%; P=0.009), reduced limb salvage (84%±2.6% vs. 93%±1.8%, P<0.0001), and survival (52%±3.5% vs. 68%±3.1%; P=0.0001). There was no difference between diabetic and nondiabetic patients with respect to assisted patency. By multivariate analysis, diabetes was associated with reduced primary patency (1.25 [1.01–1.54]; P=0.04), along with single-vessel peroneal runoff (HR, 1.54; 95% CI, 1.16–2.08; P<0.003), and dialysis dependence (HR, 1.59; 95% CI, 1.10–2.33; P<0.02). Multivariate analysis to identify those factors predicting limb loss included CLI (HR, 9.09; 95% CI, 4.17–20.00; P<0.0001) and dialysis dependence (HR, 2.94; 95% CI, 1.39–5.00; P=0.003; HR, 4.24; 95% CI, 2.80–6.45; P<0.0001) [43].

As previously noted, whether or not diabetes is an independent predictor of adverse outcome after endovascular intervention depends, to a certain extent, on the statistical models used to assess the relative contributions of various factors to patency loss. This is a

Table 9.1 Factors associated with primary patency loss by multivariate analysis

Covariate	Hazard ratio	95.0% CI for HR Lower	Upper	P
TASC C/D[a]	1.375	1.164	1.624	<0.001
CTO[b]	1.225	1.041	1.443	0.015
DM	1.243	1.056	1.463	0.009
CHF	1.204	1.011	1.434	0.038
Current smoking	1.529	1.223	1.913	<0.001
CLI[c]	2.214	1.874	2.615	<0.001

Adapted from Meltzer AJ, Shrikhande G, Gallagher KA, Aiello FA, Kahn S, Connolly P, McKinsey JF. Heart failure is associated with reduced patency after endovascular intervention for symptomatic peripheral arterial disease. J Vasc Surg. 2012;55(2):353–62. With permission from Elsevier
[a]Reference category: TASC A/B
[b]CTO = chronic total occlusion
[c]Reference category: Claudication

Table 9.2 Factors associated with secondary patency loss by multivariate analysis

Covariate	Hazard ratio	95.0% CI for HR Lower	Upper	P
TASC C/D[a]	1.400	1.111	1.764	0.004
DM	1.279	1.017	1.608	0.036
CHF	1.463	1.168	1.833	0.001
Smoking	1.789	1.338	2.392	<0.001
CLI[b]	4.007	3.106	5.169	<0.001

Adapted from Meltzer AJ, Shrikhande G, Gallagher KA, Aiello FA, Kahn S, Connolly P, McKinsey JF. Heart failure is associated with reduced patency after endovascular intervention for symptomatic peripheral arterial disease. J Vasc Surg. 2012;55(2):353–62. With permission from Elsevier
[a]Reference category: TASC A/B
[b]Reference category: Claudication

by-product of the frequent co-occurrence of diabetes and other established risk factors for adverse events (i.e., CLI and infrapopliteal disease). Therefore, statistical models may be unstable unless the frequent coexistence of diabetes and CLI is accounted for, usually by excluding one of two highly correlated variables from multivariate analysis.

From the clinical standpoint, it is not particularly important whether it is diabetes itself or the frequently coexisting comorbidities (specifically CLI) that leads to adverse outcomes after endovascular intervention. Despite some conflict in the literature, diabetes does appear to be associated with poor outcomes after endovascular therapy for PAD.

A significant problem with endovascular therapy for chronic lower extremity ischemia in diabetic patients is the anatomic distribution of disease, which characteristically involves the infrapopliteal vessels with relative sparing of pedal circulation. Moreover, diabetics frequently present with multilevel disease and a higher prevalence of CLI. In recent studies the prevalence of CLI is markedly higher in the DM population, as was the case in the MGH series (54% vs. 30%, $P<0.0001$) and our own previously reported data (52.5% vs. 36.2%, $P=0.004$) [43, 44]. The high prevalence of CLI and infrapopliteal disease found in diabetic patients has led to some studies suggesting poor limb salvage [5, 30, 43, 44].

Nonetheless, diabetes should not be considered a contraindication to endovascular therapy for PAD. To the contrary, the comorbidities that predispose endovascular interventions to accelerated failure are also associated with higher rates of adverse events after surgical bypass, as discussed elsewhere in this text.

As our understanding of the risk factors for failure of endovascular therapy improve, it may be possible to develop individualized surveillance programs post-intervention that account for a patient's comorbidities, such as diabetes, in an effort to detect restenosis prior to occlusion, thereby maintaining assisted patency and achieving durable limb salvage despite the presence of risk factors for failure.

Conclusion

The introduction of minimally invasive, endovascular techniques has revolutionized the approach to PAD. Further research is needed to identify which patients are best served by the variety of techniques available. While current evidence does suggest that diabetes places patients at higher risk for patency loss, durable results may be achieved with repeated interventions, thus providing acceptable long-term outcomes without the morbidity associated with bypass surgery.

References

1. Pande RL, Perlstein TS, Beckman JA, Creager MA. Secondary prevention and mortality in peripheral artery disease: National Health and Nutrition Examination Study, 1999 to 2004. Circulation. 2011;124(1):17–23.
2. McDermott MM. Peripheral arterial disease: epidemiology and drug therapy. Am J Geriatr Cardiol. 2002;11(4):258–66.
3. Varu VN, Hogg ME, Kibbe MR. Critical limb ischemia. J Vasc Surg. 2010;51(1):230–41.
4. LaMuraglia GM, Conrad MF, Chung T, Hutter M, Watkins MT, Cambria RP. Significant perioperative morbidity accompanies contemporary infrainguinal bypass surgery: an NSQIP report. J Vasc Surg. 2009;50(2):299–304, 304.e1–4.
5. Meltzer AJ, Shrikhande G, Gallagher KA, Aiello FA, Kahn S, Connolly P, McKinsey JF. Heart failure is associated with reduced patency after endovascular intervention for symptomatic peripheral arterial disease. J Vasc Surg. 2012;55(2):353–62.
6. Aiello FA, Khan AA, Meltzer AJ, Gallagher KA, McKinsey JF, Schneider DB. Statin therapy is associated with superior clinical outcomes after endovascular treatment of critical limb ischemia. J Vasc Surg. 2012;55(2):371–9.
7. Gallagher KA, Meltzer AJ, Ravin RA, Graham A, Shrikhande G, Connolly PH, Aiello F, Dayal R, McKinsey JF. Endovascular management as first therapy for chronic total occlusion of the lower extremity arteries: comparison of balloon angioplasty, stenting, and directional atherectomy. J Endovasc Ther. 2011;18(5):624–37.
8. Twine CP, Coulston J, Shandall A, McLain AD. Angioplasty versus stenting for superficial femoral artery lesions. Cochrane Database Syst Rev. 2009;(2): CD006767.
9. Bachoo P, Thorpe PA, Maxwell H, Welch K. Endovascular stents for intermittent claudication. Cochrane Database Syst Rev. 2010;(1):CD003228.
10. Kedora J, Hohmann S, Garrett W, Munschaur C, Theune B, Gable D. Randomized comparison of percutaneous Viabahn stent grafts vs prosthetic femoral-popliteal bypass in the treatment of superficial femoral arterial occlusive disease. J Vasc Surg. 2007;45(1):10–6.
11. McCaslin JE, Macdonald S, Stansby G. Cryoplasty for peripheral vascular disease. Cochrane Database Syst Rev. 2007;(4):CD005507.
12. Schmieder GC, Carroll M, Panneton JM. Poor outcomes with cryoplasty for lower extremity arterial occlusive disease. J Vasc Surg. 2010;52(2):362–8.
13. Spiliopoulos S, Katsanos K, Karnabatidis D, Diamantopoulos A, Kagadis GC, Christeas N, Siablis D. Cryoplasty versus conventional balloon angioplasty of the femoropopliteal artery in diabetic patients: long-term results from a prospective randomized single-center controlled trial. Cardiovasc Intervent Radiol. 2010;33(5):929–38.
14. Zeller T, Rastan A, Schwarzwalder U, et al. Percutaneous peripheral atherectomy of femoropopliteal stenoses using a new-generation device: six-month results from a single-center experience. J Endovasc Ther. 2004;11:676–85.
15. Zeller T, Rastan A, Sixt S, et al. Long-term results after directional atherectomy of femoro-popliteal lesions. J Am Coll Cardiol. 2006;48:1573–8.
16. Zeller T, Frank U, Burgelin K, et al. Initial clinical experience with percutaneous atherectomy in the infragenicular arteries. J Endovasc Ther. 2003;10: 987–93.
17. Zeller T, Rastan A, Schwarzwalder U, et al. Midterm results after atherectomy-assisted angioplasty of below-knee arteries with use of the Silverhawk device. J Vasc Interv Radiol. 2004;15:1391–7.
18. Zeller T, Sixt S, Schwarzwalder U, et al. Two year results after directional atherectomy of infrapopliteal arteries with the SilverHawk device. J Endovasc Ther. 2007;14:232–40.

19. McKinsey JF, Goldstein L, Khan HU, Graham A, Rezeyat C, Morrissey NJ, Sambol E, Kent KC. Novel treatment of patients with lower extremity ischemia: use of percutaneous atherectomy in 579 lesions. Ann Surg. 2008;248(4):519–28.
20. Scheinert D, Ulrich M, Scheinert S, Sax J, Braunlich S, Biamino G, et al. Comparison of sirolimus-eluting vs. bare-metal stents for the treatment of infrapopliteal obstructions. Eurointervention. 2006;2:169–74.
21. Duda SH, Pusich B, Richter G, Landwehr P, Oliva VL, Tielbeek A, et al. Sirolimus-eluting stents for the treatment of obstructive superficial femoral artery disease: six-months results. Circulation. 2002;106:1505–9.
22. Duda SH, Bosiers M, Lammer J, Scheinert D, Zeller T, Tielbeek A, et al. Sirolimus-eluting versus bare nitinol stent for obstructive superficial femoral artery disease: the SIROCCO II Trial. J Vasc Interv Radiol. 2005;16:331–8.
23. Duda SH, Bosiers M, Lammer J, Scheinert D, Zeller T, Oliva V, et al. Drug-eluting and bare nitinol stents for the treatment of atherosclerotic lesions in the superficial femoral artery: long-term results from the SIROCCO trial. J Endovasc Ther. 2006;13:701–10.
24. Lammer J, Bosiers M, Zeller T, Schillinger M, Boone E, Zaugg MJ, Verta P, Peng L, Gao X, Schwartz LB. First clinical trial of nitinol self-expanding everolimus-eluting stent implantation for peripheral arterial occlusive disease. J Vasc Surg. 2011;54(2):394–401.
25. Dake MD, Ansel GM, Jaff MR, Ohki T, Saxon RR, Smouse HB, Zeller T, Roubin GS, Burket MW, Khatib Y, Snyder SA, Ragheb AO, White JK, Machan LS; Zilver PTX Investigators. Zilver PTX Investigators. Paclitaxel-eluting stents show superiority to balloon angioplasty and bare metal stents in femoropopliteal disease: twelve-month Zilver PTX randomized study results. Circ Cardiovasc Interv. 2011;4(5):495–504.
26. Tepe G, Zeller T, Albrecht T, Heller S, Schwarzwälder U, Beregi JP, Claussen CD, Oldenburg A, Scheller B, Speck U. Local delivery of paclitaxel to inhibit restenosis during angioplasty of the leg. N Engl J Med. 2008;358(7):689–99.
27. Norgren L, Hiatt WR, Dormandy JA, Nehler MR, Harris KA, Fowkes FG, TASC II Working Group. Inter-Society Consensus for the Management of Peripheral Arterial Disease (TASC II). J Vasc Surg. 2007;45(Suppl S):S5–67.
28. Rutherford RB, Baker JD, Ernst C, Johnston KW, Porter JM, Ahn S, Jones DN. Recommended standards for reports dealing with lower extremity ischemia: revised version. J Vasc Surg. 1997;26(3):517–38. Erratum in: J Vasc Surg 2001;33(4):805.
29. Conte MS, Geraghty PJ, Bradbury AW, Hevelone ND, Lipsitz SR, Moneta GL, Nehler MR, Powell RJ, Sidawy AN. Suggested objective performance goals and clinical trial design for evaluating catheter-based treatment of critical limb ischemia. J Vasc Surg. 2009;50(6):1462–73.e1–3.
30. Conrad MF, Cambria RP, Stone DH, Brewster DC, Kwolek CJ, Watkins MT, Chung TK, LaMuraglia GM Intermediate results of percutaneous endovascular therapy of femoropopliteal occlusive disease: a contemporary series. J Vasc Surg. 2006;44(4):762–9.
31. Bakken AM, Protack CD, Saad WE, Hart JP, Rhodes JM, Waldman DL, Davies MG. Impact of chronic kidney disease on outcomes of superficial femoral artery endoluminal interventions. Ann Vasc Surg. 2009;23(5):560–8.
32. Apelqvist J, Elgzyri T, Larsson J, Löndahl M, Nyberg P, Thörne J. Factors related to outcome of neuroischemic/ischemic foot ulcer in diabetic patients. J Vasc Surg. 2011;53(6):1582–1588.e2.
33. O'Brien-Irr MS, Dosluoglu HH, Harris LM, Dryjski ML. Outcomes after endovascular intervention for chronic critical limb ischemia. J Vasc Surg. 2011;53(6):1575–81.
34. Haider SN, Kavanagh EG, Forlee M, Colgan MP, Madhavan P, Moore DJ, Shanik GD. Two-year outcome with preferential use of infrainguinal angioplasty for critical ischemia. J Vasc Surg. 2006;43(3):504–12.
35. DeRubertis BG, Faries PL, McKinsey JF, Chaer RA, Pierce M, Karwowski J, Weinberg A, Nowygrod R, Morrissey NJ, Bush HL, Kent KC. Shifting paradigms in the treatment of lower extremity vascular disease: a report of 1000 percutaneous interventions. Ann Surg. 2007;246(3):415–22.
36. Dormandy JA, Rutherford RB. Management of peripheral arterial disease (PAD). TASC Working Group. TransAtlantic Inter-Society Consensus (TASC). J Vasc Surg. 2000;31(1 Pt 2):S1–296.
37. Gallagher KA, Meltzer AJ, Ravin RA, Graham A, Connolly P, Escobar G, Shrikhande G, McKinsey JF. Gender differences in outcomes of endovascular treatment of infrainguinal peripheral artery disease. Vasc Endovascular Surg. 2011;45(8):703–11.
38. Pulli R, Dorigo W, Pratesi G, Fargion A, Angiletta D, Pratesi C. Gender-related outcomes in the endovascular treatment of infrainguinal arterial obstructive disease. J Vasc Surg. 2012;55(1):105–12.
39. Kim IK, Egorova N, Kahn SZ, Meltzer AJ, McKinsey JF. Comparative analysis of femoropopliteal versus tibial lesion characteristics that predict endovascular therapy success. In: Eastern Vascular Society Annual Meeting, September 2011. J Vasc Surg. 2011;54(3):923.
40. Kim IK, Egorova N, Kahn SZ, Meltzer AJ, Bush HL, McKinsey JF. Lesion characteristics that predict patency of femoral popliteal endovascular intervention: a Novel Lesion Disease Severity Score. In: New England Vascular Society Annual Meeting, September 2011. J Vasc Surg. 2011;54(4):1228.
41. Meltzer AJ, Kim IK, Khan S, Egorova N, Graham A, McKinsey JF. Comprehensive evaluation of arterial lesion characteristics and their impact on long-term patency after endovascular intervention: the creation of a Novel Lesion Severity Score for Arterial Lesions. In: Society for Vascular Surgery Annual Meeting, Chicago, IL, June 2011. J Vasc Surg. 2011;53(6):107s–8s.

42. Davies MG, Saad WE, Peden EK, Mohiuddin IT, Naoum JJ, Lumsden AB. Impact of runoff on superficial femoral artery endoluminal interventions for rest pain and tissue loss. J Vasc Surg. 2008;48(3):619–25. Discussion 625–6.
43. Abularrage CJ, Conrad MF, Hackney LA, Paruchuri V, Crawford RS, Kwolek CJ, LaMuraglia GM, Cambria RP. Long-term outcomes of diabetic patients undergoing endovascular infrainguinal interventions. J Vasc Surg. 2010;52(2):314–22.e1–4.
44. DeRubertis BG, Pierce M, Ryer EJ, Trocciola S, Kent KC, Faries PL. Reduced primary patency rate in diabetic patients after percutaneous intervention results from more frequent presentation with limb-threatening ischemia. J Vasc Surg. 2008;47: 101–8.

Surgical Treatment of Infrainguinal Occlusive Disease in Diabetes

10

Shant M. Vartanian and Michael S. Conte

Keywords

Diabetes • Claudication • Critical limb ischemia • Diabetic foot • Lower extremity bypass • Vein bypass graft • Limb salvage

Introduction

As nearly 140 million people worldwide carry the diagnosis of diabetes, it stands as a major burden to public health and the incidence will continue to rise in parallel with increasing rates of obesity [1]. In the United States, diabetes represents the seventh leading cause of death and is the fourth leading comorbid condition among hospital discharges [2, 3]. Not only is diabetes a risk factor for PAD, it accelerates the initiation and propagation of atherosclerosis throughout the body. The mechanism of vascular disease development in diabetes is multifactorial, with evidence implicating glycation of proteins and other cellular elements, abnormal lipid metabolism, changes in oxidation–reduction pathways, vascular volume shifts, alterations in platelet and endothelial function, and immune system dysfunction—among a plethora of other biochemical and cellular changes. In long-standing diabetics, specifically those that carry the diagnosis for at least 20 years, 85% will manifest some form of peripheral vascular disease and 75% will die from complications of vascular disease, such as MI or stroke [4].

In the peripheral vasculature, diabetes is the leading cause of limb loss. Nearly two-thirds of all non-traumatic lower extremity amputations occur in diabetics [5]. The pattern of peripheral vascular disease differs between diabetics and nondiabetics. In the former, a classic pattern of atherosclerosis limited to the tibial and peroneal arteries is frequently present, with relative sparing of the aortoiliac and femoral segments [6]. However, multilevel disease is not uncommon, particularly when other risk factors such as smoking or dyslipidemia coexist. In addition, neuropathy involving the sensory and motor nerves in the lower extremity results in a diabetic foot that is prone to ulceration and infection. Surgical treatment of lower extremity occlusive disease in diabetics frequently requires distal procedures for critical limb ischemia (CLI). The primary goals of surgical intervention in this patient population are the preservation of a functional limb, relief of

S.M. Vartanian, M.D. • M.S. Conte, M.D. (✉)
Department of Surgery, University of California
San Francisco, 400 Parnassus Avenue,
San Francisco, CA 94143, USA
e-mail: Michael.conte@ucsfmedctr.org

pain, clearance of infection, and promotion of wound healing. Accomplishing these goals can maintain or improve the patient's overall quality of life.

Patient Selection for Revascularization

For patients with intermittent claudication (IC)—diabetes not withstanding—the goals of treatment are secondary prevention of cardiovascular events and improvement in walking function and quality of life. Optimal medical management of risk factors, including glycemic control and smoking cessation, are primary interventions, and exercise therapy should be considered as an initial approach. Although the natural history of IC is considered fairly benign, and the lifetime risk of limb loss is low, the prognosis is more guarded in the diabetic patient [7, 8]. Several cohort studies have demonstrated that the risk of progression to CLI is significantly higher for the diabetic with IC, as is for the overall mortality [9]. Therefore, these patients warrant more aggressive risk factor management and surveillance. In a diabetic patient with peripheral neuropathy and significant hemodynamic compromise from PAD, signs of deterioration to a more critical stage may be fairly subtle. Longitudinal follow-up should include interrogation of changes in the pattern of symptoms, ankle and toe pressures, and careful inspection of the feet.

Patient selection for surgical or endovascular intervention in IC is typically reserved for disabling symptoms that have significant effect on the patients' quality of life [10]. The calculus may be slightly altered in the diabetic patient due to both the typical anatomic pattern encountered as well as the competing risks to life and limb mentioned above. The frequent involvement of infrageniculate vessels, for example, may limit the durability of an endovascular approach. In general, there is limited evidence at present to compare the effectiveness of exercise therapy versus revascularization for IC, particularly in the setting of infrainguinal disease. However the CLEVER trial, a randomized, controlled study comparing supervised exercise versus stent revascularization for patients with IC and aortoiliac disease, showed greater objective improvements for exercise and better patient-reported outcomes for stenting [11]. More clinical trials are clearly needed to develop evidence-based guidelines for the treatment of IC across all subgroups.

As the occlusive disease pattern in diabetics typically involves the infrageniculate vasculature, indications for revascularization are generally reserved for manifestations of CLI: rest pain or tissue loss, with or without infection (Rutherford classification stage 4–6). When evaluating patients with CLI, four types of treatment options exist: medical management alone, open surgical revascularization, endovascular intervention, or primary amputation. The decision on which treatment to pursue needs to be individualized for each patient, factoring in estimated life expectancy, current functional status, comorbid conditions, anesthetic risk, severity of ischemia in the foot, and the underlying vascular anatomy.

The choice between open revascularization and endovascular intervention is based on comparative estimates of risk and benefit, rather than a single dogmatic approach. For infrainguinal occlusive disease, this often boils down to weighing reduced short-term morbidity for endovascular interventions versus greater hemodynamic gain and long-term durability for bypass surgery. The principle advantages of endovascular interventions are a faster recovery and avoidance of surgical wounds and other perioperative complications. However early major cardiovascular events and peri-procedural mortality appear broadly similar between the two treatment modalities [12]. New evidence has also helped to shed light on who stands to benefit most from each intervention. The BASIL study was a prospective randomized trial that compared open surgical to endovascular interventions for advanced limb ischemia [13, 14]. In patients who survived at least 2 years from the date of the intervention, those who received a bypass procedure first had a lower mortality and an improved amputation free survival in comparison to those who were first treated by endovascular means. Furthermore, those who

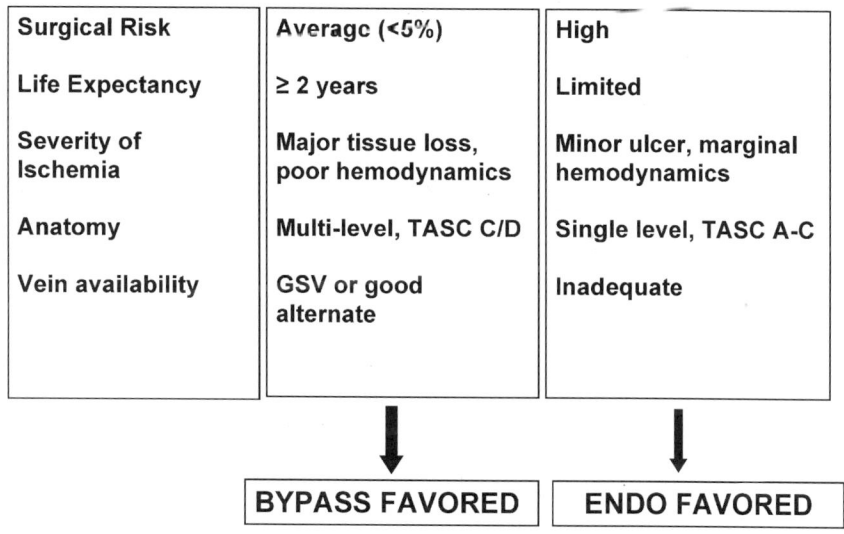

Fig. 10.1 A selective approach to the initial revascularization strategy in critical limb ischemia (CLI). Surgical risk refers to the expected perioperative (30-day) mortality

underwent a bypass procedure after a failed endovascular intervention fared worse than those who underwent a bypass initially; throwing into doubt the notion that endovascular intervention "burns no bridges." Similar to other prospective trials in CLI, 70% of the BASIL study population survived to 2 years [15, 16]. Taken together, these data and the collective literature on limb salvage revascularization suggest that most patients with CLI who are of appropriate surgical risk should preferentially be treated with a vein bypass procedure. However patients with more favorable anatomic disease patterns (e.g., non-Trans-Atlantic Inter-Society Consensus [TASC] D, single-level disease), less severe ischemia, higher surgical risk, lower functional status or those who lack adequate autogenous conduit should be considered for endovascular interventions (Fig. 10.1). More clinical trials are needed to develop evidence-based treatment algorithms for specific CLI subgroups, particularly as endovascular techniques continue to evolve and new technologies such as drug-coated balloons or stents are developed. Prosthetic bypass has performed poorly in this population and should be considered an inferior option to be used sparingly. Improvements in graft technology (e.g., heparin-coating) may alter this paradigm but remain largely unproven in this most challenging population.

Surgical Revascularization Strategy

Conduit Considerations

The single most important determinant of outcomes in infrainguinal bypass surgery is the quality of the conduit used. Autogenous vein—the great saphenous vein in particular—has been repeatedly shown to outperform all other conduits [17, 18]. Optimal preoperative planning therefore requires knowledge of the location and quality of available vein. Weighing the availability of conduit can impact decisions about the location and length of the bypass, and whether consideration should be given to the use of adjunctive procedures (e.g., hybrid techniques) to shorten the length of vein needed.

Preoperative vein mapping with ultrasonography can identify vein that is suitable as a conduit. The ideal vein will have a caliber of at least 3 mm and will not harbor noncompressible or thrombosed segments. This is particularly important when planning to use arm vein, as most of these patients had a history of multiple hospitalizations for comorbid conditions, with subsequent placement of peripheral IV's in the upper extremities. Arm veins frequently harbor thrombosed segments, sclerosed valves, webs and synechiae. Ultrasound vein mapping avoids unnecessary exploration of suboptimal conduit, resulting in less wound morbidity and a more efficient operation. However ultrasound is not infallible and marginal segments may not be reliably identified on pre-procedure imaging. The best tool to assess vein quality is intraoperative inspection with gentle distension. If sclerotic or non-distensible segments are encountered, it is far better to excise the segment and splice together two healthy ends of vein rather than retain a marginal segment that may increase the likelihood of graft failure.

Unfortunately, up to 40% of patients will not have an adequate ipsilateral great saphenous vein (GSV) [19]. In these situations contralateral GSV is generally the next best option, as it outperforms all other venous conduits. Even in the setting of symptomatic PAD, progression of disease requiring a bypass in the contralateral limb occurs in a minority, i.e., less than 25% of patients [20]. Saving the contralateral saphenous vein as a rule subjects a large number of patients who would otherwise never need contralateral revascularization or coronary bypass to a potentially compromised operation by using arm vein or composite grafts. However, in diabetic patients who present with evidence of advanced PAD in the contralateral limb, with significant symptoms or hemodynamic compromise (ABI<0.6), the use of arm vein first must be carefully considered [21].

In the absence of GSV, other sources of autogenous vein include the basilic or cephalic arm veins or the lesser saphenous vein [22]. Despite its thin walled nature, harvesting arm vein is often simpler than harvesting lesser saphenous vein when the patient is in the supine position, and arm vein harvest sites rarely have wound healing complications. The veins of the upper arm are less frequently subjected to iatrogenic trauma in comparison to the forearm. The basilic–cephalic loop graft, in which a long continuous conduit is fashioned using the basilic vein in a non-reversed fashion in continuity with reversed cephalic vein, can be a useful construct when the antecubital vein is of good quality. In the absence of a single source of adequate length vein, spliced venous grafts are favored over non-autogenous grafts (including both synthetic grafts and homografts). Autogenous vein is superior to prosthetic grafts, even when prosthetic grafts are limited to the above knee position. Though it is expected that the majority of lower extremity revascularizations for limb salvage can be performed with autogenous vein exclusively, there are circumstances where non-autogenous grafts may be necessary. Only subtle differences in outcomes have been observed amongst different prosthetics grafts in the infrainguinal position, whether using Dacron, ePTFE, ringed PTFE and more recently, heparin bonded PTFE. When forced to use prosthetic grafts for distal bypasses, modifications of the distal anastomosis, such as the Miller cuff, Taylor patch or St. Mary's boot, may improve patency [23]. Cryopreserved homografts have limited long term patency, with outcomes akin to prosthetic grafts. They are primarily used when treating graft infections, or tunneling a graft through a grossly infected field in the absence of available autogenous conduit.

Adjunctive techniques can be helpful to minimize the length of vein needed in specific circumstances. A patch angioplasty over the proximal or distal arteriotomy can move the anastomosis several centimeters in each direction. When basing the inflow from the CFA, eversion endarterectomy of the proximal SFA with subsequent placement of the proximal graft off the SFA can save additional length of vein, but the effect on long-term patency remains unclear. As the shortest distance between two points is a straight line, tunneling the vein graft anatomically rather than the more circuitous subcutaneous tunnel, minimizes the length of vein needed. In well-selected patients, hybrid open and endovascular techniques can allow for creation of distal origin grafts where no option was previously available. For example, endovascular treatment of mild or moderate SFA disease (i.e., TASC A or B lesions) can allow for a distal origin graft from the popliteal artery, dramatically reducing the length of vein needed [24]. Endovascular treatment of more severe disease (TASC C or D lesions) should be discouraged, as the unpredictable nature of these endoluminal interventions may compromise an otherwise durable lower extremity vein bypass.

Developing the Operative Strategy

Typically, preoperative imaging studies adequately assess the proximal vascular anatomy and help identify the inflow site of the vascular reconstruction. Noninvasive imaging modalities such as CT or MR angiograms are particularly good at assessing aortoiliac and femoral artery disease. Thorough investigation of the arterial anatomy helps prioritize and stratify revascularization decisions, such as selecting patients who would do well with endovascular interventions and those who need to have more proximal inflow disease treated before embarking on a lower extremity revascularization. In general, all hemodynamically significant inflow disease must be corrected before treating infrainguinal disease. In patients presenting with rest pain, correction of severe inflow disease may be enough to attenuate these symptoms. In patients with CLI, digital subtraction angiography is mandatory for delineating the anatomy of the tibial and pedal arteries for surgical planning.

The stereotypical source of inflow for lower extremity revascularizations is the CFA. This is in part a byproduct of its ease of exposure, relatively large caliber, and that the CFA is often spared of disease on its anterior surface. However, there is abundant evidence that bypass grafts taken from distal origins fare equally well over time. In general, there are multiple advantages to having shorter bypass grafts. Minimizing the length of vein needed translates into using higher quality conduit, as marginal segments are more likely to be excluded. Shorter grafts have been shown to have high rates of patency than longer grafts, even in the presence of risk factors for graft failure. And the progression of atherosclerosis proximal to the bypass grafts has not been shown to dramatically alter the fate of bypass grafts [25].

The pattern of vascular disease in diabetics makes application of distal origin grafts particularly desirable. A heavy burden of atherosclerotic disease in the infrapopliteal vessels with relative sparing of the SFA makes distal origin grafts from the SFA or popliteal to tibial or pedal vessels an excellent option for limb salvage. There is abundant evidence supporting the efficacy of this surgical approach. In fact, distal origin grafts may have even better outcomes in diabetics than non-diabetics, even in the setting of greater tissue loss [26] (Fig. 10.2). In a prospective trial, no difference was seen between CFA based and non-CFA based bypasses, and not surprisingly, shorter grafts had lower rates of re-interventions [27].

In patients who have limited conduit availability a hybrid approach—combining endovascular and open bypass—presents another potential surgical solution. As a general rule, proximal endovascular interventions fare better than distal interventions. Treating moderate SFA disease with endovascular techniques to set the stage for a distal origin graft has been well described [28]. The ideal patient is a diabetic with a heavy burden of disease in the tibial vessels, but limited, short segment disease within the SFA, consistent with TASC A or B lesions. This method may considerably shorten the length of conduit needed to treat distal disease. The reverse situation, of bypassing proximal disease and employing endovascular interventions for more distal lesions to treat CLI, should only be used in extreme cases.

A detailed understanding of the vascular anatomy of the foot and ankle is requisite for decision making in distal target selection. When treating tissue loss or frank necrosis, the optimal result is not only pulsatile flow to the foot but also adequate perfusion of the angiosome supplying the ischemic areas in question. The angiosome principle separates the body into distinct three dimensional blocks of tissue perfused by a source artery [29]. Cadaveric studies have detailed the six distinct but overlapping angiosomes of the foot and ankle, derived from each of the three crural vessels. In broad terms, branches of the posterior tibial artery supplies the plantar foot, the peroneal artery perfuses the lateral ankle and heel, and the anterior tibial artery supplies the dorsum of the

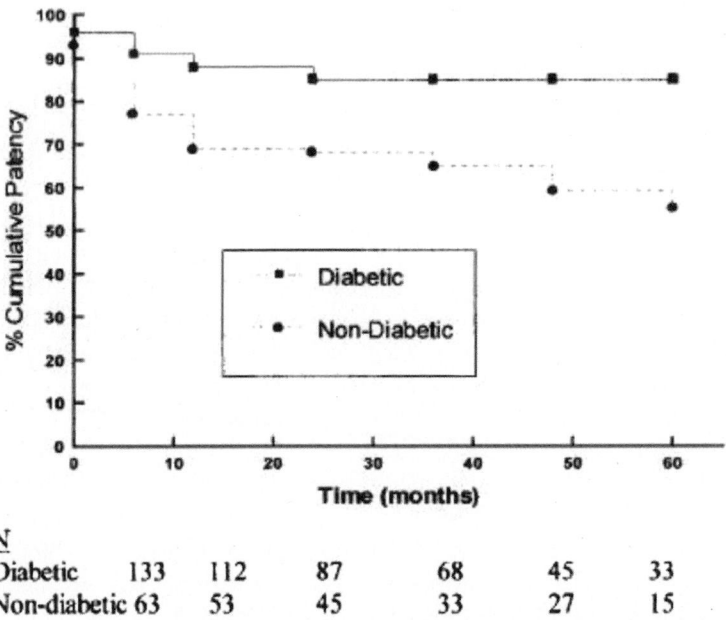

Fig. 10.2 Distal origin grafts, using either the SFA or popliteal artery for inflow, perform particularly well in diabetic patients. Not only is diabetes not a risk factor for vein graft failure, but cumulative graft patency has also been shown to be superior in diabetics who receive distal origin grafts when compared to nondiabetics (reprinted from Reed AB, et al. Usefulness of autogenous bypass grafts originating distal to the groin. J Vasc Surg. 2002;35(1):48–54; With permission from Elsevier)

foot [30] (Fig. 10.3). Pulsatile flow within the foot or ankle angiosome that harbors the wound has been shown to hasten wound healing when compared to distal bypasses to outflow vessels that are not in direct continuity with the angiosome in question [31].

Nevertheless, the blood flow to the foot is redundant and angiosomal territories frequently overlap. The practical utility of this principle in clinical practice remains an open question. In clinical situations where performing a bypass to the crural artery supplying the angiosome in question is not possible, bypassing to the tibial vessel that is continuous with the foot should be chosen as the outflow site, as the distal collateral circulation may be enough to promote wound healing. This is particularly true if the pedal arch is continuous through the foot. In situations where no tibial vessel is continuous to the foot, a robustly collateralized peroneal artery has been repeatedly shown to be an adequate outflow vessel. Neither graft patency nor limb salvage rates have been shown to be inferior when comparing peroneal to tibial artery outflow grafts in critical limb ischemia [32]. The peroneal artery is the most frequently spared of the crural vessels in diabetes. A shorter bypass to the peroneal artery may be particularly useful in situations where conduit availability is limited.

In diabetics, where there is often a heavy burden of atherosclerotic disease within the infrapopliteal vessels, inframalleolar bypasses are an important option for revascularizing the foot and ankle. Some groups have enthusiastically embraced bypasses to pedal and tarsal arteries and the technique has been shown to be equally effective at salvaging limbs specifically in diabetics [33, 34]. Even in circumstances where a dorsalis pedis artery is not visualized on angiography, but a Doppler signal is present over the vessel, exploration often reveals an adequate outflow site for the bypass graft [35]. The superficial location

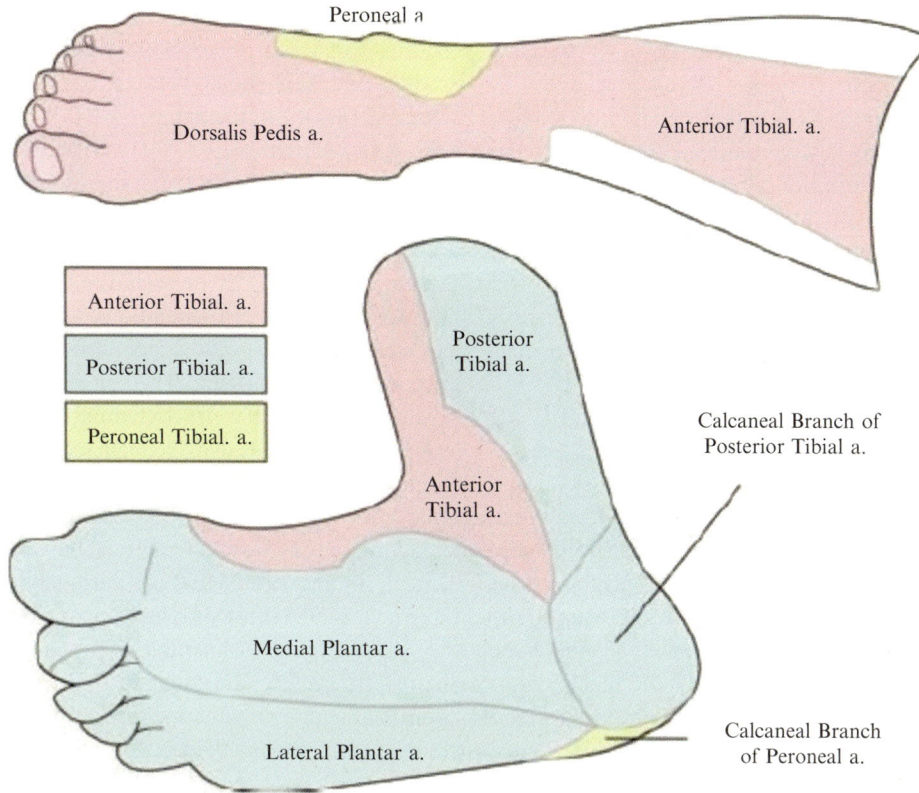

Fig. 10.3 "Angiosomes" of the foot. The angiosome concept defines the vascular contribution of each source artery to the foot and ankle. In this simplified diagram, 5 of the 6 angiosomes of the foot are visible. However, vascular supply to each territory is not isolated. Redundant perfusion and collateral circulation permit successful revascularization of the foot despite bypassing to neighboring angiosomes (reprinted from Iida O, et al. Importance of the angiosome concept for endovascular therapy in patients with critical limb ischemia. Catheter Cardiovasc Interv. 2010;75(6):830–6. With permission from John Wiley & Sons, Inc.)

of the pedal vessels—the dorsalis pedis in particular—simplifies the surgical exposure. However, careful thought must be put into the location of the incision and coverage of the graft so as to not contribute to the wounds in the foot or develop postoperative wound breakdown that exposes a superficial bypass graft.

In patients without any suitable outflow target, bypass to an isolated popliteal segment can be considered in selected cases. Patients with rest pain or ulceration but without extensive tissue loss are particularly well suited for this type of procedure. Bypassing to well collateralized isolated popliteal segments with saphenous vein grafts have yielded surprisingly good results, both in terms of graft patency and limb salvage, despite the presence of a disadvantaged runoff [36, 37].

Surgical Technique of Infrainguinal Bypass

The choice of anesthetic is largely dependent upon the patients' comorbid conditions and operator preference. In patients with significant pulmonary disease, epidural anesthesia mitigates postoperative pulmonary complications. Regional anesthesia has the additional benefit of vasodilating the peripheral vasculature, resulting in a distended venous system which can simplify procuring the saphenous vein. Postoperative pain control is also simplified with the addition of regional anesthesia as patients with long standing rest pain may have a tolerance to narcotic analgesia. Adding epidural to a general anesthetic provides excellent perioperative analgesia for lower extremity surgery. In patients where there are questions about the quality of the lower extremity vein as conduit, general anesthesia is preferred should there develop a need for harvesting arm vein.

As the quality of the venous conduit is the most important—and yet most variable—determinant of outcomes in lower extremity bypass surgery, our preference is to expose the vein first. As detailed previously, preoperative vein mapping is important for operative planning, but repeating the study by the operating team in the room prior to draping helps with planning the location of incisions. Typically, the saphenofemoral junction is exposed first, 2 cm inferior and lateral to the pubic tubercle. The skin is opened with a scalpel, taking care not to form wide subcutaneous flaps during exposure of the saphenous. Flaps undermine skin perfusion and relative subcutaneous ischemia may lead to wound necrosis. Large flaps by definition harbor large potential spaces, which are more likely to develop seromas or hematomas. We often leave one or more bridges of intact skin along the course of the exposure and at the knee joint, each about 3 cm in length. This small additional step helps with the lining up the wound at closure.

A "minimal touch" technique of handling the saphenous vein is used. Even gentle manipulations, such as grasping the vein with vascular forceps, have been shown to traumatize the underlying endothelium and damage to the endothelium may set the stage for future vein graft stenosis. Gentle traction on the adventitia helps with dissection of the surrounding tissues away from the vein. Only sharp dissection is used around the vein, as electrocautery used in close proximity to the vein can result in uncontrolled discharge of current with subsequent unrealized injury to the vein wall.

The saphenofemoral junction is fully mobilized by ligating its multiple branches. This enables the saphenous vein to be transected with a small cuff of the anterior wall of the femoral vein, which helps to create a generous anastomotic patch when using the saphenous in a non-reversed fashion. All other vein branches are ligated 2 mm off the saphenous vein itself, so that upon distention of the vein the ligatures do not restrict its ability to distend. The vein is left in situ until the arterial inflow and outflow sites are exposed and confirmed. This step minimizes potentially harmful warm ischemia time to the vein and also ensures that adequate length of vein has been exposed. Though the ideal site for the arteriotomy is suggested by palpating the artery, an additional 2–3 cm of vein is harvested to account for unexpected findings during the arteriotomy. A small Satinsky-style clamp is applied to the saphenofemoral junction and the vein is sharply transected. The stump of femoral vein is controlled with a running mattress polypropylene suture, taking care not to narrow the femoral vein. Once the vein has been isolated, it is flushed with a neutral buffered crystalloid solution (Plasmalyte) containing heparin sodium (2 units/mL) and papaverine hydrochloride (0.12 mg/mL). Gentle, controlled distention can break spasmed segments and facilitates identification of uncontrolled branches and leaks.

Orienting the vein graft reversed, non-reversed or in situ works equally well and the decision is largely a matter of surgeon preference [38]. For distal bypass in particular, if a large size discrepancy is present between the two ends of the conduit, using the vein in a non-reversed orientation avoids the technical challenge of sewing a large patulous vein segment into a smaller caliber tibial vessel. We find that translocation of the vein generally reduces the length of conduit needed in comparison to an in situ approach.

When lysing valves in the non-reversed orientation, the most proximal valve just beyond the saphenofemoral junction is often easily excised under direct vision with fine scissors. Either a self-centering (Le Maitre) or a retrograde valvulotome (Mills) is then used for the remainder of the vein.

Valve lysis is a simple but critical skill that requires training and experience. Our preference is to use a retrograde Mills valvulotome. Prograde flow is needed to coapt the bivalved leaflets, simplifying capture. This can be achieved either by flushing the vein solution by hand via an angled cannula, or after the proximal anastomosis has been fashioned. Regardless, distention of the vein is a key part of ensuring adequate lysis of all valves while simultaneously protecting the vein from inadvertent injury. For long segments of vein, rather than intussuscepting the entire length of the vein on a long valvulotome, inserting a shorter valvulotome via branches along its length allows for a more controlled lysis. Branch points are particularly susceptible to injury and the resulting venotomy can be difficult to fix without narrowing the vein. Successful lysis is demonstrated when vigorous pulsatile flow is present at the end of the graft. If this is not the case, a retained valve cusp is likely present and the entire graft should be re-interrogated.

The vein graft can be tunneled anatomically or subcutaneously and each method has its own merits and deficiencies. In subcutaneous tunnels, the saphenous vein is either left in its own wound bed, or if the distal target is the anterior tibial or dorsalis pedis artery, a new lateral subcutaneous tunnel is made. The advantage of a subcutaneously located graft is that if a mid graft stenosis develops over time, the subsequent exposure and revision are simplified. The principle drawback is that wound breakdown can expose the graft and its superficial location can make subsequent graft coverage somewhat challenging. Anatomic tunneling in the thigh is through a sub-sartorial plane into the popliteal fossa. For infrapopliteal targets, the graft is tunneled between the medial and lateral head of the gastrocnemius muscle. The anterior compartment of the lower leg can be accessed following division of the interosseus membrane. Advantages of tunneling anatomically are that the route is more direct than the circuitous subcutaneous tunnel, which minimizes the length of vein graft needed. Wound complications are also less likely to involve the graft. However, in the event of a subsequent graft stenosis, open surgical revision is more challenging for anatomically located conduits. In the case of distal origin grafts for CLI, we favor using the proximal vein (i.e., from saphenofemoral junction) to minimize the harvest incisions in the more ischemic distal extremity and to allow for tunneling of the graft under intact skin in the lower leg.

Prior to arterial occlusion, heparin sodium is given (100 U/kg) and allowed to circulate for 3 min. When using arterial clamps for control, only the minimal occlusive force is used. The proximal anastomosis is always performed first so that the graft can be oriented and tunneled under arterial pressure. This minimizes the risks of a kink or twist during tunneling, and maintains excess length at this stage. The graft should never be trimmed until the distal arteriotomy has been finalized.

For infrageniculate arterial exposures, using a thigh tourniquet has numerous advantages. Exposure of the distal target is simplified as circumferential control is unnecessary. Collateral vessels at the outflow site can be left unexposed and unharmed. Using a tourniquet leaves the operative field unobstructed by arterial clamps and a crush injury to heavily calcified vessels is avoided. For inframalleolar exposures, thigh tourniquets are still generally effective and calf tourniquets should be applied with caution. Rarely, a peroneal nerve injury can develop from compression against the fibular head. Extensive calcification can present a technical challenge. Sometimes a combination of techniques, such as both tourniquet and fine clamps (Yasergil or bulldog style), are required. Gentle crushing of circumferential calcification can render the vessel clampable, but should be done cautiously, particularly on the outflow side. All loose debris must be removed from the luminal surface, and care must be taken to avoid creating a dissection which may propagate. Newer alloys have been used to develop strong, penetrating needles for suturing calcified vessels which can be helpful.

Assessing the function of the bypass begins with simple observation. A pulse should be palpable in the operative field, distal to the anastomosis. However, in a cold, vasoconstricted leg, distal pulses are often difficult to appreciate by palpation, though capillary refill should be noticeably improved. Doppler flow assessment is routinely preformed and occlusion of the bypass graft should diminish the signal. However, Doppler evaluation affords only a crude assessment of the overall function of the graft. We employ completion imaging studies in all cases—generally both duplex ultrasound as well as contrast angiography, to ensure the technical outcome.

Early graft failure occurs in 5% of lower extremity bypasses and most are due to technical issues at the time of surgery [39]. There are numerous pitfalls during the construction of a lower extremity bypass: location of the arteriotomy, imperfect anastomosis, dissections from clamp injuries or endarterectomies, retained valves, kinks in the graft during the tunneling process, unappreciated sclerosed segments or webs, or any one variety of other technical issues. The best opportunity to fix imperfections that would otherwise lead to early graft failure is at the time of the original operation. More sensitive completion studies, such as angiography or duplex ultrasonography, help the surgeon to identify such imperfections.

Intraoperative angiography is simple and efficient. Even in the absence of a C-arm imaging, flat plate radiographs can add valuable information about the appearance of the graft. In one large series of lower extremity bypasses, completion angiograms led to intraoperative revisions of 8% of grafts [40]. Distal bypass were particularly likely to need revision. Completion duplex ultrasonography is a complementary method, which adds physiologic information to the anatomic assessment. Direct injection of papaverine (60–90 mg) into the graft relieves spasm and should demonstrate vasolidation and improved diastolic flow. Segments of increased velocity should be addressed intraoperatively, with either a patch angioplasty or segmental revision. As in the case of completion angiography, studies have shown that completion ultrasonography predicts which grafts are at highest risk for early graft failure.

In one large series of intraoperative duplex imaging, 15% of vein grafts needed some form of revision [41].

Postoperative Care

Optimizing long-term outcomes from lower extremity bypass surgery requires a commitment from both the patient and the practitioner to manage the patient's systemic diseases, wound care, and for surveillance of the vascular reconstruction. In the early postoperative period, patients are encouraged to walk but they should otherwise keep their operated leg elevated. Nearly all patients develop significant lower extremity edema that can last for 1 or 2 months. The putative etiology of the edema includes autonomic dysfunction from chronic ischemia, postoperative inflammation and interruption of lymphatics during the surgical exposure. Leg elevation alone is typically enough to control symptoms of edema, however some patients may need a compressive bandage when not elevating the leg. Unchecked edema adds to 15% of patients who develop minor wound complications.

Though vein grafts have intrinsic anti-thrombotic properties, patients are typically maintained on antiplatelet therapy with low-dose aspirin (81 mg/day). Routine use of anticoagulants has not been consistently shown to improve long-term outcomes of lower extremity vein bypass surgery. We reserve anticoagulation for patients with previous graft failure, poor runoff or other features that place the graft at high risk. As the leading cause of mortality in this patient population is cardiovascular events, all patients should be treated according to practice guidelines for management of their underlying coronary artery disease, hyperlipidemia, hypertension and diabetes. Typically, this involves statin therapy and a number of studies have suggested to improve mortality in patients who undergo lower extremity bypass surgery while on statin therapy [42]. Other potential salutary effects of stain therapy, such as those on vein graft stenosis and graft failure, are less clear and need additional study.

Vein graft stenosis develops in 30–40% of patients, typically within the first 18 months. Surveillance should include regular visits with specific attention paid to a recurrence of symptoms or a change in the physical exam. A change in the ABI of >0.2 warrants further investigation. As salvage of a previously thrombosed vein graft has poor long-term outcomes, ultrasound surveillance aims to identify vein graft stenosis early and gives an opportunity to maintain patency before grafts fail. A surveillance program should include duplex ultrasonography of the entire graft with measurements of peak systolic velocities and calculation of velocity rations across all lesions. Studies should be performed at 1, 3, 6, and 12 months following surgery, and then every 6 months thereafter. Abnormal findings, such as increased peak systolic velocities of >300 cm/s, a velocity ration of >3.5, or very low velocities (<40 cm/s) should prompt angiography and possible re-intervention, even in the absence of a change in symptoms or ABIs [43].

Postoperative care in the setting of CLI or the diabetic foot also revolves around management of the foot itself. Aggressive debridement, control of infection, and staged reconstruction procedures are frequently used to achieve efficient wound healing and maintain functional status. Postoperative footwear should minimize trauma from weight bearing to any areas of wounds or incisions. A dedicated multidisciplinary team, including vascular surgeons and podiatrists as the critical elements, has been shown to improve functional outcomes in diabetic patients with limb-threatening conditions [44].

Expected Outcomes

A variety of outcome measures help place the importance of lower extremity bypass surgery into perspective. The most basic measure of outcome is graft patency (Table 10.1). By far, the most important factor in determining the longevity of the bypass is the quality of the conduit.

Table 10.1 Estimated 5 year secondary patency for infrainguinal vein graft bypass procedures

Bypass type	Diabetics (%)	Non-diabetics (%)
Common femoral above knee popliteal with vein [10]	75	75
Common femoral below knee popliteal with vein [10]	75	75
Common femoral tibial with vein [45]	75	75
Popliteal pedal with vein [33–35]	65	65
Distal origin graft with vein [26]	70	50

Autogenous vein outperforms all other conduits, but even within this group, a variety of risk factors affect the overall outcome, including a vein graft that is of suboptimal size (less than 3 mm in diameter), non-saphenous and spliced vein grafts, and to a lesser degree longer bypass grafts and the quality of the outflow. However, multiple studies have demonstrated that diabetes per se is not a risk factor for vein graft failure, including both single center series and prospectively accrued data from multicenter trials (Fig. 10.4) [45]. Furthermore it is important to note, particularly given the anatomic pattern that exists in diabetes, that the level of distal anastomosis is a much weaker predictor than conduit quality. In fact, grafts comprised of a single segment GSV of good caliber (≥3.5 mm) perform equally well for popliteal, tibial, or pedal targets (Fig. 10.5).

Although graft patency per se is unaltered in diabetics, amputation free survival is lower and mortality is higher in this patient population [46–48]. Limb salvage is also affected by race, gender and other comorbid conditions [49]. Chronic renal disease for example, frequently the result of diabetes, is an independent risk factor for limb loss and mortality. Up to 15% of lower extremity bypass patients with end stage renal disease (ESRD) may go on to major amputation despite having a patent bypass graft [50]. In fact,

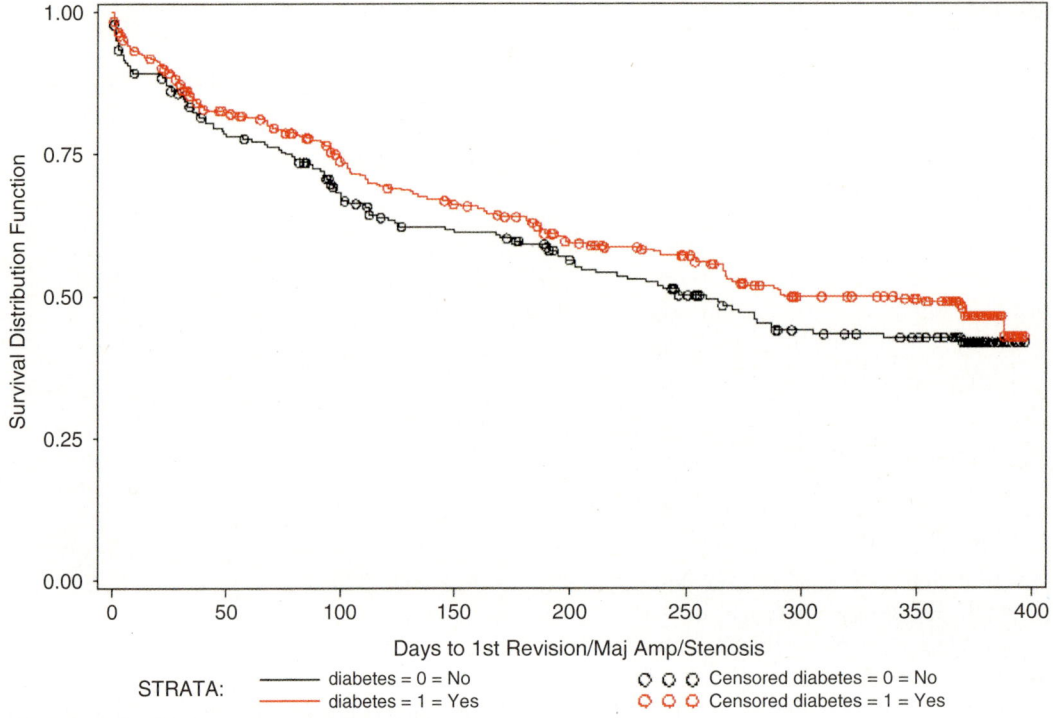

Fig. 10.4 Diabetes has not been shown to be a significant risk factor for vein graft failure. Amongst several key outcomes reported in the Society for Vascular Surgery's objective performance goals for CLI, freedom from re-intervention, amputation, or stenosis (RAS) was no different amongst diabetics and non-diabetics for the open surgical dataset (reprinted from Critical Limb. http://www.criticallimb.org/ with permission from the Society of Vascular Surgery)

there is a nearly linear relationship between the degree of chronic renal insufficiency and mortality amongst patients undergoing lower extremity bypass surgery, and the relationship develops well before the onset of ESRD [51].

Possibly more important that amputation free survival is the functional outcome after lower extremity bypass surgery—namely ambulatory status, ability to live independently, improved quality of life, and complete wound healing. A minority of patients undergoing bypass for CLI meet all of these functional goals, underscoring the severity of the systemic disease in this patient population [52]. The most predictive factor for high functional outcomes for limb salvage is preoperative ambulatory status [53]. Successful bypass surgery has been shown to improve quality of life in CLI, but maintaining that benefit depends upon avoiding re-interventions and achieving complete wound healing [54]. Multiple studies have demonstrated that recrudescence of ulceration in the diabetic foot is high, up to 80% within 1 year of an index ulceration. This underscores the importance of selecting and performing a durable and effective revascularization in this otherwise high risk patient population.

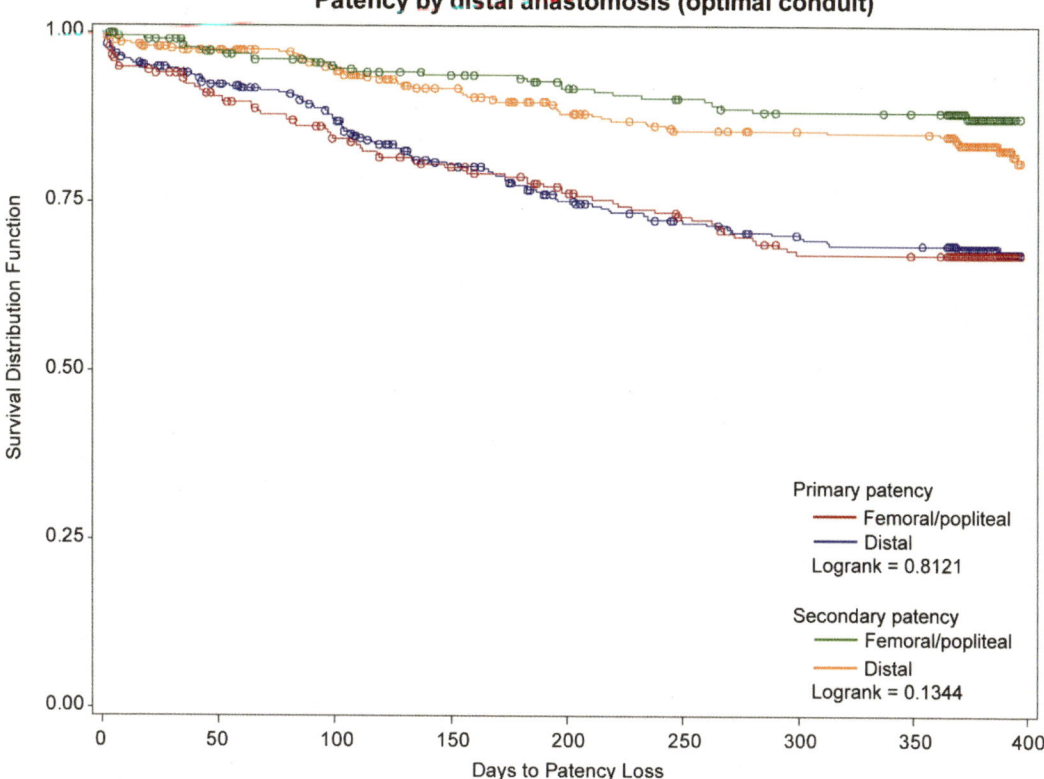

Fig. 10.5 For good quality venous conduit, the outcomes are not affected by the level of the distal anastomosis in infrainguinal bypass surgery. Data from the PREVENT III trial were used to examine the performance of bypass grafts employing a single segment of great saphenous vein with minimal diameter ≥ 3.5 mm, in a CLI-only population

References

1. Pinhas-Hamiel O, Zeitler P. The global spread of type 2 diabetes mellitus in children and adolescents. J Pediatr. 2005;146(5):693–700.
2. Heron M, et al. Deaths: final data for 2006. Natl Vital Stat Rep. 2009;57(14):1–134.
3. Umpierrez GE, et al. Management of hyperglycemia in hospitalized patients in non-critical care setting: an endocrine society clinical practice guideline. J Clin Endocrinol Metab. 2012;97(1):16–38.
4. Hu FB, et al. The impact of diabetes mellitus on mortality from all causes and coronary heart disease in women: 20 years of follow-up. Arch Intern Med. 2001;161(14):1717–23.
5. Ramsey SD, et al. Incidence, outcomes, and cost of foot ulcers in patients with diabetes. Diabetes Care. 1999;22(3):382–7.
6. Conrad MC. Large and small artery occlusion in diabetics and nondiabetics with severe vascular disease. Circulation. 1967;36(1):83–91.
7. Hooi JD, et al. The prognosis of non-critical limb ischaemia: a systematic review of population-based evidence. Br J Gen Pract. 1999;49(438):49–55.
8. Jonason T, Ringqvist I. Diabetes mellitus and intermittent claudication. Relation between peripheral vascular complications and location of the occlusive atherosclerosis in the legs. Acta Med Scand. 1985;218(2):217–21.
9. Hooi JD, et al. Incidence of and risk factors for asymptomatic peripheral arterial occlusive disease: a longitudinal study. Am J Epidemiol. 2001;153(7):666–72.
10. Hirsch AT, et al. ACC/AHA 2005 Practice Guidelines for the management of patients with peripheral arterial disease (lower extremity, renal, mesenteric, and abdominal aortic): a collaborative report from the American Association for Vascular Surgery/Society for Vascular Surgery, Society for Cardiovascular Angiography and Interventions, Society for Vascular Medicine and Biology, Society of Interventional Radiology, and the ACC/AHA Task Force on Practice Guidelines (Writing Committee to Develop Guidelines for the Management of Patients With Peripheral

Arterial Disease): endorsed by the American Association of Cardiovascular and Pulmonary Rehabilitation; National Heart, Lung, and Blood Institute; Society for Vascular Nursing; TransAtlantic Inter-Society Consensus; and Vascular Disease Foundation. Circulation. 2006;113(11):e463–654.
11. Murphy TP, et al. Supervised exercise versus primary stenting for claudication resulting from aortoiliac peripheral artery disease: six-month outcomes from the claudication: exercise versus endoluminal revascularization (CLEVER) study. Circulation. 2012; 125(1):130–9.
12. Bradbury AW, et al. Bypass versus Angioplasty in Severe Ischaemia of the Leg (BASIL) trial: an intention-to-treat analysis of amputation-free and overall survival in patients randomized to a bypass surgery-first or a balloon angioplasty-first revascularization strategy. J Vasc Surg. 2010;51(5 Suppl):5S–17.
13. Bradbury AW, et al. Bypass versus Angioplasty in Severe Ischaemia of the Leg (BASIL) trial: a description of the severity and extent of disease using the Bollinger angiogram scoring method and the TransAtlantic Inter-Society Consensus II classification. J Vasc Surg. 2010;51(5 Suppl):32S–42.
14. Bradbury AW, et al. Bypass versus Angioplasty in Severe Ischaemia of the Leg (BASIL) trial: analysis of amputation free and overall survival by treatment received. J Vasc Surg. 2010;51(5 Suppl): 18S–31.
15. Conte MS, et al. Results of PREVENT III: a multicenter, randomized trial of edifoligide for the prevention of vein graft failure in lower extremity bypass surgery. J Vasc Surg. 2006;43(4):742–51. Discussion 751.
16. Brass EP, et al. Parenteral therapy with lipo-ecraprost, a lipid-based formulation of a PGE1 analog, does not alter six-month outcomes in patients with critical leg ischemia. J Vasc Surg. 2006;43(4):752–9.
17. Monahan TS, Owens CD. Risk factors for lower-extremity vein graft failure. Semin Vasc Surg. 2009;22(4):216–26.
18. Twine CP, McLain AD. Graft type for femoropopliteal bypass surgery. Cochrane Database Syst Rev. (5):CD001487.
19. Taylor Jr LM, et al. Autogenous reversed vein bypass for lower extremity ischemia in patients with absent or inadequate greater saphenous vein. Am J Surg. 1987;153(5):505–10.
20. Chew DK, et al. Bypass in the absence of ipsilateral greater saphenous vein: safety and superiority of the contralateral greater saphenous vein. J Vasc Surg. 2002;35(6):1085–92.
21. Faries PL, et al. The use of arm vein in lower-extremity revascularization: results of 520 procedures performed in eight years. J Vasc Surg. 2000;31(1 Pt 1): 50–9.
22. Londrey GL, et al. Infrainguinal reconstruction with arm vein, lesser saphenous vein, and remnants of greater saphenous vein: a report of 257 cases. J Vasc Surg. 1994;20(3):451–6. Discussion 456–7.
23. Stonebridge PA, Prescott RJ, Ruckley CV. Randomized trial comparing infrainguinal polytetrafluoroethylene bypass grafting with and without vein interposition cuff at the distal anastomosis. The Joint Vascular Research Group. J Vasc Surg. 1997;26(4):543–50.
24. Norgren L, et al. Inter-Society Consensus for the Management of Peripheral Arterial Disease (TASC II). Eur J Vasc Endovasc Surg. 2007;33 Suppl 1:S1–75.
25. Walsh DB, et al. The natural history of superficial femoral artery stenoses. J Vasc Surg. 1991;14(3):299–304.
26. Reed AB, et al. Usefulness of autogenous bypass grafts originating distal to the groin. J Vasc Surg. 2002;35(1):48–54. Discussion 54–5.
27. Ballotta E, et al. Prospective randomized study on reversed saphenous vein infrapopliteal bypass to treat limb-threatening ischemia: common femoral artery versus superficial femoral or popliteal and tibial arteries as inflow. J Vasc Surg. 2004;40(4):732–40.
28. Schanzer A, et al. Superficial femoral artery percutaneous intervention is an effective strategy to optimize inflow for distal origin bypass grafts. J Vasc Surg. 2007;45(4):740–3.
29. Taylor GI, Palmer JH. The vascular territories (angiosomes) of the body: experimental study and clinical applications. Br J Plast Surg. 1987;40(2):113–41.
30. Attinger CE, et al. Angiosomes of the foot and ankle and clinical implications for limb salvage: reconstruction, incisions, and revascularization. Plast Reconstr Surg. 2006;117(7 Suppl):261S–93.
31. Neville RF, et al. Revascularization of a specific angiosome for limb salvage: does the target artery matter? Ann Vasc Surg. 2009;23(3):367–73.
32. Darling 3rd RC, et al. Choice of peroneal or dorsalis pedis artery bypass for limb salvage. Semin Vasc Surg. 1997;10(1):17–22.
33. Hughes K, et al. Bypass to plantar and tarsal arteries: an acceptable approach to limb salvage. J Vasc Surg. 2004;40(6):1149–57.
34. Pomposelli Jr FB, et al. Dorsalis pedis arterial bypass: durable limb salvage for foot ischemia in patients with diabetes mellitus. J Vasc Surg. 1995;21(3):375–84.
35. Pomposelli FB, et al. A decade of experience with dorsalis pedis artery bypass: analysis of outcome in more than 1000 cases. J Vasc Surg. 2003;37(2):307–15.
36. Samson RH, Showalter DP, Yunis JP. Isolated femoropopliteal bypass graft for limb salvage after failed tibial reconstruction: a viable alternative to amputation. J Vasc Surg. 1999;29(3):409–12.
37. Kram HB, et al. Late results of two hundred seventeen femoropopliteal bypasses to isolated popliteal artery segments. J Vasc Surg. 1991;14(3):386–90.
38. Wengerter KR, et al. Prospective randomized multicenter comparison of in situ and reversed vein infrapopliteal bypasses. J Vasc Surg. 1991;13(2):189–97. Discussion 197–9.

39. Schanzer A, et al. Technical factors affecting autogenous vein graft failure: observations from a large multicenter trial. J Vasc Surg. 2007;46(6):1180–90. Discussion 1190.
40. Mills JL, Fujitani RM, Taylor SM. Contribution of routine intraoperative completion arteriography to early infrainguinal bypass patency. Am J Surg. 1992;164(5):506–10. Discussion 510–1.
41. Johnson BL, et al. Intraoperative duplex monitoring of infrainguinal vein bypass procedures. J Vasc Surg. 2000;31(4):678–90.
42. Schouten O, et al. Fluvastatin and perioperative events in patients undergoing vascular surgery. N Engl J Med. 2009;361(10):980–9.
43. Tinder CN, Bandyk DF. Detection of imminent vein graft occlusion: what is the optimal surveillance program? Semin Vasc Surg. 2009;22(4):252–60.
44. Sumpio BE, et al. The role of interdisciplinary team approach in the management of the diabetic foot: a joint statement from the Society for Vascular Surgery and the American Podiatric Medical Association. J Am Podiatr Med Assoc. 2010;100(4):309–11.
45. Akbari CM, et al. Lower extremity revascularization in diabetes: late observations. Arch Surg. 2000;135(4):452–6.
46. Wolfle KD, et al. Graft patency and clinical outcome of femorodistal arterial reconstruction in diabetic and non-diabetic patients: results of a multicentre comparative analysis. Eur J Vasc Endovasc Surg. 2003;25(3):229–34.
47. Axelrod DA, et al. Perioperative cardiovascular risk stratification of patients with diabetes who undergo elective major vascular surgery. J Vasc Surg. 2002;35(5):894–901.
48. Hamdan AD, et al. Lack of association of diabetes with increased postoperative mortality and cardiac morbidity: results of 6565 major vascular operations. Arch Surg. 2002;137(4):417–21.
49. Nguyen LL, et al. Disparity in outcomes of surgical revascularization for limb salvage: race and gender are synergistic determinants of vein graft failure and limb loss. Circulation. 2009;119(1):123–30.
50. Lantis 2nd JC, et al. Infrainguinal bypass grafting in patients with end-stage renal disease: improving outcomes? J Vasc Surg. 2001;33(6):1171–8.
51. Owens CD, et al. Refinement of survival prediction in patients undergoing lower extremity bypass surgery: stratification by chronic kidney disease classification. J Vasc Surg. 2007;45(5):944–52.
52. Golledge J, et al. Critical assessment of the outcome of infrainguinal vein bypass. Ann Surg. 2001;234(5):697–701.
53. Abou-Zamzam Jr AM, et al. Functional outcome after infrainguinal bypass for limb salvage. J Vasc Surg. 1997;25(2):287–95. Discussion 295–7.
54. Nguyen LL, et al. Prospective multicenter study of quality of life before and after lower extremity vein bypass in 1404 patients with critical limb ischemia. J Vasc Surg. 2006;44(5):977–83. Discussion 983–4.

Managing Complications of Vascular Surgery and Endovascular Therapy

11

Salvatore T. Scali and Timothy C. Flynn

Keywords
Complications • Bypass • Endovascular • Infrainguinal • Surgery • Management

Complications of Open Peripheral Arterial Reconstruction

General Considerations and Etiology of Autogenous Graft Failure

The natural history leading to late failure of an autogenous infrainguinal graft is inextricably linked to the impact of neointimal hyperplasia and/or progression of atherosclerotic disease within the native arteries. Over time, a significant decline in primary patency is frequently observed and the incidence of the development of these lesions is 20–30% in both reversed saphenous and in situ bypasses [1, 2]. Mechanisms of vein graft failure outside of the perioperative (postoperative days 0–>30) interval are frequently secondary to anastomotic or vein conduit stenosis resulting from negative graft adaptation [3]. The process of vein adaptation takes up to 2 years, and consequently, the anatomic and hemodynamic sequelae of this remodeling leads to a 5% per year risk of need for remediation [4]. The failing or "threatened" bypass will have significantly worse long-term patency if prophylactic secondary intervention or revision is not undertaken prior to thrombosis [4]. The long-term patency of a thrombosed vein graft is dismal and 3-year patency rates of revised thrombosed in situ or reversed saphenous vein grafts are only 15–47% [1, 5, 6]. In situations where the bypass has been undertaken for limb salvage, amputation-free survival and overall patient survival can be negatively impacted by these complications, so attempts to minimize the risk of failure and prediction models to identify patients at greatest risk for thrombosis are needed [7]. In sharp contrast, failing grafts that undergo revision prior to thrombosis can have equivalent patency to grafts that never required intervention [8]. The impact of graft thrombosis on outcome highlights the importance of developing strategies to avoid this dreaded complication. Probably, the most important factors determining success are the

S.T. Scali, M.D. (✉) • T.C. Flynn, M.D., F.A.C.S.
Division of Vascular Surgery and Endovascular Therapy,
Department of Surgery, University of Florida College of Medicine, Shands Hospital at the University of Florida,
Health Sciences Center, 1600 SW Archer Road,
PO Box 100128, Gainesville, FL 32610-0128, USA
e-mail: Salvatore.Scali@surgery.ufl.edu;
Timothy.Flynn@surgery.ufl.edu

Table 11.1 Factors reported to be associated with early lower extremity bypass graft failure (<30 days postoperatively)

Technical factors (e.g. clamp injury, dissection, hematoma, pseudoaneurysm, florid outflow disease, untreated inflow disease, nonsingle segment saphenous vein graft, composite graft, vein < 3.5 mm in diameter)
Young age (<60)
African American status
Crural target
Diabetes
Hypercoaguable state
Poor distal run-off (Rutherford run-off score or distal graft EDV < 5 cm/s)
Compromised conduit (ePTFE below the knee, cadaveric products)
End-stage renal disease
General anesthesia
Tobacco abuse
Operative indication (critical limb ischemia)

preoperative decision making around patient selection, identification of optimal inflow and outflow vessels, and evaluation and selection of conduit. Intraoperative factors such as meticulous dissection, careful handling of tissues, and technically perfect construction of the anastomosis are the sine qua non of success. Vigilant intraoperative and postoperative surveillance protocols will lead to improved outcomes in the long-term management of an infrainguinal bypass [9].

Early Lower Extremity Bypass Graft Complications

Perioperative bypass graft failures are traditionally grouped into early and late causes. Early or acute failure (≤30 days) occurs in 4–12% of cases and is generally believed to be related to technical issues or problems related to inflow–outflow arteries and the adequacy of the conduit [10]. Numerous other factors have been reported to impact early failure of lower extremity bypass grafts such as young age (<60), African-American race, use of tibial targets, poor distal run-off (as measured by Rutherford run-off score or distal bypass end-diastolic velocity; EDV), compromised conduit choice, use of general anesthesia, and preexisting hypercoaguable states (Table 11.1) [11–14]. Saltzberg and colleagues [15] reported that early graft thrombosis can occur in up to 11% of young, diabetic patients; however, many of these failures were thought to be secondary to an aggressive limb salvage policy in the face of poor conduit, targets, or both. Technical errors that can lead to early bypass failure include dissecting and clamping the inflow and outflow arteries leading to intimal flaps which can subsequently lead to luminal stenosis and/or thrombosis. Errors that occur during the construction of the proximal or distal anastomosis include suture line bleeding, pseudoaneurysm formation, or suture line stricture. Likewise, untreated proximal aortoiliac or femoral occlusive disease can lead to premature graft failure. Intraoperative conduit manipulation and unanticipated vein imperfections such as luminal thrombus, synechiae, webs, sclerotic segments, platelet aggregates, graft torsion, kinking, entrapment, inadequate side branch ligation, and direct vein injury from distension, traction, or valve ablation may all lead to early graft complications and/or failure.

In our practice, we employ several strategies in an effort to reduce the risk of developing technical problems leading to early graft complications, including routine use of preoperative vein mapping (≥3 mm conduit), gentle distension and manipulation of the graft, utilization of physiologic/heparinized flush solutions (e.g., heparinized plasmalyte ± papaverine), liberal use of angioscopy, minimization of warm ischemia time to the vein graft endothelium, and routine completion imaging (arteriography and/or completion duplex ultrasound). Gentle handling of the target vessels, particularly in the infragenicular circulation, is critical to avoiding vessel dissection. Any questionable inflow or outflow lesion above or below the bypass should be investigated or remediated either at the time of the bypass operation or preoperatively. Many pitfalls of angiogram interpretation can lead to the classic example of the seemingly "normal" two-dimensional preoperative arteriogram that underestimates the degree of iliofemoral occlusive disease. Measuring intraarterial femoral pressures (with or without vasodilators) *after* bypass reconstruction can be helpful in determining if there are any untreated proximal lesions that may compromise long-term patency of the graft. A significant hemodynamic gradient (greater than 20 mmHg between the brachial systolic pressure and the femoral pressure or 10 mmHg mean arterial pressure difference) should trigger further intervention (e.g., proximal aortic bypass, extra-anatomic bypass, iliofemoral endarterectomy, or intraoperative balloon angioplasty and/or stenting).

Our preferred conduit is the ipsilateral greater saphenous vein (GSV); however, over 50% of the patients in our practice do not have this option due to prior coronary bypass procedure(s), failed arterial reconstruction attempts, or small vein conduit diameters, which is consistent with other reports [16]. Consequently, the use of contralateral saphenous vein or arm vein is preferred to nonautologous options such as prosthetic or cadaveric products. In the setting of a reoperative field with active wound infection, we prefer cadaveric products over heparin-bonded expanded polytetrafluoroethylene (hePTFE) when an autogenous option is not available. If revascularization below the popliteal trifurcation is required with nonautogenous conduit, we frequently employ an autogenous vein patch to both simplify the technical construction of the distal anastomosis and reduce the compliance differential that exists between a nonautogenous bypass and the native tibial vessel [17]. In this way, the development of subsequent fibrointimal hyperplasia may be ameliorated and potentially lead to a 15–20% augmentation in long-term patency of prosthetic crural bypass grafts [18]. A variety of other techniques have been described in the literature, including construction of Miller cuffs, Wolfe boots, and arteriovenous fistula; however, the evidence for these adjuncts is limited to primarily retrospective, single-center experiences and have not been routinely adopted in our practice [19].

If a high-risk conduit is utilized (hePTFE below the knee, cadaveric products, venovenostomy, arm vein, or inadequate arterial outflow), the graft is considered disadvantaged, and lifelong warfarin and aspirin are initiated in the perioperative recovery period. Thereafter, postoperative surveillance with duplex ultrasound and ankle–brachial indices (ABI) are then performed at 1, 3, 6, 9, 12, 18, and 24 month intervals. If, after 2 years, the graft has not required reintervention, no peak-systolic velocity step-up ratio greater than 3.5 exists or, deterioration in ABI>0.15 has been observed, annual surveillance for life is then advocated in our practice. Indefinite surveillance is recommended since up to 30% of infrainguinal bypass grafts followed over a 13-year interval required salvage procedures, despite being "normal" after the initial 24 months of implantation [20]. Moreover, the importance of a surveillance protocol to reduce complications of lower extremity bypass procedures is further underscored by the fact that only about a third of patients will manifest symptoms suggestive of a failing graft (e.g., claudication, rest pain, new tissue loss), despite evidence of hemodynamic failure by duplex ultrasound [6, 8, 9].

If the dreaded complication of early graft thrombosis occurs, the operating surgeon should have made the determination at the initial operation if a return trip to the operating would be warranted. Many surgeons have been faced with a high-risk patient with compromised conduit and/or targets and a discussion with the operative team combined with judicious patient and family counseling about the anticipated outcome of the bypass procedure should be made prospectively. If the graft is thought to be salvageable, systemic heparinization and an expeditious return to the operating room are indicated. Initial strategies include reexploration of the distal anastomosis, graftotomy, thromboembolectomy, and subsequent digital subtraction arteriography. The differential diagnosis of possible causes of failure is legion (outlined above) and each may trigger a number of different interventions (see Fig. 11.1).

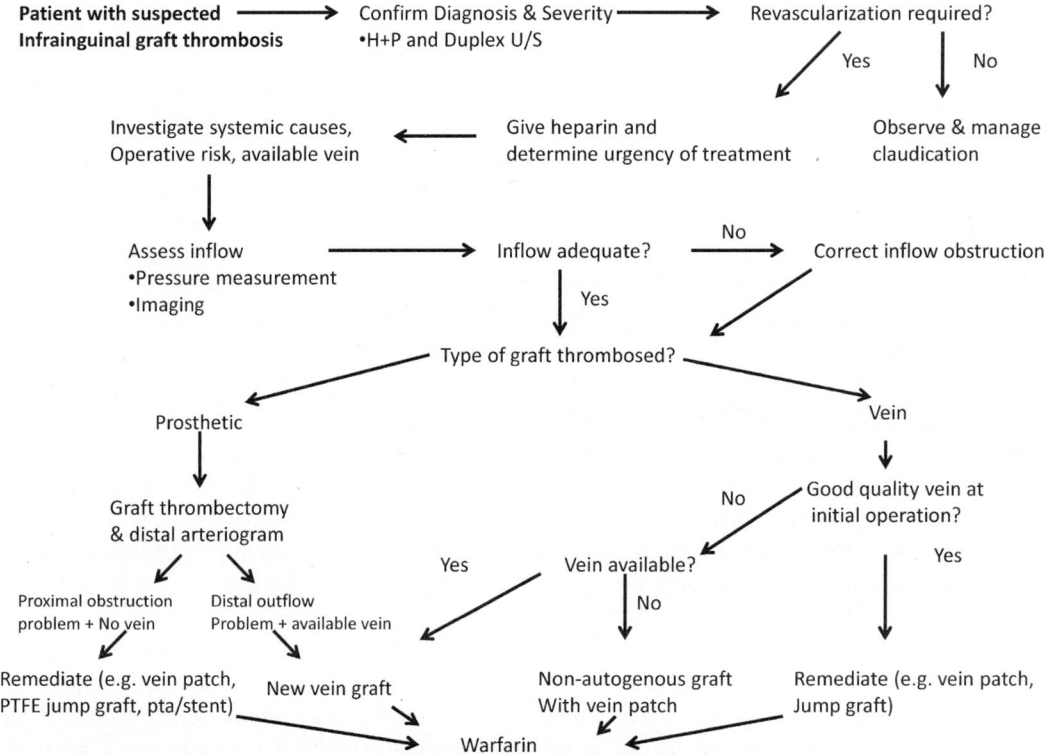

Fig. 11.1 Algorithm for management of early lower extremity bypass failure (adapted from Walsh DB. Infrainguinal graft thrombosis. In: Cronenwett JL & Rutherford RB, editors. Decision making in vascular surgery. Philadelphia, PA: W.B. Saunders; 2001. With permission from Elsevier)

Operative Management of the Patent but Failing Graft

The primary goals in the management of a patent but failing lower extremity bypass graft are correction of the anatomic abnormality, restoration of normal hemodynamics of the autogenous graft, and maintenance of long-term graft patency. Clinical and hemodynamic assessment of patients in the postoperative setting with the use of noninvasive vascular lab imaging is essential to the surveillance protocol. A variety of different duplex criteria have been reported to be associated with the threatened or failing graft [8] (Table 11.2).

Graft revisions require a clear understanding of the cause, location, and extent of the lesion. Traditionally, these lesions have been repaired with open surgical (OS) revision, including patch angioplasty, interposition bypass, or jump grafts.

Table 11.2 Duplex criteria for a failing LEB

Recurrence of symptoms of limb ischemia
Peak systolic velocity elevation >3.5
Low peak systolic graft velocity (<45 cm/s)
Decrease in flow velocity >30 cm/s
Decrease in ankle/brachial index >0.15 on serial examination

LEB lower extremity bypass
Adapted from Bandyk DF, Schmitt DD, Seabrook GR, et al. Monitoring functional patency of in situ saphenous vein bypasses: the impact of a surveillance protocol and elective revision. J Vasc Surg. 1989;9(2):286–96. With permission from Elsevier

Anticipation of retained valve leaflets, sclerotic segments, missed inflow or outflow lesions, and neointimal hyperplastic stenosis is required when planning open secondary procedures of the patent but failing graft. Indeed, the assisted primary patency achieved by repairing a graft stenosis is generally better than the secondary patency that results when repair is performed after the graft has occluded [21]. Nguyen et al. [22] demonstrated that OS of infrainguinal vein grafts resulted in a 5-year patency rate of 49% and a secondary patency rate of 80%. Landry et al. [23] demonstrated an 87% primary-assisted patency at 5 years after OS revision of vein bypass grafts and Bandyk et al. [6] found an 85% primary-assisted patency rate at 5 years.

Although surgical revision is generally well tolerated, occasional deaths or serious perioperative morbidity has been reported in the literature [24, 25]. Additional concerns regarding open graft revision include need for additional conduit, dissection through scar tissue to achieve an anastomosis with either an inflow or outflow artery may be necessary, and surgical wound healing may delay recovery. Although these operations are not typically associated with significant morbidity, a stay in the hospital is usually required. Because of these concerns, several authors have reported on the role of endovascular salvage of infrainguinal bypass grafts over the past 10 years. A variety of secondary endoluminal procedures have been reported such as plain balloon angioplasty, cutting balloon angioplasty, and self-expanding stent (or stent-graft) placement [26]. Notably, the first description of percutaneous balloon angioplasty (PTA) to treat vein graft stenosis was reported by Alpert et al. [27] and has been utilized with increasing frequency in the management of failing infrainguinal bypass grafts. This strategy remains controversial with widely varying post-angioplasty patency rates of 30–80% at 12 months, suggesting that individual patient or graft factors may influence outcome [28]. Anatomic and temporal factors that may predict favorable outcome of angioplasty of infrainguinal vein grafts include single, less than 2-cm lesions in grafts older than 3 months [28]. In general, most historical series demonstrate superiority of OR compared to PTA of failing grafts with regard to long-term patency; however, with correct patient and anatomic selection, satisfactory results can be anticipated.

If any clinical or hemodynamic abnormalities are detected postoperatively (see Table 11.2), our practice is to have patients undergo repeat vein mapping followed by digital subtraction arteriography. Lesions with favorable anatomic characteristics are treated with balloon angioplasty. Because the etiology of these stenotic lesions is frequently neointimal hyperplasia, cutting balloon angioplasty is often employed as a first-line therapy in these circumstances, and high insufflation pressures for extended periods (60 s) may be required to achieve technical success [26]. We have not incorporated the use of vein graft stenting due to the unacceptable results reported in the literature. Once an adequate angiographic result is achieved, the patient is placed on clopidogrel (75 mg daily) for a month after the intervention and the surveillance duplex protocol is reestablished as if this was a new bypass graft. For those patients who fail initial angioplasty of their bypass or those with poor predictors of angioplasty salvage (immature graft; <3 months, >2-cm-long stenosis, or multiple tandem stenoses), open surgical reconstruction of the bypass is performed.

Operative Management of Late Infrainguinal Graft Occlusions

The consequence of late graft thrombosis is usually a recrudescence of the patient's original limb ischemia symptoms (disabling claudication, rest pain or new/persistent ulceration) or may be evidenced by frank, acute limb-threatening ischemia. Up to 10–20% of patients may receive major amputation as their secondary procedure for late graft thrombosis if the original operation was performed for critical limb ischemia [11]. When confronted with a patient who suffers late thrombosis of their vein graft, a frequent strategy surgeons attempt is restoration of patency and salvage of the graft. This may be achieved by direct open surgical thrombectomy followed by angiography and/or duplex ultrasonography with subsequent repair of the underlying anatomic defects that are the etiology of failure. Unfortunately, thrombectomy of vein grafts has seldom proved to be a durable strategy with patency rates of only 19–28% at 5 years after intervention [29, 30]. The recognition of the limitations of bypass thrombectomy led to considerable enthusiasm for the use of thrombolytic therapy. Thrombolytic therapy offers several potential advantages, including more complete thrombus dissolution from the outflow vessels and preoperative recognition of the lesions responsible for vein graft occlusion. Some groups have espoused that this technique also may allow avoidance of balloon catheter-induced trauma to the vein graft wall.

Despite these potential advantages, thrombolytic therapy has not been proven to be a particularly useful strategy for restoring patency to vein grafts. Belkin and associates [30] reported that only 23% of vein grafts remained patent 3 years after successful thrombolysis and open surgical revision. Interestingly, a series by Nackman et al. [31] reported on 44 thrombosed vein grafts managed with thrombolysis and subsequent revision; subgroup analysis identified mature vein grafts (>12 months) as having more durable patency rates than those that have failed within a year of the original operation. Given the limitations of thrombolytic therapy for restoring durable vein graft patency, we have not readily adopted this into our management algorithm. Currently, we attempt thrombolytic salvage only for patients with no evidence of Rutherford IIb/III ischemia and limited autogenous conduit, possessing a mature (>12 months) vein graft, with significant thrombus in the outflow vessels, and/or those with advanced comorbidities that preclude a major reoperation. In general, our preferred approach for intermediate to late vein graft failure is to proceed with an entirely new infrainguinal reconstruction in those of whom revascularization is clinically indicated.

The challenges of secondary infrainguinal bypass surgery after a previous failed reconstruction are well known to vascular surgeons. Management strategies vary with the time interval from bypass, the functional status of the patient, the degree of ischemia, and the availability of autogenous vein. Severe scarring in the operative field and the lack of ipsilateral GSV necessitating use of alternative vein conduits presents technical challenges to the surgeon. Furthermore, by virtue of the fact that these patients have suffered failure of a previous reconstruction, graft thrombosis sub-selects a group of patients who frequently

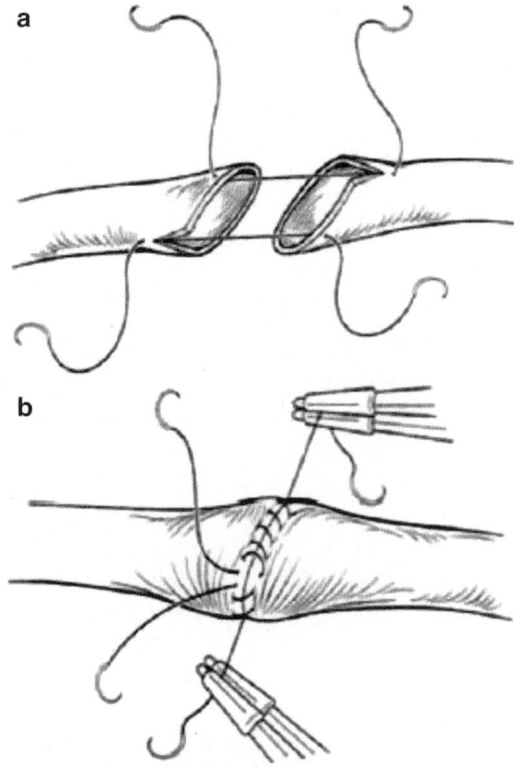

Fig. 11.2 Schematic representation of technique utilized to perform a veno-venostomy with equally sized bevels in each conduit and anchoring each corner with a 6-0 or 7-0 monofilament suture (**a**). Gentle distraction is maintained to prevent "purse-stringing" as the sides are sutured (**b**) (adapted from Belkin M. Secondary bypass after infrainguinal bypass graft failure. Semin Vasc Surg. 2009;22(4):234–239. With permission from Elsevier)

manifest more severe atherosclerosis, a marked intimal hyperplastic response, poor-quality venous conduits, and hypercoaguable states [32]. Given these attributes, it is not surprising that the outcome of secondary bypass operations is generally inferior to those achieved with primary bypass procedures. Tenets of reoperative lower extremity bypass surgery include strict adherence to basic surgical principles, utilization of autogenous conduit, and resourcefulness in adapting the operative plan to the patient's specific anatomy.

Whenever possible, autogenous vein should be the preferred bypass conduit even if multiple arm-vein segments with venovenostomy are required (Fig. 11.2). Careful sharp dissection of arterial targets must be undertaken and avoidance of the so called "exarterectomy" should be the rule. Reexposure of tibial target vessels can be quite challenging due to extensive scarring, obliteration of normal anatomic relationships, and tenacious adherence of robust tibial collateral veins. Attempts to resite the bypass to alternative bypass targets should be made and alternative anatomic exposures (e.g., lateral peroneal artery exposure with fibulectomy; trans-interosseous anterior tibial access) may be particularly useful in these complex situations. A bloodless field is often required, so the use of proximal tourniquets and/or intraluminal tibial balloon occluders may further facilitate the technical conduct of reoperative crural revascularization. Alternative conduits such as arm veins or the lesser saphenous vein have proven to be useful and durable conduits in the absence of GSV. Andros et al. [33] reported a 57% secondary patency rate at 5 years after surgery in a series of 88 arm-vein bypass grafts. Similarly, Hayward and associates [34] reported a 64% secondary patency rate at 3 years in a series of 43 patients who received operations with arm-vein grafts.

Management of Graft Infection, Wound Complications (Dressings, Muscle Flaps, VAC, Cadaveric Products)

Although the subject of wound complications is beyond the scope of this chapter, an important component to the perioperative management of lower extremity revascularization in diabetic patients is wound management. Surgical site infections (SSI) are a common complication with open lower extremity revascularization occurring in 11–15% of patients and is associated with a more than twofold increased risk of early graft loss and reoperation [35, 36]. Several basic strategies are advocated to reduce the risk of SSI, including control of ongoing foot sepsis (e.g., preoperative antibiotics and diabetic foot abscess drainage), avoidance of undermining or tissue flap creation, consideration of transverse groin incisions in obese patients, utilization of skip incisions for saphenous harvest, employment of multiple-layered, tension-free closure of lower extremity wounds, and judicious perioperative normothermia. Simple strategies such as the use of an absorbent silver-eluting dressing system can further reduce lower extremity revascularization wound complications [37]. Preoperative metabolic derangements such as hypoalbuminemia, hyponatremia, severe azotemia, and hyperglycemia all increase the risk of SSI after lower extremity arterial bypass or thromboendarterectomy, so prudent evaluation and patient optimization is required prior to infrainguinal revascularization [35].

In the dreaded situation of an early postoperative deep SSI, wound debridement, irrigation, deep tissue coverage, VAC dressing application, and broad-spectrum intravenous antibiotics may salvage a lower extremity bypass. If a patient presents with systemic sepsis as a result of their early postoperative SSI, particularly in the setting of a prosthetic infrainguinal graft, consideration of a staged revascularization strategy can be made. Initial wound debridement and graft inspection to ensure anastomotic integrity is required followed by temporary closure and admission to the surgical intensive care unit. Groin wound "blow-out" precautions are instituted (NPO status, large bore IV access, bed rest, serial examination, and reservation of blood products), which may facilitate physiologic resuscitation and secondary operative planning with patient and family counseling. Complex wounds, late graft infections with mycotic degeneration, or the presence of gram negative organisms may necessitate utilization of extra-anatomic bypass circuits, aggressive wound debridement, and utilization of myocutaneous tissue flaps [38]. It has been our practice to remove all prosthetic conduits within an infected field and use autogenous or cadaveric products, depending on availability. If in-line anatomic reconstruction is not possible, extra-anatomic revascularization strategies are employed. Because each patient scenario is so unique due to patient comorbidities and complex anatomic considerations, consultation with other members of the group is frequently undertaken in these challenging cases. Despite the hostile environment and increased perioperative morbidity and mortality that can be anticipated with management of lower extremity revascularization wound complications, good outcomes may be anticipated when a multi-modal, multi-disciplinary approach is employed.

Complications of Peripheral Endovascular Intervention

General Considerations

It is has been estimated that 40–70% of all peripheral vascular procedures performed in the United States have some element of endoluminal therapy as a component of the management algorithm [39]. Indeed, the current mantra in most practices is to embrace an "endo first" strategy in the treatment of disabling claudication or critical limb ischemia. A desire to improve patient outcomes, as well as, free market forces have led to a veritable explosion of endovascular therapies to treat peripheral artery disease in the last two decades, despite little Level 1 evidence to support superiority over traditional open surgical methods. Notwithstanding the challenges faced by attempting to determine a judicious and prudent algorithm for the application of the myriad of endoluminal technologies in the lower extremity, these interventions are inextricably linked to contemporary vascular surgery practice. Consequently, diagnostic or therapeutic procedures should be undertaken only when a thoughtful analysis of the indications, risk, benefits, and alternatives has been completed and an informed discussion held with the patient and family. Similarly, vigilance needs to be maintained when performing these procedures, so that early recognition of complications occurs.

If complications of an endovascular procedure are not recognized in a timely manner, access across the treatment site may be lost, leading to further difficulty in treating the problem. Further, challenging the management of endovascular complications is the potential limitation of the available tools and the remote nature of the access site. Bearing these limitations in mind, operators should always remind themselves about the role of open surgical salvage and restrain from prolonged attempts at endoluminal remediation which may lead to further complications, higher cost, increased procedural time, and greater contrast exposure. One must develop and pay particular attention to tactile feedback from wires and catheters and not simply follow the procedure visually on the monitor.

A recurrent trend in the literature is that higher procedural morbidity rates are reported with therapeutic, as opposed to diagnostic interventions [40]. This usually is a result of the need for larger sheath access, complexity of the treated lesions, and required manipulations, as well as the frequent need for perioperative anticoagulation/antiplatelet therapy [40]. Moreover, the impact of obesity, vessel calcification, tortuosity, lesion morphology, thrombus, and the patients overall medical comorbidities further influences the potential for technical complications of endovascular therapies in the management of peripheral arterial disease in the diabetic patient and must be considered when performing these techniques.

Access Complications (Puncture Site and Catheter Induced): Pseudoaneurysm, Hematoma, AVF, Manual Pressure vs. Closure Devices

It is estimated that the overall incidence of access site complications for arterial interventions is between 1 and 6% [41, 42]. The true rate of complications is probably underestimated because of the heterogeneity of definitions used for access site complications for peripheral interventions; for example, the definition of "hematoma" has been quite variable in the literature [43] (Table 11.3). Furthermore, because of the outpatient nature of many interventions, many authors believe that there is underrecognition or underreporting of arterial access morbidity. Like many complications in surgery, the best management is frequently prevention. The routine execution of endovascular procedures in daily practice may lead proceduralists to become complacent about the initial steps of a peripheral intervention. Although limb-threatening or life-threatening complications are rare, complications of vascular access can often lead to increased procedure time, wound morbidity, cost, length of stay, need for surgical revision, and patient dissatisfaction. A number of different complications may result from arterial access so it is crucial that familiarity and anticipation with these possible outcomes occurs even with routine peripheral vascular intervention.

Table 11.3 Indicators and thresholds for complications in diagnostic and therapeutic arteriography

	Overall reported rates (%)	Major adverse event threshold (%)
Puncture site complications		
Hematoma (requiring transfusion, surgery, or delayed discharge)	1.2–8.9	0.5
Occlusion	0.0–0.76	0.2
Pseudoaneurysm/arteriovenous fistula	1.1–7.7	0.2
Catheter-induced complications (other than puncture site)		
Distal emboli	0.0–0.1	0.5
Arterial dissection/subintimal passage	0.43	0.5
Subintimal injection of contrast	0.0–0.44	0.5
Major contrast reactions	0.0–3.58	0.5
Contrast-associated nephrotoxicity	0.2–1.4	0.2

Adapted from Singh H, Cardella JF, Cole PE, et al. Quality improvement guidelines for diagnostic arteriography. J Vasc Interv Radiol. 2003;14:S283. With permission from Elsevier

General Approach to Arterial Access

The initial assessment should be with the physical exam paying particular attention to the quality and symmetry of the femoral and brachial pulses. If patients have inguinal scar, the vascular surgeon needs to be acutely aware of the presence of a bypass, as well as the impact that scar may have on tractability for sheath access. If asymmetry or absence of a pulse in the femoral position is documented, it has been our practice to evaluate the patient with spiral arterial-phased computed tomography (CTA). In this way, determination of the burden of aortoiliac or common femoral occlusive disease can be made and appropriate surgical access planning is further clarified. Frequently, the patient may have significant inflow occlusive disease on the CTA and preoperative planning for endovascular, hybrid, or open surgical reconstruction may be considered without digital subtraction angiography. Drawbacks of this strategy are the exposure to contrast agents, additional costs, potential for additive radiation if subsequent intervention is required, need to clarify the impact of calcification on imaging interpretation, and poor resolution of tibial imaging for distal bypass planning.

When attempting arterial puncture, particular attention should be paid to achieving anterior wall puncture and avoiding the so-called "through and through" or double wall technique. In this way, avoidance of puncturing the posterior atherosclerotic plaque that frequently is encountered in lower extremity ischemia patients is achieved and reduction in the risk of femoral access dissection assured. The obese patient can present particular challenges since typical surface anatomy landmarks are distorted so reliance on ultrasound and/or fluoroscopic guidance may be required. Avoiding a "high" or "low" puncture is of paramount importance so referencing the position of the inguinal ligament by surface anatomy and localizing the top of the femoral head on fluoroscopy is recommended. Indeed, many surgeons recommend routine use of ultrasound guidance to further reduce access site complications. Micropuncture techniques using a 0.014 introducer wire should be the rule and particular attention is payed to the behavior of the microwire. If the wire bends back on its self in anyway, the operator needs to recognize this immediately so as to avoid initial subintimal dissection which is further exacerbated by subsequent sheath and catheter manipulations. When attempting antegrade puncture, attention must be payed to the presence of significant femoral bifurcation disease, patient obesity, and the possibility of a high profunda origin. Higher complication rates have been reported with antegrade approaches but with appropriate patient selection, optimal pushability, catheter, and wire control, as well as distal tibial vessel access can be achieved.

Hematoma, Pseudoaneurysm, and Arteriovenous Fistula

A variety of different risk factors have been reported to be associated with higher rates of access site complications, including larger sheath access, arteriotomy site and approach, interventional procedures, low body mass index, female gender, uncontrolled hypertension, excessive anticoagulation, utilization of glycoprotein IIb/IIIa inhibitors, and advanced age [43] (Fig. 11.3). Keeping these covariates in mind, endovascular surgeons should be alerted to this high-risk cohort of patients and implement preemptive maneuvers to reduce the risk of morbidity. Fitts and colleagues reported an almost threefold reduction in pseudoaneurysm (PSA) formation and a significantly lower risk of all arterial injuries (1.9% versus 0.7%, $P<0.01$) by simply identifying the femoral head fluoroscopically prior to puncture [44]. Utilization of periprocedural adjuncts like duplex ultrasound may further delineate anatomic landmarks, elucidate vessel morphology, calcification, and plaque burden; thereby, providing additional information about anticipated difficulty with arterial access. Several reports have described the utility of ultrasound guidance when performing femoral puncture for endovascular intervention, which may further reduce the risk of access site complications [41, 44–46].

A summary of the various access vessel complications are outlined in Table 11.4 and explanations of presentation and management are provided. Oweida and associates [45] reported on postcatheterization vascular complications and found an overall complication rate of 1% with pseudoaneurysms being the most common complication to require operative repair, occurring in almost 60% of patients with this complication. McCann et al. found a similar incidence of ischemic and hemorrhagic complications in a study of 16,350 patients undergoing diagnostic

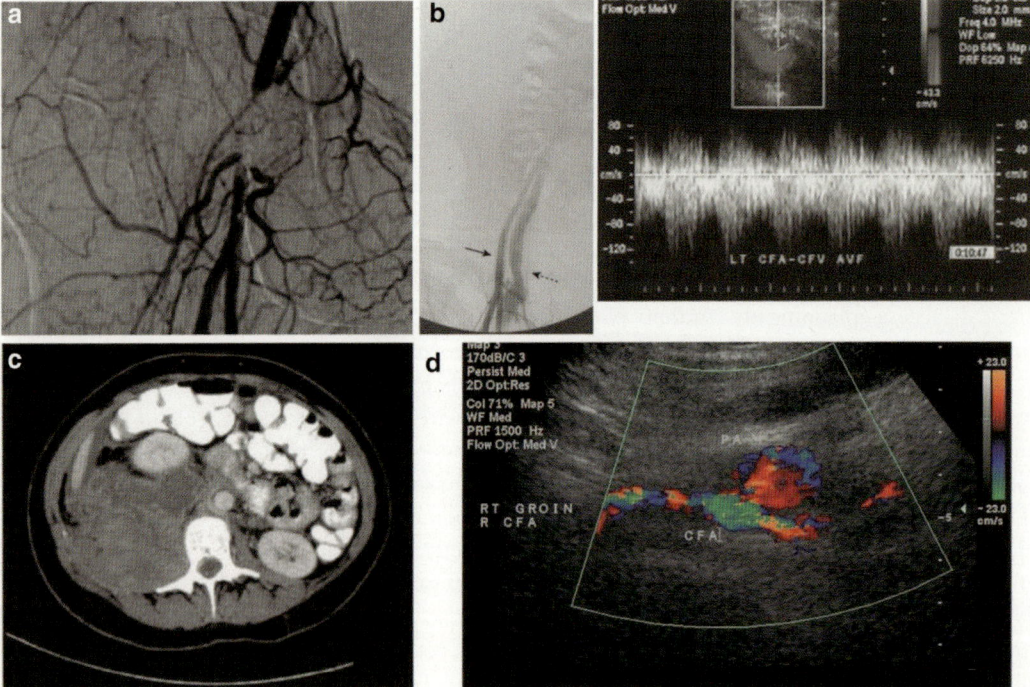

Fig. 11.3 Depiction of various access-related complications from femoral puncture. (**a**) Femoral occlusion due to closure device complication. (**b**) Angiographic and duplex demonstration of an AVF between the common femoral vein and femoral artery bifurcation. (**c**) Retroperitoneal hematoma. (**d**) Duplex evidence of femoral pseudoaneurysm

Table 11.4 Description of different access site complications, risk factors, clinical manifestation and diagnosis, and corresponding management strategies

Complication	Risk factors	Manifestation and diagnosis	Management
Access site hematoma	Female gender, age >65, IIb/IIIa inhibitor use, multiple access attempts	• Swelling, pain, ecchymosis, bleeding, neuropathy, anemia, hypotension, shock • Physical exam, duplex	Observation, bed rest, correct coagulopathy, manual compression, transfusion, surgery
Retroperitoneal hematoma	"High puncture"	• Asymptomatic, groin or flank pain, neuropathy, hypotension, anemia, shock • Grey-Turner sign, CT scan	Observation, bed rest, transfusion, endovascular or open surgical repair
Arteriovenous fistula	"Low puncture"	• Asymptomatic, groin pain, limb swelling, cardiac failure • Bruit, duplex	Observation, endovascular or surgical repair
Pseudoaneurysm	Anticoagulation, obesity, ≥7 Fr sheath, inadequate compression, simultaneous artery-vein catheterization, Ca2+, hypertension, ESRD	• Pulsatile mass, neuropathy, skin ecchymosis or necrosis • Bruit, duplex	Observation, U/S-guided compression, Thrombin injection, endovascular or surgical repair

Based on data from Sambol E, McKinsey J. Local complications: endovascular. In: Cronenwett J, Johnston W, editors. Rutherford's vascular surgery. 7th ed. Philadelphia, PA: W.B. Saunders; 2010

and therapeutic cardiac catheterization [46]. In a multivariate analysis, congestive heart failure, female gender, and therapeutic catheterization were found to be significantly predictive of vascular injury. A spectrum of management schemes are employed for each of these unique complications and may range from observation and serial examination to major vascular reconstruction (see Table 11.4). The decision to intervene is based on the physiologic status of the patient, impact of the complication on lower extremity perfusion, and local tissue effects of the lesion.

Closure Devices

Besides the initial complications that may result from arterial access, difficulties can be encountered when attempting to achieve hemostasis with sheath removal. Arterial closure following percutaneous coronary intervention has received considerable attention; however, relatively little investigation has occurred in patients with peripheral vascular disease. Much enthusiasm has been reported in the utilization of arterial closure devices in an effort to minimize patient discomfort with manual compression, as well as attempting to reduce pseudoaneurysm and hematoma formation rates. Starnes et al. evaluated a suture-mediated closure device specifically in vascular surgery patients with femoral artery calcification in a randomized trial comparing manual compression with suture-mediated closure device in 102 patients [47]. While they achieved hemostasis with a suture-mediated closure device in 49 of 52 attempts, six complications occurred, two of which were major and required reoperative intervention. Mackrell et al. described a 95% deployment success rate in 500 patients undergoing peripheral vascular interventions; however, seven patients suffered a major complication, including one death from a retroperitoneal hematoma, and three episodes of limb ischemia, all of which required operative or lytic intervention [48]. Wilson et al. described complications occurring in ten patients following use of percutaneous arterial closure devices in a vascular surgery practice, noting six arterial infections, all of which required operative drainage, and four patients required arterial reconstruction [49]. Lastly, while not focusing on vascular surgery patients specifically, a systematic review of arterial puncture closure devices performed in 2004 studied the results from randomized trials of several different closure devices compared to manual compression [50]. This meta-analysis assimilated data from over 4,000 patients across 30 randomized trials, although many of these trials were judged to be of poor methodologic quality. While time to hemostasis was overall shorter if patients received a closure device (mean difference of 1 min, range 14–19 min), the risk of hematoma was nearly twice as high (relative risk [RR] 1.89, 95% confidence interval [CI] 1.13–3.15) and risk of pseudoaneurysm was over five times as high (RR 5.40, 95% CI 1.21–24.5) in patients who received a closure device compared with those who received manual compression.

In an attempt to standardize and improve outcomes resulting from percutaneous arterial access, Goodney et al. described implementation of a percutaneous arterial closure protocol that led to a decrease in complications after endovascular interventions in vascular surgery (Fig. 11.4) [51]. Interestingly, despite an overall reduction in the use of closure devices pre- and postimplementation of the protocol (57–32%, $P<0.01$), the closure device failure rate also decreased from 23 to 7% ($P<0.01$), underscoring the utility of a selective approach in the application of these new technologies. The influence of arterial calcification, vessel tortuosity, and previous groin scar may have significant impact on the success or failure of a suture-mediated or collagen-plug closure device [51].

Lesion Treatment Complications: Thrombosis, Dissection, Embolization, Perforation

In many cases of peripheral vascular intervention, the most treacherous part of the procedure is crossing the lesion, whether it is stenotic or occlusive. In cases of stenotic lesions, attempts to gain wire access may result in dissection, in situ thrombosis, embolization, or perforation. Dissection or thrombosis may convert a stenosis into an occlusion, potentially precipitating a change in treatment plan. Intentional subintimal angioplasty with distal vessel reentry (with or without reentry catheters) is increasingly being performed due to the treatment of TASC II C/D lesions [52]. This can lead to perforation or "shearing off" important collateral vessels, leading to diminished pedal perfusion. If a guide-wire perforation occurs, this can safely be observed in most cases; however, some reports of stent grafting, balloon tamponade, coil embolization, and direct open surgical repair have been described to manage this complication. Peripheral microembolization from wire manipulation of friable aortoiliac or superficial femoral atherosclerotic plaque may cause "trash foot" or blue-toe syndrome. Small fragments of clot may form in situ and embolize; this situation is frequently not amenable to endovascular salvage. Anticoagulation with or without thrombolysis and supportive measures are often required. If larger particles are recognized in the peripheral arterial bed, attempts at suction embolectomy can be made through the existing arterial access. If these attempts are unsuccessful, surgical embolectomy and occasional open surgical bypass may be needed to restore pedal perfusion. This dreaded complication emphasizes the need for caution when attempting to cross lesions and limiting repeated attempted intervention when initial treatment is unsuccessful.

The frequency of peripheral embolization during superficial femoral artery (SFA) intervention is probably underreported or not readily recognized in most cases. This point is highlighted in a study by Muller-Hulsbeck and colleagues who treated 29 patients for disabling claudication with the intent to evaluate the safety and efficacy of a debris-capture distal embolic protection system (FilterWire EZ EPS, Boston Scientific, Mountain View, CA). Of the 30 filters placed, 27 (90%) had macroscopic debris with particle sizes ranging from 90 to 2,000 μm (mean 1,200 ± 640 μm) [52]. Fortunately, there is little to no clinical impact on patency rates and limb salvage if distal embolization events are recognized and managed successfully with endovascular techniques [53].

Complications of PTA/Stent: Deployment Failure, Inappropriate Sizing, Jailing Collaterals, Fracture, Restenosis

Because of the enthusiasm from short- and mid-term outcome data of endovascular revascularization in the lower extremity, practitioners are

11 Managing Complications of Vascular Surgery and Endovascular Therapy

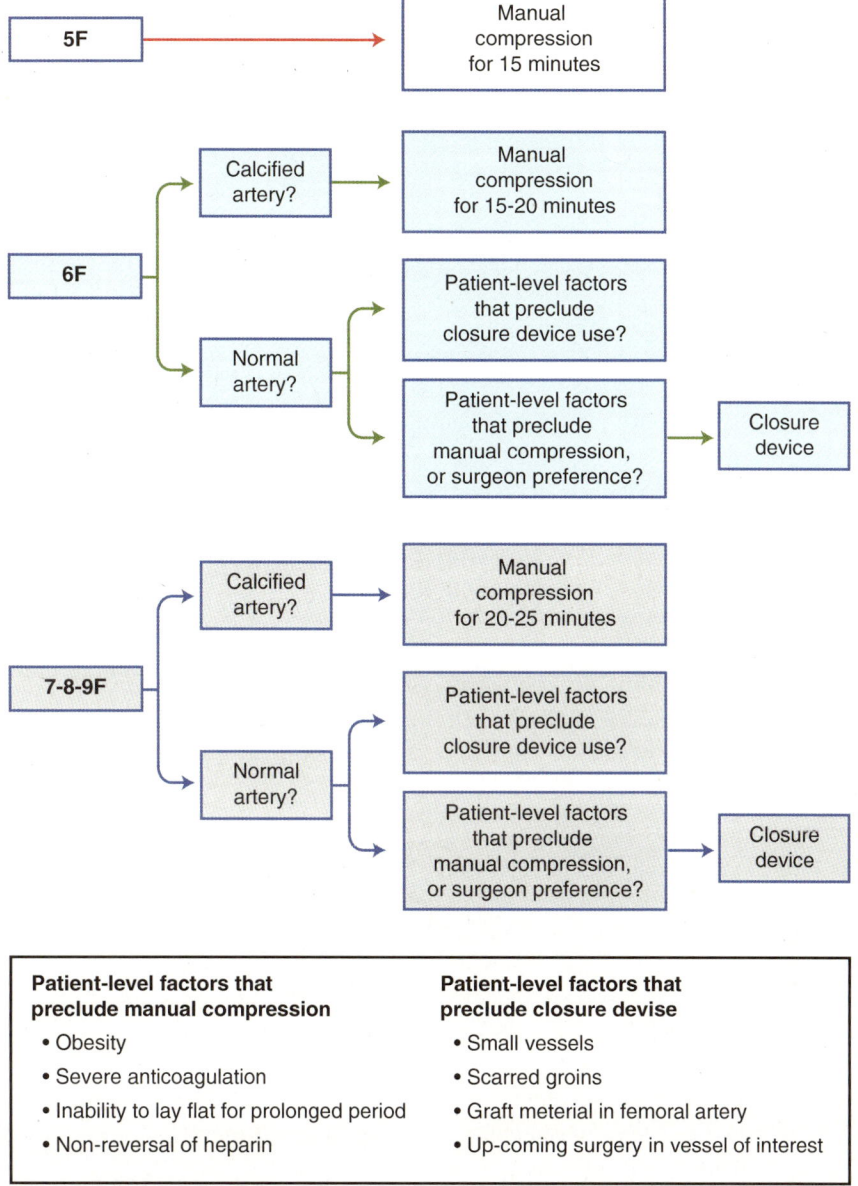

Fig. 11.4 Algorithm depicting a proposed vascular surgery arterial closure protocol to reduce arterial access complications with peripheral vascular intervention (reprinted from Goodney PP, Chang RW, Cronenwett JL. A percutaneous arterial closure protocol can decrease complications after endovascular interventions in vascular surgery patients. J Vasc Surg. 2008;48(6):1481–8. With permission from Elsevier)

attempting to treat more complex lesions. Increasing lesion complexity often leads to the need for endoluminal stent placement [53]. Some providers advocate a primary stent placement strategy, particularly in the SFA, which invites the potential for additional technical considerations and resultant complications [54] (Fig. 11.5).

Larger sheath access and crossing profiles may increase the risk of access-related or lesion treatment complications (see above). Inappropriate sizing, deployment failure, and stent fracture (in up to 10% of cases; range 2–65%) are all additional complications that can occur with endovascular revascularization of the lower extremity

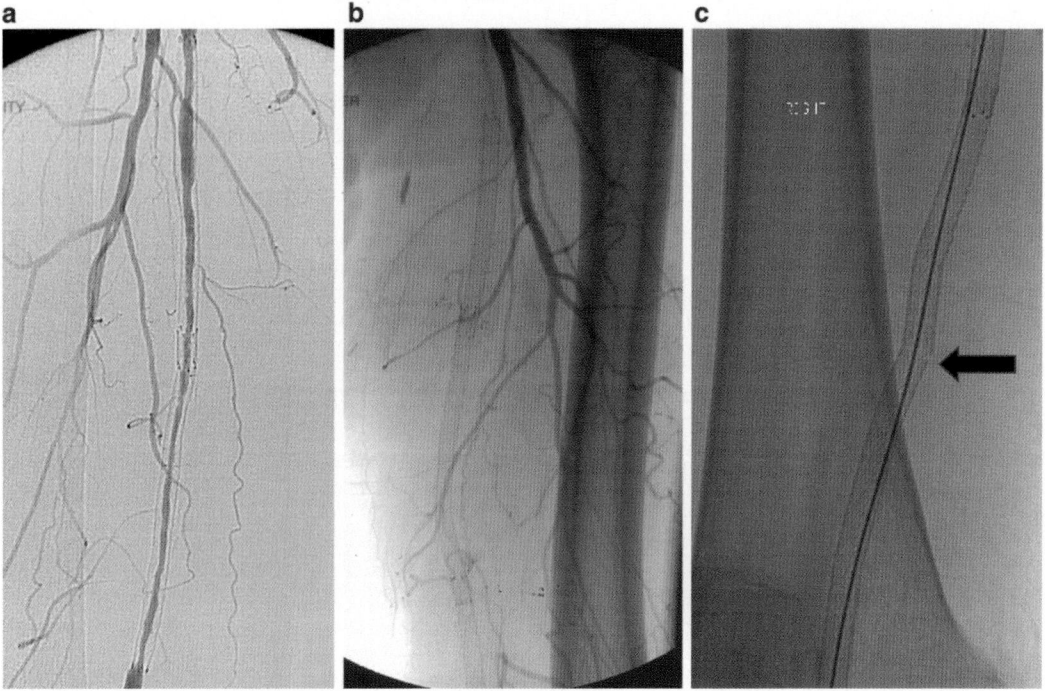

Fig. 11.5 Examples of complications resulting from stent placement. This figure demonstrates common complications of SFA stent placement, including: (**a**) Neointimal hyperplasia with resultant in-stent restenosis. (**b**) Thrombosed SFA stent. (**c**) Stent fracture

[52]. In the rare event of stent maldeployment, frequently as a result of vessel tortuosity and/or calcification, attempts at balloon retrieval, endoluminal snaring, or placement into relatively normal vessel can be made. If the stent cannot be salvaged and stent embolization occurs, a second stent to trap or crush the stent can sometimes be used or open stent retrieval may be required.

Another troubling complication of stent placement is the loss of collateral blood flow as a result of "jailing" the orifice of these vessels. This can be particularly problematic in the scenario of stent thrombosis. A common perception is that the mechanism of stent thrombosis, not unlike prosthetic bypass thrombosis, leads to a more virulent clinical presentation than autologous bypass failure. Due to the quaternary referral pattern of our practice, we are particularly sensitive to this issue and advocate using the shortest stent possible that avoids large collateral vessel coverage when possible. Preoperative CT angiography or duplex interrogation in conjunction with careful intraoperative decision making can lead to avoidance of sacrificing these important collateral perfusion beds.

The most common complication of peripheral intervention is late failure as a result of neointimal hyperplasia. Two-year primary patency of SFA stent placement for disabling claudication ranges from 44 to 58%; however, excellent primary-assisted patency (92%) can be anticipated with an aggressive surveillance protocol [55]. Many factors have been reported to be associated with stent restenosis in the femoral–popliteal segment, including female gender, low ABI (<0.6), TASC II C/D lesions, and stent fracture [56]. There is an emerging literature to support the use of duplex surveillance, as well as pharmacologic adjuncts such as clopidogrel and/or cilostazol, to mitigate the impact of neointimal hyperplasia development after endoluminal stent placement; however, prospective validation is lacking. Promising reports demonstrating the feasibility of drug-eluting balloons and stents has begun to emerge, however, comparative effectiveness studies will be needed to validate their efficacy and define their role in the contemporary treatment paradigm of infrainguinal artery occlusive disease in the diabetic patient.

Amputation and Other Considerations

For many vascular surgeons, major amputation is considered a failure, and the merits of limb salvage require little discussion. Although the literature is replete with descriptions of techniques and results, few series describe the functional outcomes of lower extremity revascularization. The fundamental consideration of determining good patient selection that will gain the best long-term functional outcome is undertaken with relatively little guidance. Indeed, it is important to point out that if one begins the decision-making process without understanding if the patient will derive benefit with limb salvage attempts, revascularization leads to accumulation of cost, hospitalization, and attendant morbidity and mortality without reward. Simply stated, the goal of revascularization should be to optimize the patient's ability to ambulate and live independently. A sobering reminder of the frequency of failure to achieve "success" with infrainguinal revascularization in the setting of diabetic patients with ischemic tissue loss is a report from Taylor and colleagues [57] that sited an 85.2% probability of failure to achieve patient-oriented outcome measures of clinical success (as defined by patency of reconstruction until wound healing, limb salvage at 1 year, maintenance of ambulation at 1 year, and survival for 1 year). Frequently, the success or failure of infrainguinal arterial reconstruction is not determined by the method of revascularization or defined by surgeon-centered outcomes of amputation-free survival and reintervention rates. With these data in mind, improved patient and family counseling can be undertaken prior to an attempt at lower extremity revascularization so that optimal patient outcomes can be achieved.

References

1. Bergamini TM, et al. Experience with in situ saphenous vein bypasses during 1981 to 1989: determinant factors of long-term patency. J Vasc Surg. 1991;13(1):137–47. Discussion 148–9.
2. Sladen JG, Gilmour JL. Vein graft stenosis. Characteristics and effect of treatment. Am J Surg. 1981;141(5):549–53.
3. Berceli SA, et al. Surgical and endovascular revision of infrainguinal vein bypass grafts: analysis of midterm outcomes from the PREVENT III trial. J Vasc Surg. 2007;46(6):1173–9.
4. Bandyk DF, et al. Durability of the in situ saphenous vein arterial bypass: a comparison of primary and secondary patency. J Vasc Surg. 1987;5(2):256–68.
5. Cohen JR, et al. Recognition and management of impending vein-graft failure. Importance for long-term patency. Arch Surg. 1986;121(7):758–9.
6. Bandyk DF, et al. Durability of vein graft revision: the outcome of secondary procedures. J Vasc Surg. 1991;13(2):200–8. Discussion 209–10.
7. Rzucidlo EM, et al. Prediction of early graft failure with intraoperative completion duplex ultrasound scan. J Vasc Surg. 2002;36(5):975–81.
8. Bandyk DF, et al. Monitoring functional patency of in situ saphenous vein bypasses: the impact of a surveillance protocol and elective revision. J Vasc Surg. 1989;9(2):286–96.
9. Seeger JM, et al. Potential predictors of outcome in patients with tissue loss who undergo infrainguinal vein bypass grafting. J Vasc Surg. 1999;30(3):427–35.
10. Stept LL, et al. Technical defects as a cause of early graft failure after femorodistal bypass. Arch Surg. 1987;122(5):599–604.
11. Donaldson MC, Mannick JA, Whittemore AD. Causes of primary graft failure after in situ saphenous vein bypass grafting. J Vasc Surg. 1992;15(1):113–8. Discussion 118–20.
12. Raffetto JD, et al. Differences in risk factors for lower extremity arterial occlusive disease. J Am Coll Surg. 2005;201(6):918–24.
13. Gibson KD, et al. Identification of factors predictive of lower extremity vein graft thrombosis. J Vasc Surg. 2001;33(1):24–31.
14. Woodburn KR, et al. Clinical, biochemical, and rheologic factors affecting the outcome of infrainguinal bypass grafting. J Vasc Surg. 1996;24(4):639–46.
15. Saltzberg SS, et al. Outcome of lower-extremity revascularization in patients younger than 40 years in a predominantly diabetic population. J Vasc Surg. 2003;38(5):1056–9.
16. Taylor Jr LM, Edwards JM, Porter JM. Present status of reversed vein bypass grafting: five-year results of a modern series. J Vasc Surg. 1990;11(2):193–205. Discussion 205–6.
17. Neville RF, Tempesta B, Sidway AN. Tibial bypass for limb salvage using polytetrafluoroethylene and a

distal vein patch. J Vasc Surg. 2001;33(2):266–71. Discussion 271–2.
18. Neville RF, et al. Distal vein patch with an arteriovenous fistula: a viable option for the patient without autogenous conduit and severe distal occlusive disease. J Vasc Surg. 2009;50(1):83–8.
19. Moawad J, Gagne P. Adjuncts to improve patency of infrainguinal prosthetic bypass grafts. Vasc Endovascular Surg. 2003;37(6):381–6.
20. Erickson CA, et al. Ongoing vascular laboratory surveillance is essential to maximize long-term in situ saphenous vein bypass patency. J Vasc Surg. 1996;23(1):18–26. Discussion 26–7.
21. Rhodes JM, et al. The benefits of secondary interventions in patients with failing or failed pedal bypass grafts. Am J Surg. 1999;178(2):151–5.
22. Nguyen LL, et al. Infrainguinal vein bypass graft revision: factors affecting long-term outcome. J Vasc Surg. 2004;40(5):916–23.
23. Landry GJ, et al. Long-term outcome of revised lower-extremity bypass grafts. J Vasc Surg. 2002;35(1):56–62. Discussion 62–3.
24. Pomposelli FB, et al. A decade of experience with dorsalis pedis artery bypass: analysis of outcome in more than 1000 cases. J Vasc Surg. 2003;37(2):307–15.
25. Sullivan Jr TR, et al. Clinical results of common strategies used to revise infrainguinal vein grafts. J Vasc Surg. 1996;24(6):909–17. Discussion 917–9.
26. Schneider PA, Caps MT, Nelken N. Infrainguinal vein graft stenosis: cutting balloon angioplasty as the first-line treatment of choice. J Vasc Surg. 2008;47(5):960–6. Discussion 966.
27. Alpert JR, et al. Treatment of vein graft stenosis by balloon catheter dilation. JAMA. 1979;242(25):2769–71.
28. Simosa HF, et al. Predictors of failure after angioplasty of infrainguinal vein bypass grafts. J Vasc Surg. 2009;49(1):117–21.
29. Whittemore AD, et al. Secondary femoropopliteal reconstruction. Ann Surg. 1981;193(1):35–42.
30. Belkin M, et al. Observations on the use of thrombolytic agents for thrombotic occlusion of infrainguinal vein grafts. J Vasc Surg. 1990;11(2):289–94. Discussion 295–6.
31. Nackman GB, et al. Thrombolysis of occluded infrainguinal vein grafts: predictors of outcome. J Vasc Surg. 1997;25(6):1023–31. Discussion 1031–2.
32. Belkin M. Secondary bypass after infrainguinal bypass graft failure. Semin Vasc Surg. 2009;22(4):234–9.
33. Andros G, et al. Arm veins for arterial revascularization of the leg: arteriographic and clinical observations. J Vasc Surg. 1986;4(5):416–27.
34. Harward TR, et al. The use of arm vein conduits during infrageniculate arterial bypass. J Vasc Surg. 1992;16(3):420–6. Discussion 426–7.
35. Greenblatt DY, Rajamanickam V, Mell MW. Predictors of surgical site infection after open lower extremity revascularization. J Vasc Surg. 2011;54(2):433–9.
36. Giles KA, et al. Body mass index: surgical site infections and mortality after lower extremity bypass from the National Surgical Quality Improvement Program 2005-2007. Ann Vasc Surg. 2010;24(1):48–56.
37. Childress BB, et al. Impact of an absorbent silver-eluting dressing system on lower extremity revascularization wound complications. Ann Vasc Surg. 2007;21(5):598–602.
38. Alkon JD, et al. Management of complex groin wounds: preferred use of the rectus femoris muscle flap. Plast Reconstr Surg. 2005;115(3):776–83. Discussion 784–5.
39. Veith FJ. Presidential address: Charles Darwin and vascular surgery. J Vasc Surg. 1997;25(1):8–18.
40. Messina LM, et al. Clinical characteristics and surgical management of vascular complications in patients undergoing cardiac catheterization: interventional versus diagnostic procedures. J Vasc Surg. 1991;13(5):593–600.
41. Nowygrod R, et al. Trends, complications, and mortality in peripheral vascular surgery. J Vasc Surg. 2006;43(2):205–16.
42. Hoffer EK, Bloch RD. Percutaneous arterial closure devices. J Vasc Interv Radiol. 2003;14(7):865–85.
43. Singh H, et al. Quality improvement guidelines for diagnostic arteriography. J Vasc Interv Radiol. 2003;14(9 Pt 2):S283–8.
44. Fitts J, et al. Fluoroscopy-guided femoral artery puncture reduces the risk of PCI-related vascular complications. J Interv Cardiol. 2008;21(3):273–8.
45. Oweida SW, et al. Postcatheterization vascular complications associated with percutaneous transluminal coronary angioplasty. J Vasc Surg. 1990;12(3):310–5.
46. McCann RL, Schwartz LB, Pieper KS. Vascular complications of cardiac catheterization. J Vasc Surg. 1991;14(3):375–81.
47. Starnes BW, et al. Percutaneous arterial closure in peripheral vascular disease: a prospective randomized evaluation of the Perclose device. J Vasc Surg. 2003;38(2):263–71.
48. Mackrell PJ, et al. Can the Perclose suture-mediated closure system be used safely in patients undergoing diagnostic and therapeutic angiography to treat chronic lower extremity ischemia? J Vasc Surg. 2003;38(6):1305–8.
49. Wilson JS, et al. Management of vascular complications following femoral artery catheterization with and without percutaneous arterial closure devices. Ann Vasc Surg. 2002;16(5):597–600.
50. Koreny M, et al. Arterial puncture closing devices compared with standard manual compression after cardiac catheterization: systematic review and meta-analysis. JAMA. 2004;291(3):350–7.
51. Goodney PP, Chang RW, Cronenwett JL. A percutaneous arterial closure protocol can decrease complications after endovascular interventions in vascular surgery patients. J Vasc Surg. 2008;48(6):1481–8.
52. Muller-Hulsbeck S, et al. Final results of the protected superficial femoral artery trial using the FilterWire EZ system. Cardiovasc Intervent Radiol. 2010;33(6): 1120–7.

53. Shrikhande GV, et al. Lesion types and device characteristics that predict distal embolization during percutaneous lower extremity interventions. J Vasc Surg. 2011;53(2):347–52.
54. Scali ST, et al. Long-term results of open and endovascular revascularization of superficial femoral artery occlusive disease. J Vasc Surg. 2011;54(3):714–21.
55. Gallagher KA, et al. Endovascular management as first therapy for chronic total occlusion of the lower extremity arteries: comparison of balloon angioplasty, stenting, and directional atherectomy. J Endovasc Ther. 2011;18(5):624–37.
56. Iida O, et al. Long-term outcomes and risk stratification of patency following nitinol stenting in the femoropopliteal segment: retrospective multicenter analysis. J Endovasc Ther. 2011;18(6):753–61.
57. Taylor SM, et al. Clinical success using patient-oriented outcome measures after lower extremity bypass and endovascular intervention for ischemic tissue loss. J Vasc Surg. 2009;50(3):534–41. Discussion 541.

Diabetes and Lower Extremity Amputation

12

Roman Nowygrod and Nii-Kabu Kabutey

Keywords

Amputation • Rehabilitation • Complications • Transmetatarsal • Below-knee amputation • Above-knee amputation • Diabetes • Syme's • Charcot's • LisFranc's

Introduction

In the United States, the full extent of the diabetic foot problem is unknown. Many of the estimated 14 million diagnosed and undiagnosed diabetics will experience vascular and/or soft tissue lower extremity complications, which when combined with trauma and infection may lead to minor amputation or limb loss. Patients with diabetes have a 15–60 times greater risk than nondiabetics of requiring a lower extremity amputation. Over the past 10 years there has been a 32% increase in the prevalence of diabetes [1]. Dillingham and colleagues reported that diabetic amputees are more likely to be severely disabled, have their initial amputation at a younger age, require more proximal levels of lower extremity amputations, and die at a younger age [2]. Indications for elective lower extremity amputations in diabetics include gangrene, infection, rest pain, and non-healing ulcers. Emergent amputation can be a life-saving procedure especially in diabetics with uncontrolled ascending infections or wet gangrene.

There are between 30,000 and 50,000 new lower extremity amputations performed in the United States each year. It is estimated that two-thirds of lower limb amputations in the United States occur in diabetic patients. Clinical epidemiologic studies suggest that foot ulcers precede approximately 85% of nontraumatic lower extremity amputations in individuals with diabetes [3].

Between 5 and 15% of all diabetics will eventually require a lower extremity amputation during their lifetime. Nearly 50% of patients receiving a lower extremity amputation will require a contralateral amputation [4]. Lower-level amputations (toe, foot, and ankle) were more common in individuals with diabetes than without diabetes. Amputation rates are greater with increasing age, in males compared to females, and among members of racial and ethnic minorities compared to whites [5].

R. Nowygrod, A.B., M.S., M.D. (✉)
Department of Surgery, Columbia University Medical Center, 161 Ft. Washington Ave., New York, NY 10032, USA
e-mail: rn5@columbia.edu

N. Kabutey, M.D.
Department of Surgery, Columbia University Medical Center/Weill Cornell, New York, NY, USA

Brief History of Amputation

Amputations are considered to be one the oldest of surgical procedures. Hand-drawn figures with amputated fingers and limbs on cave walls in France and Spain date back to 5000 BC. Skeletal figures with amputated limbs have been found in Peru that date back to 300 BC. Amputations were performed for a number of indications, including trauma, frostbite, and leprosy. In the Middle East a common reason for amputation was punishment for criminal activities. Early on amputations for medical reasons may have been limited because it was believed that individuals would be deprived of the amputated body part in both this life and the afterlife, it is believed most individuals would have preferred to die with the diseased limb intact.

The first writings on amputation and prosthetic usage were recorded in Sanskrit in the book of Vedas. The leg of Queen Vishpala was amputated in battle and fitted with an iron leg, which allowed her to eventually return to the battlefield [6].

Hippocrates described the use of ligatures to obtain hemostasis. He also advocated amputation at the level of devitalized and angrenous tissue to limit the amount of bleeding. Other methods used to achieve hemostasis throughout history have included boiling oil, turpentine, cautery, vitriol, or crushing of the surgical stump [6].

The technique of early amputations was certainly crude when compared to today's standards. Although Hippocrates had described the use ligatures for hemostasis, this was rarely practiced. Surgeons often worked alone and did not have skilled assistants to help with the timely placement of ligatures. When performing amputations speed was of the essence, especially before the advent of surgical anesthesia. Amputations were performed in a guillotine fashion. Famed Napoleonic era surgeon Dominque Jean Larrey's (1776–1842) average amputation time was three minutes; during one battle he reportedly performed 200 amputations in the first 24 h [6].

Ambroise Paré (1510–1590), a French military surgeon, is noted for important advancements in surgical technique for amputation surgery. He championed the use of vascular ligatures, tourniquets, and developed guidelines to determine the level of amputation. Paré recommended retracting skin and muscle proximally before cutting the bone to allow for additional coverage of the bone [6].

With the advancement of antiseptic techniques and surgical anesthesia, further technical improvements were made with amputations, particularly the amputation stump. Antisepsis and anesthesia allowed more time and more attention for the operative surgeon to concentrate on the stump. The first true simple flap amputation is credited to James Younge of England in 1679. As the construction of the surgical amputation stump improved, prosthetic design and function followed. A mosaic from the Cathedral of Lescar in France dating back to the Roman era shows an amputee supported by a wooden pylon. Peruvian figurines from the second century AD show amputees with cup-like prostheses on their stumps [6].

The oldest recovered prosthesis was made from wood and copper and dates back to 300 BC. During the American Civil War over 30,000 amputations were performed by the Union Army Medical Corps alone; Marks and Hanger helped to develop more functional lower limb prostheses. In 1863, Dubois Parmelee developed the prosthesis suction socket. Marked improvements in postoperative rehabilitation with early fitting of artificial limbs have led to improved function and outcome [6].

Current Amputation Trends

With the advent and increased application of endovascular therapies for the management of peripheral vascular disease, there has been a notable change in the amputation rates performed in the United States. More than 50,000 lower extremity amputations are performed yearly in the United States, with a majority being performed for complications of diabetes and arterial insufficiency. Data from the Nationwide Inpatient Sample and the National Discharge Survey examined between 1998 and 2003 demonstrated a progressive decrease in the national per capita rate of amputations. But both nationally and regionally, mortality rates have declined only slightly [7].

The number of major amputations nationally and the number of major and minor amputations regionally have both declined. For the period 1998–2003, regional state data revealed a 5.8% decrease in volume; nationally, the decrease over the same period was 6.6%. More significantly, however, there has been a 15.6% (state) and 15.2% (national) decrease in major amputations in what continues to be a high-risk group of patients, i.e., those with diabetes (65.9%), hypertension (57.4%), large-vessel peripheral vascular disease (73.1%), coronary artery disease (32.5%), renal insufficiency (22.1%), cerebrovascular disease (10.2%), and COPD (16.3%). Overall mortality is declining, but slowly, and remains more than 6% for major amputations nationally [7].

In the same study, National Inpatient Sample (NIS) data sets and New York State inpatient hospitalizations and outpatient surgeries discharge databases from 1998 through 2007 were used to identify major amputations. The number of major amputations declined by 38% from 59 (95% CI, 54–65) in 1998 to 37 (95% CI, 33–41) per 100,000 population in 2007. This trend was statistically significant [8]. Mortality has declined from 6.9 to 5.3% for major amputation. Mortality for revascularization with major amputation remains quite high but has declined from 12.8% in 1998 to 8.2% in 2007.

Methods

Determining Level

There is no single diagnostic test nor clinical indicator that can alone best determine the optimal level of surgical amputation in diabetic patients. Physician judgment and experience has been shown in studies to be moderately accurate in helping to determine the level of amputation [9].

Accurate physical examination is essential in helping to determine the viability of ischemic tissue and likelihood of healing in diabetic patients. When planning to perform an amputation a careful history and physical examination should be obtained. Surgical scars indicating the presence of metallic knee implants or orthopedic rods can facilitate appropriate procedural planning. Knowledge of the location of stents and patent peripheral bypass grafts may minimize intraprocedural blood loss and help determine levels of amputation as does visual assessment of areas of ischemia, infection, dependent rubor, and erythema. The absence or presence of palpable peripheral pulses can determine the likelihood of postsurgical wound healing. In the study by Dwars et al., a palpable pulse immediately proximal to level of amputation led to a nearly 100% probability of successful wound healing [10].

Intraoperatively, there are a number of indicators that may help determine the viability of the tissue and the likelihood of successful wound closure. Pale discoloration of the subcutaneous fat and muscle may suggest the tissue is malperfused. Lack of muscle bleeding after incision with a scalpel or minimal signs of muscular twitching during contact with electrocautery provide additional clues of poor perfusion.

Accepted goals of amputation surgery include the preservation of limb length, and the removal of all infected or gangrenous tissue to allow for adequate wound healing and to assist in postoperative rehabilitation efforts. The importance of limb length preservation should not be underestimated. Below-knee amputations require a 10–30% increase in energy expenditure, in comparison to 50–70% energy expenditure for above-knee amputations for ambulation [11]. Numerous reports have shown increased successful prosthetic rate usage and rehabilitation for patients with below-knee amputations compared to patients with above-knee amputations. Mobility capability is also a predictor for increased quality of life for patients who have undergone lower limb extremity amputation [12].

Significant mortality rate increases also occur with more proximal levels of amputation with reported rates of 6–10% for below knee amputations, compared to 13–19% for above knee amputations [3, 13].

Noninvasive testing methods have been employed to help to accurately determine amputation levels. Toe pressures of less than 40 mmHg have demonstrated poor healing rates in diabetic patients [14]. Segmental pressures can aid in the prediction of wound healing in below-knee amputations, with absolute ankle pressures above 60 mmHg having an accuracy of 50–90%. However, these methods alone may prove inadequate. ABI's as the major parameter has failed in as many as 50% of predicting Syme's amputation success and any level success in 10–20% of diabetics with calcified noncompliant arteries [15].

Transcutaneous oxygen measurement has been shown by some authors to have high accuracy in predicting wound healing rates, while others have not been able to come to any consensus regarding a consistent transcutaneous oxygen threshold that guarantees wound healing [2]. Factors such as edema, infection, and inflammation will affect measurements.

Additional noninvasive methodologies include a novel diagnostic tool: optical tomographic imaging which is currently under investigation, as well as systemic parameters. Given known impaired wound healing and lymphocytic functional pathophysiology in diabetics, the use of parameters, including albumin levels and lymphocyte counts, has been advocated as useful adjuncts to perfusion determinations [15].

Particularly in diabetics with presumed "small vessel disease," it is important to maximize perfusion prior to debridement or amputation. Interventions which might otherwise be deferred for claudication or even rest pain are essential to help maximize successful outcomes.

Toe Amputation

Amputations of the toe are the most common amputation performed for diabetic patients. Closed amputations of the toes are performed for gangrene, ischemia, or isolated infection not involving bone, soft tissue, or skin at the base of the digit. Determination of extremity vascular examination should be charted, and noninvasive imaging such as an X-ray or magnetic resonance imaging (MRI) should be obtained to document soft tissue infection or bony involvement. Although a number of tests are available to aid in determining the appropriate level of amputation, few of these have been well studied to differentiate the proper operation for forefoot disease.

Ankle or digital nerve block anesthesia is often sufficient for pain control. Incisions may need to be modified based on the extent of compromised tissue. Either a transverse or vertical fish mouth or racket incision can be used as long as there is sufficient tension-free coverage of the transected bone with healthy viable tissue and skin.

All nonhealthy tissue is debrided; deep tissue cultures should be obtained to assist with the determination of appropriate antibiotic coverage for wound care management and infection control. Both the flexor and extensor digit tendons are placed under traction and cut to allow them to retract into the soft tissue so they will not be incorporated into the closure. A bone cutter is next used to disarticulate the phalanx, and the exposed poorly vascularized articular cartilage is removed with rongeurs. Bony sharp edges are removed and the bone edges are smoothened to ensure there is no compression against the suture line or any superficial soft tissue. The wound is copiously irrigated and incision is closed in one layer using nonabsorbable monofilament suture or staples. Care is taken during closure to minimize electrocautery and rough handling of the tissue edges.

Bulky circumferential dressings are used to protect the incision, and weight bearing is minimized until the wound is completely healed. Sutures are left in place for 2–4 weeks to minimize dehiscence. Especially after first toe amputations neuropathic diabetic patients are prone to pressure ulcerations of the interphalangeal joints of the second toe due to varus deformity and hyperextension. Patients often require orthotic fitting to allow for distributive weight bearing of the forefoot. With amputation of the other digits, toe separators can be used to retard migration of the adjacent toes medially to the empty space left by the amputated toe or toes [15].

Ray Amputations

For more extensive infection, gangrene, or ischemia involving the proximal phalanx, a ray amputation involving removal of part or all of the corresponding metatarsal is required. Due to variability in presentation of forefoot lesions, the surgeon must carefully plan his or her incision to ensure that adequate wide debridement is performed to rid the wound of devascularized and infected tissue. In addition, adequate soft tissue coverage is required to allow for tension-free wound closure. A racket incision allows for adequate proximal metatarsal bone exposure. Both the flexor and extensor tendons are divided under tension to allow for retraction. The metatarsal shaft is then divided with a bone cutter or oscillating saw, and sharp bone edges are cleared from the wound. A small periosteal elevator applied parallel to the metatarsal shaft is used to circumferentially separate the soft tissue attachments along the metatarsal shaft, being careful to limit injury to the associated adjacent neurovascular bundles. Incisions are closed with nonabsorbable monofilament suture or staples and dressed with bulky dressings. All patients are nonweight bearing until incisions are well healed, and often they will require specialized footwear or insoles.

Additional cautions include avoidance of resecting more than one ray because of subsequent difficulties with prosthetic fitting; with first toe amputations, proximal phalangeal preservation is important for maintaining pedal stability [15].

Transmetatarsal Amputation

Indications for transmetatarsal amputations include extensive gangrene or ischemia involving the forefoot. When three or more digits require a ray amputation a transmetatarsal amputation may be more desirable due to improved healing rates and rehabilitation. Advantages of transmetatarsal amputations in comparison to more proximal amputations include preservation of the attachments of the tibialis anterior and peroneous brevis tendons, allowing for active dorsiflexion during ambulation and near-normal ambulatory mechanics. Additionally, if a long stump can be fashioned, most patients can use regular footwear.

A plantar flap is created by incising the skin at the level of distal metatarsal heads. The flap must be vascularized and long enough to cover the metatarsal bone transections. The dorsal incision is made across the foot at the distal or midmetatarsal level. Both the flexor and extensor tendons are sharply cut under tension to allow for retraction. The bone is divided with an oscillating power saw; sharp edges are contoured with rongeurs and raspers to ensure there is no tension on the closure. The wound is irrigated and bleeding is controlled with judicious electrocautery usage and suture ligatures. The myofascial layer is generally closed with interrupted absorbable sutures, but may be left open to avoid tension or tissue necrosis. The skin is closed with interrupted nonabsorbable monofilament sutures or staples. A bulky dressing is applied and the patient is non-weight bearing for the treated extremity until flap integrity and wound healing is attained. Flap ischemia for all foot level amputations may not be manifest for several days, so close sustained scrutiny during the postoperative period is necessary.

LisFranc's Amputation (Tarsometatarsal Disarticulation)

A Lisfranc amputation should be considered when there in not enough skin or soft tissue coverage to adequately cover a transmetatarsal amputation without undue tension. A plantar soft tissue flap is constructed to overlie the tarsometatarsal disarticulation plane. Excision occurs through the first, third, fourth, and fifth tarsometatarsal joints, preserving 1–2 cm of the second metatarsal distal to the medial cuneiform. The plantar ligaments attached to the second metatarsal provides stability to the medial cuneiform. In order to reduce the development of equinovarus deformity, care is taken to retain the base of the fifth metatarsal to maintain the attachments of peroneus brevis and peroneus tertius tendons. An option to help avoid the occurrence of equinus deformity is performance of an Achilles tendonectomy after wound irrigation and closure [15].

Chopart's Amputation

This amputation is a disarticulation through the talonavicular and calcaneocuboid joints often together with an associated Achilles tendonectomy to help prevent equinus deformities. Historically, Chopart's amputation was associated with a high failure rate due to the development of equinovarus deformity and poor rehabilitative outcomes. Recent procedural modifications have significantly improved clinical outcomes and reduced complication rates. A posterior flap can provide adequate wound coverage. After incision and soft tissue debridement, the extensor digitorum longus tendons are divided under tension. The anterior tibial tendon and extensor hallucis longus tendons may be reattached to the talus and an Achilles tendonectomy is performed [16] (Figs. 12.1, 12.2, and 12.3).

Syme's Amputation

Syme's amputation is disarticulation at the level of the ankle joint. It is a technique that is indicated for diabetic patients with suitable vascular perfusion and intact skin, soft tissue, and bone at the level of the hindfoot. Major advantages of the technique include preservation of limb length, which can facilitate patient's lateral transfer when compared to a below-knee amputation. The tough plantar heel surface allows for partial weight bearing. Disadvantages of the procedure include leg length discrepancy, which may lead to proximal or contralateral joint stress, or inadequate perfusion leading to flap ischemia or ulceration.

The dorsal skin incision is made just distal to the medial and lateral malleolus across the ankle. The incision is extended vertically towards the plantar surface at the level of the malleolar tips to join at the sole. The dorsalis pedis artery is identified and ligated. The dorsal incision is extended to the dome of the talus bone. Extensor tendons are sharply ligated and allowed to retract. The collateral ligaments of the ankle are divided, ensuring the posterial tibial artery is not injured during dissection. Care must also be taken when freeing the heel pad from its calcaneal attachment to ensure the skin is not disrupted. Disarticulation of the joint can be performed with a broad bone elevator. The malleoli are divided with an oscillating saw at the tibial plateau. The heel pad is stabilized to the undersurface of the tibia by stitching it the anterior tibia and fibular surfaces. The incision is closed in layers and dressed with a bulky dressing. The patient is nonweight bearing until adequate wound healing, which usually occurs in 4–6 weeks [15].

Below-Knee Amputation

Transtibial amputations are indicated for diabetic patients with extensive ischemia, pain, or gangrene of the lower extremity deemed to have sufficient blood supply and viable tissue flaps to heal the stump. There are several flap reconstruction techniques which have been used to close the incisions

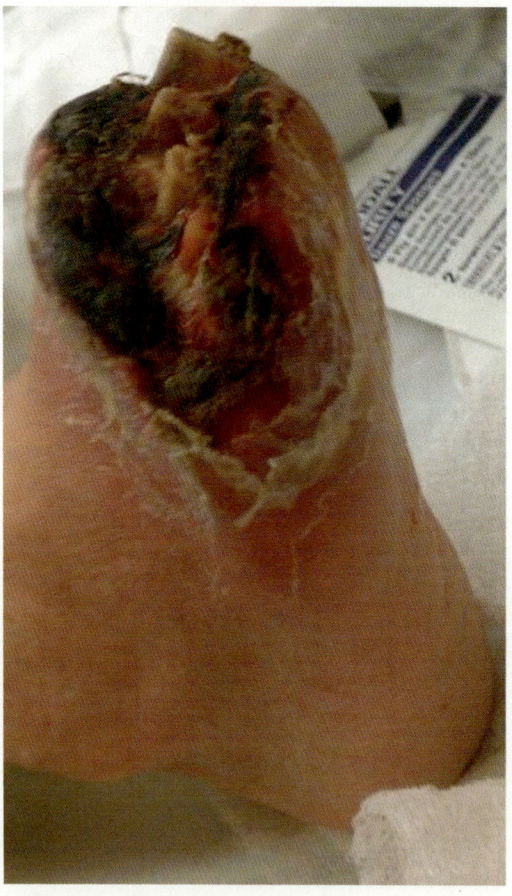

Fig. 12.1 Failed closed transmetatarsal amputation may still be salvageable with a Lisfranc or Chopart amputation if perfusion is adequate and infection is treated

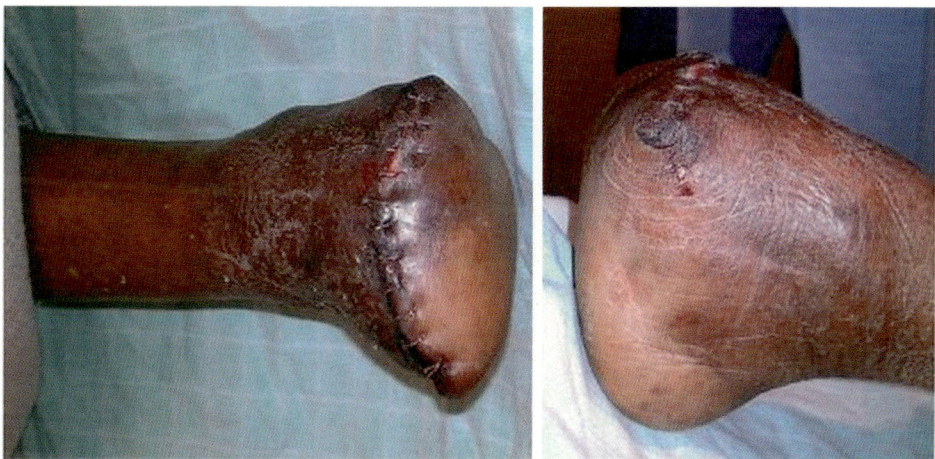

Fig. 12.2 Proximal Chopart and Lisfranc amputations with heel platform preservation, are preferable to major above- or below-knee amputations for ambulatory rehabilitation

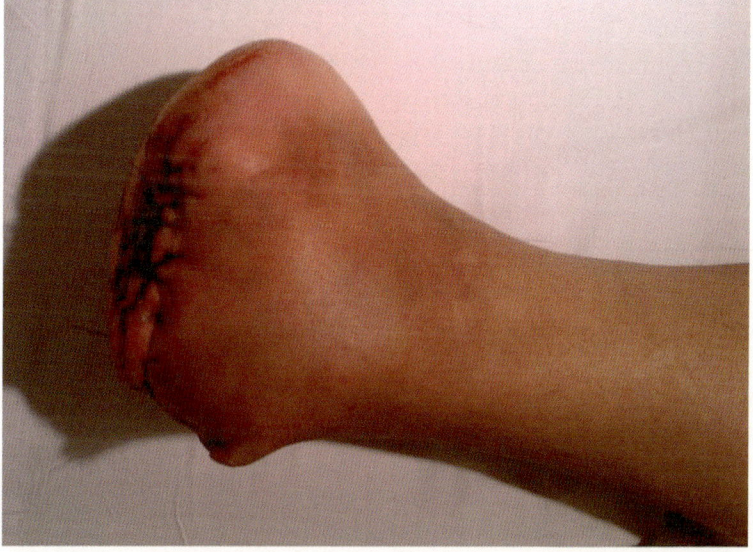

Fig. 12.3 Patient with extensive mid plantar foot wound. Standard flap construction may require modification to achieve adequate coverage, but can still lead to pedal preservation

and ultimately aid in prosthetic fitting and rehabilitation. The below-knee stump is more prone to decubitus ulceration and may not be the most appropriate therapeutic option for patients with knee contractures or patients confined to bedrest.

A posterior myocutaneous flap that utilizes soleus and gastrocnemius muscle fibers to cover the tibia and fibula bone fragments is a commonly used technique. The tibial tuberosity is used as a landmark to help determine where the anterior incisions should begin, optimally tibia should be divided approximately 10–12 cm below the tuberosity, or 14 cm below the knee joint. Depending on swelling, edema, and the size of the patient's leg, the diameter of the anterior incision should be approximately half to two-thirds the circumference of the leg. The length of the posterior flap should be approximately one-third the leg's circumference. After careful incision planning, the anterior skin subcutaneous tissue and fascia are incised to the tibia. The greater saphenous vein is ligated. The tibia and fibula are circumferentially stripped of periosteum 1–2 cm above the edge of the skin flap. The tibia is transected in a beveled fashion to reduce the direct pressure of sharp edges against the anterior flap. The fibula is transected proximal to the level of the tibial transection. To reduce blood loss during dissection, the neurovascular bundles are individually identified, and the anterior tibial artery, posterior tibial artery, and peroneal artery are clamped and ligated or suture ligated under direct visualization. The tibial and peroneal nerves are placed under traction and sharply divided to help avoid neuroma formation.

Incision of the posterior flap is completed. The transition point between the anterior and posterior flap should be gently curved to help decrease the formation of dog ears. Careful construction of the posterior flap is essential to ensure that there is sufficient coverage of the tibia. Proper shaping of the stump also allows for earlier prosthetic fitting and rehabilitation. However, flap perfusion is paramount and should not be compromised for immediate operative appearance. Bulky flaps will subsequently mold over time with resolution of edema and muscle atrophy.

The gastrocnemius muscle provides cushioning and coverage for tibial bone, the soleus muscle is transected near the level of the tibia osteotomy. The wound is copiously irrigated and both the fascial layer and skin are closed without tension. To help prevent postoperative knee flexion, which can severely hamper timely rehabilitation and utilization of a prosthetic device, the use of a knee immobilizer and early aggressive physical therapy are important therapeutic adjuncts.

Knee Disarticulation

Through-knee amputation is a surgical option for selected patients. The operation results in a longer lever arm than the above-knee amputations, facilitating patient rehabilitation. The broadly shaped stump allows for the construction of an end weight-bearing prostheses, which provides greater comfort and stability than the ischial weight bearing above-knee prostheses.

The operation can be performed under regional or local anesthesia. Equal length anterior and posterior flaps are constructed at the level of the tibial tuberosity. The patellar tendon is transected from its tibial attachment. The knee joint capsule is circumferentially incised, followed by transection of the medial and lateral collateral ligaments and the anterior and posterior collateral ligaments. The popliteal artery and vein are identified and doubly ligated or sutured ligated. The tibial nerve is sharply incised and allowed to retract to prevent neuroma formation. The gastrocnemius muscle and all remaining extensor attachments are divided prior to knee disarticulation. The femoral condyles are transected. In the modified Gritti–Stokes amputation, the patellar tendon is sutured to the underside of the transected femoral condyles. The wound is irrigated and closed in layers [17].

Above-Knee Amputation

The level chosen for an above-knee amputation can be quite variable depending on the patient's presenting pathology, symptoms, and clinical examination. For postoperative ambulation and rehabilitation, longer limb length is facilitative. Fish mouth or circular incisions are the commonly used techniques for wound closure. The skin and subcutaneous tissue and fascia are incised. The greater saphenous vein and superficial femoral artery and vein are dissected and ligated or suture ligated. Periosteal elevators are used to circumferentially elevate the periosteum 2–4 cm above the skin incision. An oscillating saw is used to transect the femur and sharp edges are smoothened with a rasp. Care must be taken to factor in postoperative anatomical changes that may occur that can change the stump configuration such as muscle atrophy and resolution of edema. Bone transection too distally will increase the potential for dependent flap tension and may lead to operative revision if the stump flap becomes compromised. The sciatic nerve is sharply transected under tension. The wound is copiously irrigated, the fascia is closed with absorbable suture, and the skin is closed with nonabsorbable monofilament or staples.

Hip Disarticulation

Hip disarticulation is rarely performed procedure accounting for only 0.5% of lower extremity amputations in the United States. The procedure is primarily performed for resection of musculoskeletal malignancies, but occasionally severe infection or gangrene may necessitate hip disarticulation [18]. Hip disarticulation is an amputation through the hip joint. The anterior incision is started medial to the anterior superior iliac spine, descending medially over the pubic bone to the gluteal crease. The posterior incision descends from the anterior superior iliac spine to the greater trochanter and then extends posterior to the gluteal crease. The skin, soft tissue, and fascia are excised and the femoral neurovascular bundle is identified below the inguinal ligament. The femoral artery and vein are doubly ligated and the femoral nerve is sharply transected under tension to allow for the nerve to retract proximally. One technique which can be useful in controlling hemorrhage in selected cases is the use of percutaneous iliac artery occlusion by intraluminal balloon tamponade [19]. The sartorius muscle is transected from its proximal anterior superior iliac spine attachment. The gracilis, iliopsoas, pectineus, and adductors are divided at their origin. The obturator neurovascular vessel is identified near the adductor brevis muscle; these vessels must be controlled and ligated. The flexor muscles are divided at the ischial tuberosity. The hip is flexed to allow for adequate posterior exposure. The tensor fascia lata, gluteus maximus, and rectus femoris muscles are transected with electrocautery. The hip joint is exposed and the joint capsule is incised. The sciatic nerve is sharply transected to allow for retraction into the soft tissue. Once the specimen is removed, the wound is copiously irrigated. The acetabulum is covered by approximating the obturator externus and gluteus medius to one another. The quadratus femoris is sutured to the iliopsoas. The glueal fascia is secured to the inguinal ligament. The skin is closed with suture or staples [3].

Guillotine and Open Amputations

Open amputations and guillotine amputations of the foot and leg are indicated for patients with severe uncontrolled ascending infections, wet gangrene, and metabolic or hemodynamic compromise directly related the compromised extremity. A guillotine amputation is defined as a circular cut through the skin, soft tissue, and bone at the same anatomical level, with no attempt of wound closure at the time of initial operation. The initial guillotine amputation can be more quickly performed minimizing operative time, blood loss, and sepsis. Pedal guillotine amputations are usually performed at the level of the ankle just proximal to the malleoli. This distal incision will allow for construction of flaps and potential wound closure once the acute infectious process has subsided. The skin and soft tissue are incised with a scalpel down to the level of the tibia and fibula bone. Vascular control is obtained with suture ligation to minimize blood loss. An oscillating saw is used to transect the bone. Once hemostasis is obtained the wound is covered with a moist sponge and a bulky dressing. Conversion to a below-knee amputation can be performed after an appropriate length of treatment with antibiotics and resolution of systemic toxicity. For infection or wet gangrene that has extended beyond the level of the hindfoot, a high level of guillotine amputation may be required and conversion to either an above knee amputation may be necessary.

An open amputation removes the gangrenous or infected tissue with no attempt at surgical closure during the initial procedure. Adjunctive therapies that may aid in open wound closure and decrease the time to closure and subsequent rehabilitation include negative pressure vacuum-assisted closure and skin grafting. The vacuum-assisted closure system promotes wound healing and tissue granulation by creating a localized controlled subatmospheric environment. A sealed foam is placed over the wound and connected to a vacuum pump. In a large multicenter randomized trial comparing negative pressure

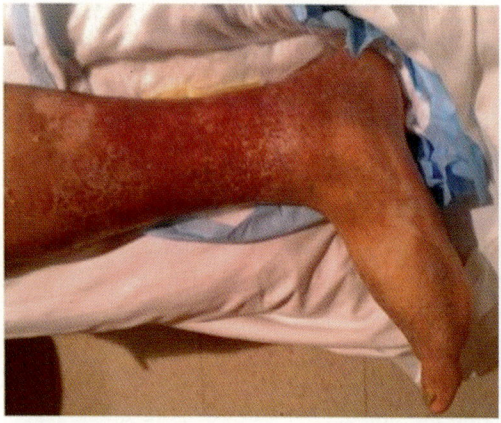
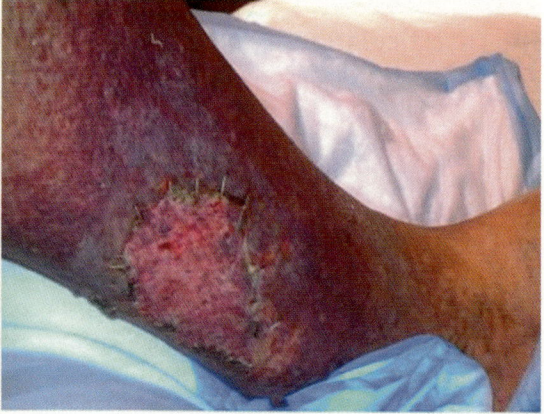

Fig. 12.4 In the presence of both arterial and venous insufficiency, with appropriate revasularization, control of edema, and venous hypertension, debridement and skin grafting may preclude the need for amputation

wound therapy to advanced moist wound therapy, negative pressure wound therapy was shown to be safe and efficacious for the treatment of diabetic foot wounds. A greater proportion of foot ulcers achieved complete wound closure in a shorter period of time with vacuum assisted closure [20]. In another multicenter trial specifically examining the use of negative pressure wound therapy for partial diabetic foot amputations, Armstrong et al. demonstrated more patients had complete healing in the negative pressure wound therapy group (56%) than the control group (39%). The rate of healing was also faster in the negative pressure wound therapy group [21].

Split thickness skin grafting is also a useful technique that can be implemented to obtain skin coverage over granulated tissue open amputation wounds (Fig. 12.4). Consideration must be taken for patients with diabetic neuropathy to ensure skin grafts does not overlie weight-bearing surfaces as these areas will be prone to reulceration.

Complications

There are numerous reported complications associated with lower extremity amputations. These include postoperative bleeding, wound infections, pain, flap necrosis, reamputation, and death.

Diabetic patients undergoing lower extremity amputations often have preexisting comorbidities which to the morbidity and mortality attributed to the surgical procedures. Despite continued improvements in the perioperative treatment and care of patients undergoing major amputation, the mortality and complication rates still remain quite high. Interestingly, in a recent NSQIP-based survey of several thousand patients of risk factors for below-knee amputation, diabetes alone if not associated with sepsis, renal or cardiac disease was not an independent predictor increased morbidity or mortality [1].

Several reports in the literature reveal that as the level of lower extremity amputation progresses more proximally, the operative mortality rate increases. Pollard and colleagues retrospectively examined transmetatarsal amputations in 90 patients. The 30-day perioperative mortality rate was 1.98% [22]. A study using the National Surgical Quality Improvement Program database examined 30-day postoperative mortality of 2,911 patients who underwent below-knee amputations. The authors reported a 7% 30-day mortality rate with 1,627 complications in 1,013 patients. Multivariate logistic regression analysis demonstrated that renal insufficiency, preoperative sepsis, COPD, increased age, and cardiac pathology all were independent risk factors for increased mortality rates [1]. Operative mortality for above-knee amputations range 10–18% [2].

Bleeding, infection, ischemia, and poor judgment or surgical technique can all lead to wound complications. Diabetic patients often have poor blood supply and compromised healing, making them prone to wound complications. The rate of wound complications has been documented to be as high as 30%. Data from the National Surgical Quality Improvement Program database has demonstrated that wound complications occurred in approximately 10.4% of below-knee amputations and 7.2% of above-knee amputations [1]. Amputation stump infection is a common complication in diabetics. Some studies have demonstrated that prophylactic antibiotic therapy significantly reduces the rate of stump infection and reamputation [23].

Diabetic patients are more likely to require reamputation. In a retrospective cohort study examining the risk of reamputation in 277 diabetic patients, the 1-year, 3-year and 5-year cumulative reamputation rate were respectively 26.7%, 48.3%, and 60.7%. A majority of patients required reamputation of the ipsilateral limb within 6 months or primary amputation [24].

In addition to poor initial surgical site selection and technique, multiple factors may contribute to the need for reamputation, including infection, progressive ischemic changes, and failure of patients to comply with off-loading instructions [25] (Figs. 12.5 and 12.6).

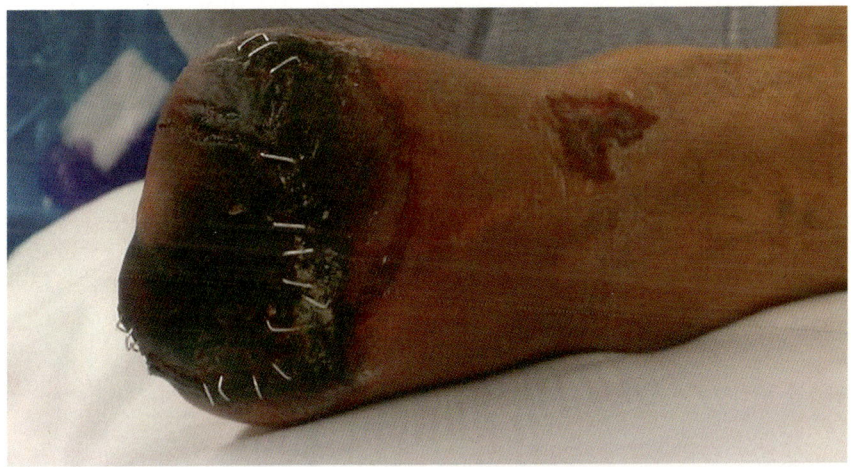

Fig. 12.5 Flap necrosis can be avoided with appropriate preoperative assessment

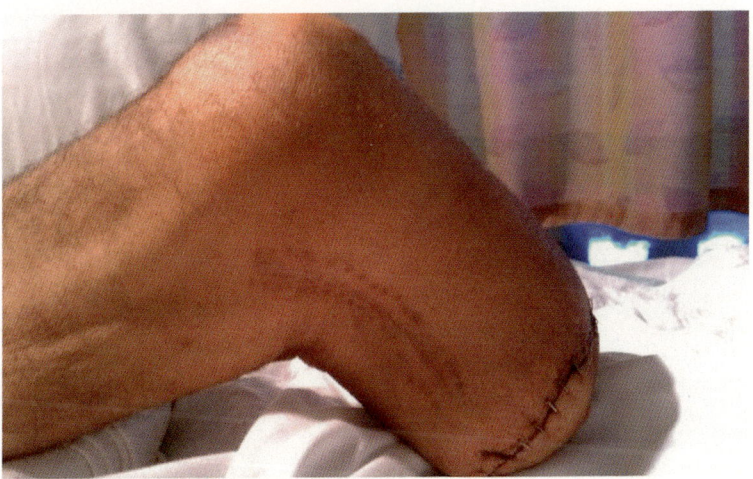

Fig. 12.6 Persistent knee flexion is problematic, not only for subsequent prosthetic usage, but sustained pressure on the posterior flap can lead to reulceration as well

Rehabilitation

The goal after amputation is successful rehabilitation to help improve transfers or ambulatory function. Preserving limb length ultimately aids in the patient rehabilitation potential and likelihood of ambulation. Patients with a below-knee amputation have a much better chance of returning to ambulation than patients with above-knee amputations. There are multiple factors which influence rehabilitation potential, including, age, preoperative ambulatory, and mental status. Immediately after amputation, the focus must turn toward wound healing, bulky dressings, and in some situations cast may be applied to ensure the operative site is well protected from pressure ulcers or abrasions. Sufficient pain control is crucial and consultation by a pain specialist may help to reduce postoperative recovery time. Physiotherapy should being as early as clinically tolerable, and arrangements should begin for prosthetic fitting. Specialized exercises can be performed to maintain muscle proprioception and strength. Lower extremity amputations can cause considerable psychological strain, symptoms of depression may require counseling and possibly pharmacological treatment. A multidisciplinary team approach can improve the rehabilitative potential of lower extremity amputees.

It is important to recognize that despite the general inclination to aggressively preserve limbs, there are degrees of tissue necrosis and advanced ischemia where quality of life and realistic rehabilitation expectations favor primary amputation [15] (Figs. 12.7 and 12.8).

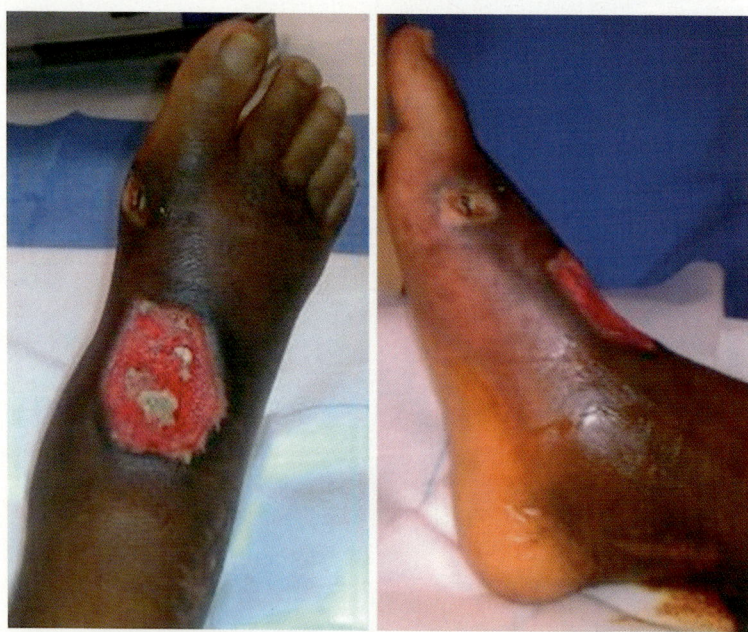

Fig. 12.7 Despite adequate pedal perfusion, delayed wound care with extensive necrosis to the joint space can preclude limb salvage and necessitate a major amputation

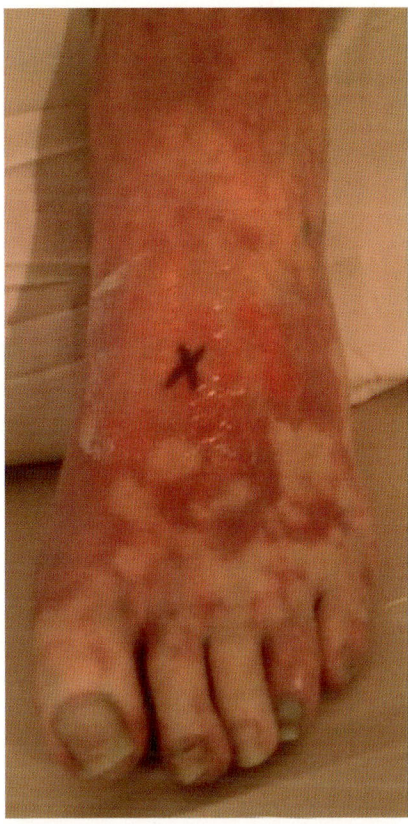

Fig. 12.8 Advanced ischemia with no avert gangrene, for which primary amputation should be considered after appropriate patient counseling

References

1. Belmont PJ, Davey S, Orr JD, Ochoa LM. Risk factors for 30-day postoperative complications and mortality after below-knee amputation: a study of 2911 patients from the National Surgical Quality Improvement Program. J Am Coll Surg. 2011;213:370–8.
2. Dillingham TR, Pezzin LE, Shore AD. Reamputation, mortality, and health care costs among person with dysvascular lower-limb amputations. Arch Phys Med Rehabil. 2005;86(3):480–6.
3. Cronewett JL, Johnston W. Rutherford's vascular surgery. 7th ed. Philadelphia, PA: Elsevier; 2010.
4. Ashry HR, Lavery LA, Murdoch DP, Frolich M, Lavery DC. Effectiveness of diabetic insoles to reduce foot pressures. J Foot Ankle Surg. 1997;36(4):268–71.
5. Reiber GE, Boyko EJ, Smith DG. Diabetes in America. 2nd ed. Bethesda, MD: National Diabetes Data Group of the National Institute of Diabetes and Digestive and Kidney Diseases, National Institute of Health; 1995.
6. Sellegren KR. An early history of lower limb amputations and prostheses. Iowa Orthop J. 1982;2:13–27.
7. Nowygrod R, Egorova N, Greco G, Anderson P, et al. Trends, complications, and mortality in peripheral vascular surgery. J Vasc Surg. 2006;43:205–16.
8. Egorova NN, Guillerme S, Gelijins A, Morrissey N, et al. An analysis of the outcome of a decade of experience with lower extremity revascularization including limb salvage, lengths of stay and safety. J Vasc Surg. 2010;51:878–85.
9. Keagy BA, Schwartz JA, Kotb M, Burnham SJ, Johnson G. Lower extremity amputation: the control series. J Vasc Surg. 1986;4:321–6.
10. Dwars BJ, van den Broek TA, Rauwerda JA, Bakker FC. Criteria for selection of the lowest level of amputation in peripheral vascular disease. J Vasc Surg. 1992;15:536–42.
11. DeFrang RD, Taylor LM, Porter JM. Basic data related to amputations. Ann Vasc Surg. 1991;5:202–7.
12. Asano M, Rushton P, Miller WC, Deathe BA. Predictors of quality of life among individuals who have a lower limb amputation. Prosthet Orthot Int. 2008;32(2):231–43.
13. Campbell WB, Marriott S, Eve R, Mapson E, Sexton S, Thompson JF. Amputations for acute ischaemia is associated with increased comorbidity and higher amputation level. Cardiovasc Surg. 2003;11:121–3.
14. Vitti MJ, Robinson DV, Hauer-Jensen M, Thompson BW, Ranval TJ, Barone G et al. Wound healing in forefoot amputations: the predictive value of toe pressure. Ann Vasc Surg. 1994;8:99–106.
15. Pinzur MS. Outcomes oriented amputation surgery. Plast Reconstr Surg. 2011;127(Suppl):241–7.
16. Yoho RM, Wilson PK, Gerres JA, Freschi S. Chopart's amputation: a 10-year case study. J Foot Ankle Surg. 2008;47(4):326–31.
17. Newcombe JF, Marcuson RW. Through-knee amputation. Br J Surg. 1972;59(4):260–6.
18. Zalavras CG, Rigopoulos N, Ahlmann E, Patzakis MJ. Hip disarticulation for severe lower extremity infections. Clin Orthop Relat Res. 2009;467:1721–6.
19. Azzoni R, Nano G, Dalainas I, Bianci P, Stegher S. Endovascular balloon assistance during hip disarticulation. Curr Orthop Pract. 2009;20(1):92–3.
20. Blume PA, Ayala J, Walter J, Lantis J, Payne W. Comparison of negative pressure wound therapy using vacuum assisted closure with advanced moist wound therapy in the treatment of diabetic foot ulcers. Diabetes Care. 2008;31(4):631–6.
21. Armstrong DG, Lavery LA. Negative pressure wound therapy after partial diabetic foot amputation: a multicenter, randomized controlled trial. Lancet. 2005;366:1704–10.
22. Pollard J, Hamilton GA, Rush SM, Ford LA. Mortality and morbidity after transmetatarsal amputation:

retrospective review of 101 cases. J Foot Ankle Surg. 2006;45(2):91–7.
23. McIntosh J, Earnshaw JJ. Antibiotic prophylaxis for the prevention of infection after major amputation. Eur J Vasc Endovasc Surg. 2009;37:696–703.
24. Izumi Y, Lee S, Satterfield K, Harkless LB. Risk of reamputation in diabetic patients stratified by limb and level of amputation. Diabetes Care. 2006;29: 566–70.
25. Hasanadka R, McLafferty RB, Moore CJ, Hood DB, Ramsey DE, Hodgson KJ. Predictors of wound complications following major amputation for critical limb ischemia. J Vasc Surg. 2011;54: 1374–82.

Diabetic Considerations in Cerebrovascular Disease

13

Christine Chung, Sharif Ellozy, Michael L. Marin, and Peter L. Faries

Keywords

Diabetes • Stroke • Cerebrovascular disease • Risk factor • Management • Carotid disease • Biomarker

The Burden of Disease

Diabetes is a major public health concern with formidable healthcare ramifications. In 2007, the American Diabetes Association estimated the cost of diabetes to be $174 billion in the United States, with $116 billion in excess medical expenditures and $58 billion in decreased national productivity [1]. According to the Centers for Disease Control and Prevention (CDC), 25.8 million people, or 8.3% of Americans, are afflicted with diabetes, with 1.9 million new cases diagnosed in 2010 [2]. Globally, more than 220 million people suffer from diabetes, with a projected rise in prevalence from 171 million people in 2000 to over 366 million by 2030 [3].

The increased cardiovascular complications associated with diabetes have been well recognized, estimated to comprise 65% of all diabetes-related morbidity and mortality [4]. Although coronary events have been the primary focus of diabetic complications, cerebrovascular disease is the most common long-term cause of morbidity in type 1 and type 2 diabetes [5]. Strokes represent the third leading cause of mortality in the Western world, affecting more than 600,000 people in the United States annually [6]. Diabetes is an established risk factor for stroke, for the risk of cerebral infarction is increased by two to four times in diabetic individuals compared to that of the nondiabetic population [7].

Not only does diabetes affect the incidence of stroke, but it also impacts outcomes after stroke. Diabetic patients were demonstrated to have longer hospital stays, increased neurological deficits, and increased mortality following strokes [8, 9]. Diabetes also doubles the risk of recurrent stroke, which is associated with poorer outcomes and increased mortality compared to the initial occurrence [10].

Pathophysiology of Cerebrovascular Disease in Diabetics

Diabetes is as much a vascular disease as it is a metabolic condition. In this complex disease, multiple mechanisms interact to cause cerebrovascular

C. Chung, M.D. (✉) • S. Ellozy, M.D. •
M.L. Marin, M.D., F.A.C.S. • P.L. Faries, M.D., F.A.C.S.
Department of Vascular Surgery, Mount Sinai School of Medicine, 5 East 98th Street, Rm 415, New York, NY 10029, USA
e-mail: Christine.chung@mssm.edu

impairment and progressive endothelial dysfunction [11]. Diabetes and chronic hyperglycemia have been associated with vascular smooth muscle proliferation, insidious inflammation, endothelial cell degeneration, thickening of the capillary basement membrane, and increased platelet aggregation and adhesion to the vascular endothelium [12].

Diabetes also places individuals at increased thromboembolic risk through various mechanisms. A hypercoagulable state is promoted by increased levels of clotting factors and fibrinogen, inhibition of fibrinolysis, and higher levels of plasminogen activator inhibitor-1 (PAI-1), a major fibrinolysis antagonist [13, 14]. Diabetics have also been demonstrated to possess impairments in the autoregulation of blood flow within the cerebral vasculature, which may further predispose these individuals to cerebral infarction [15].

Diabetes rarely exists in isolation, and often coexists with other well-recognized risk factors, such as hypertension and dyslipidemia, which act synergistically to increase the risk for stroke (Fig. 13.1) [16]. Although there are several explanations for the complex interaction among risk factors and vascular changes observed in diabetics, further investigations are necessary to better elucidate the pathological basis for this relationship.

Diabetic Presentation of Cerebrovascular Disease

The primary manifestation of cerebrovascular disease in the diabetic population is ischemic stroke [17, 18]. The incidence of hemorrhagic strokes, however, remains controversial in this group. In one study, the proportion of ischemic strokes compared to that of hemorrhagic strokes was found to be significantly greater in diabetics than in the general population (11:1 vs. 5:1) [19]. In addition, this study demonstrated that 88% of diabetics with strokes had ischemic infarctions, while 8% sustained intracerebral and subarachnoid hemorrhage; the type of stroke in the remaining 4% could not be determined. In the Honolulu Heart Study, the incidence of ischemic strokes in diabetics was more than twice that of the general population, with 44.9 vs. 20.7 per 1,000 strokes occurring in each group, respectively [20]. The rate of hemorrhagic strokes was nearly equal in both groups (10.1 vs. 9.6 per 1,000 strokes, respectively). In contrast, the Copenhagen Stroke Registry demonstrated hemorrhagic strokes to occur six times less frequently in diabetics compared to nondiabetic subjects [21].

Ischemic strokes in diabetics are predominantly of the lacunar subtype, which results from microatheroma formation in the cerebral microvasculature [5]. Studies have shown that 28–43% of patients with lacunar infarcts have diabetes [22, 23]. Though often clinically silent, lacunar strokes may represent markers of widespread vascular disease. Specific imaging techniques are required to recognize lacunar strokes. Recent investigations using CT and MRI imaging have shown that diabetic patients may be at greater risk for these microinfarctions [21, 24, 25].

Although strokes occur more frequently in diabetic subjects, transient ischemic attacks (TIA) occur less frequently in these patients [17, 26]. Interestingly, diabetes is less prevalent among individuals with TIA than among patients with ischemic stroke [27]. Furthermore, studies have demonstrated that diabetics are predisposed to stroke within the 90-day period following prior TIA; no predisposition to recurrent TIA was observed during this time [28]. These findings may be explained by the greater severity of atherosclerotic disease in the cerebral circulation of diabetics, which may make ischemia less likely to be reversible in this population [26]. Given the same insult, diabetics may sustain permanent cerebral damage, while nondiabetics may only experience temporary deficits with complete resolution of any impairments [29].

Unlike stroke or TIA, the presence of cognitive impairment has received little attention in the setting of diabetes. This particular presentation of diabetes has been relatively uncommon, usually only seen in the elderly diabetic population. With earlier diagnosis and improved management, the mortality related to diabetes has been decreasing. Therefore, longer lifespans have unmasked a greater population of patients experiencing

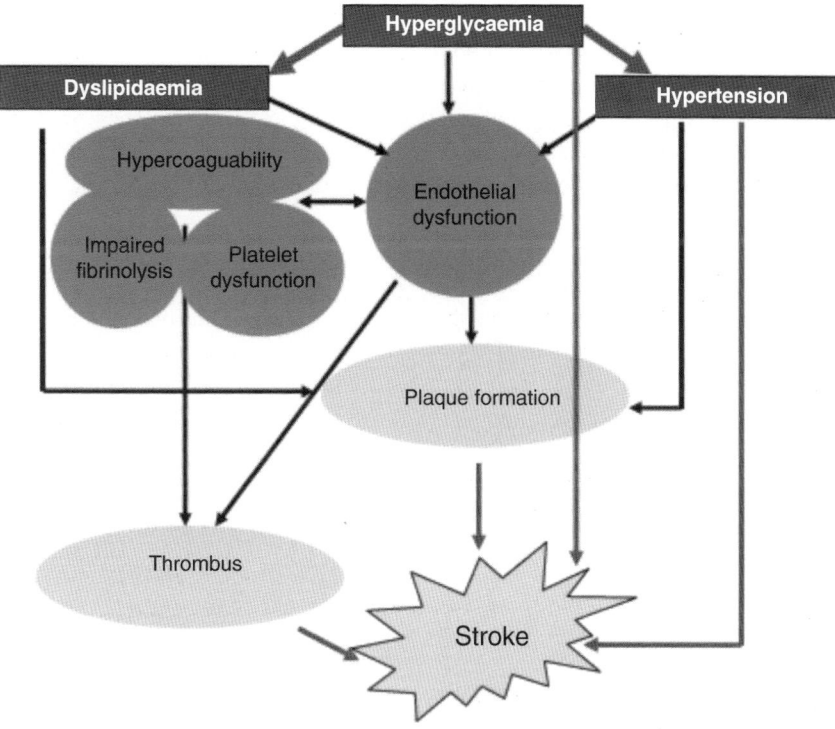

Fig. 13.1 Mechanisms underlying hyperglycemia and stroke risk. Dyslipidemia, hyperglycemia, and hypertension interact to promote endothelial dysfunction and plaque and thrombus formation, which increases risk for stroke (reprinted from Quinn TJ, Dawson J, Walters MR. Sugar and stroke: cerebrovascular disease and blood glucose control. Cardiovasc Ther. 2010;1–12. With permission from John Wiley and Sons, Inc.)

cognitive decline due to diabetes. Several factors have been implicated in this relationship, including chronic hyperglycemia, advanced cerebrovascular disease, repeated hypoglycemic episodes, insulin resistance, longer duration of diabetes, and age-related changes in metabolism [11]. Furthermore, the elderly diabetic population has been shown to possess greater cortical and hippocampal atrophy along with increased accumulation of advanced glycation end products as compared to non-diabetics [30–32].

Several studies have demonstrated the increased risk for cognitive impairment and future dementia in the diabetic population [33, 34]. Furthermore, elderly type 2 diabetics have been found to be at greater risk for amnestic mild cognitive impairment, the transition between normal cognition and Alzheimer's disease, compared to elderly nondiabetics [35].

Hyperglycemia and Stroke in Diabetics

Glucose control has been the foundation of appropriate diabetic management. Impaired glucose tolerance and insulin resistance has been demonstrated to increase the risk of stroke. Hyperglycemia is present in 20–50% of patients upon presentation and is associated with poor outcomes following ischemic stroke. Patients with hyperglycemia with no history of diabetes possess an especially dismal prognosis, found to be worse than that of diabetics [36]. In addition to high glucose levels on admission, the development of elevated glucose levels during hospitalization is associated with worse outcomes [37, 38].

Hyperglycemia has been demonstrated to extend the ischemic penumbra, or hypoperfused area of the brain, which predisposes the patient to neurological complications [39]. This penumbra can either suffer irreparable damage or be completely restored. Hyperglycemia and hypoxia leads to lactic acidosis, which further decreases perfusion and leads to enlargement of the infarct [40]. Increased glucose levels also increases vasogenic edema, impairs collateral flow, and increases the hyperthrombotic state. Thus, the circulation of the cerebral vasculature and the autoregulation of blood flow are impaired [38].

With the robust connection between hyperglycemia and ischemic stroke, it has been hypothesized that tight glycemic control may decrease the incidence of cardiovascular events, including that of ischemic strokes. Major randomized controlled trials have evaluated this hypothesis. These studies include the Action to Control Cardiovascular Risk in Diabetes (ACCORD) [41], Action in Diabetes and Vascular Disease: Preterax and Diamicron Modified Release Controlled Evaluation (ADVANCE) trial [42], Veterans Affairs Diabetes Trial (VADT) [43], and the United Kingdom Prospective Diabetes Study (UKPDS) [44]. Although differences in the definition of intense glucose control versus standard glucose control exist among these studies and various methods were used to attain glycemic control, these trials showed no benefit of intensive therapy on the primary endpoint of cardiovascular death, nonfatal MI, or nonfatal stroke compared with standard glucose control. The posttrial results of the UKPDS study, however, did show a significant reduction of risk for myocardial infarction and all-cause mortality in newly diagnosed diabetics compared with nondiabetics [45]. Additionally, the UKPDS study demonstrated the benefit of strict glucose control on reducing diabetic microvascular complications, such as nephropathy, retinopathy, and peripheral neuropathy, although it did not effect the incidence of stroke. A more detailed comparison of these randomized controlled trials are outlined in Table 13.1 [46].

A recent meta-analysis, which included six randomized controlled trials with 150,000 patient-years of follow-up further supported previous unremarkable findings regarding glycemic control and stroke prevention [47]. This analysis also demonstrated that intensive glucose management was not superior to conservative treatment in reducing stroke risk in diabetic individuals. As is shown in Fig. 13.2, the only statistically significant finding regarding macrovascular events (myocardial infarction, stroke, and death) was a 14% relative risk reduction in the rate of nonfatal myocardial infarction.

Based on available data, there appears to be no compelling evidence that meticulous reduction in glucose levels decreases the risk of cerebrovascular events in diabetics [48]. Thus, diabetes is a multifaceted disease that extends beyond the simple impairment of glucose regulation alone. In their most recent guidelines, the American Diabetes Association has recommended a general HbA1c target of <7.0% to prevent long-term complications [49]. Further investigations are underway to determine whether this threshold actually reduces the long-term risk of cardiovascular events and stroke.

Hypertension and Stroke in Diabetics

Hypertension is a key risk factor for stroke in diabetic patients. The presence of diabetes in hypertensive individuals has been associated with advanced brain damage, characterized by diminished functional neuronal mass and decreased cerebrovascular reserve [50]. Therefore, the management of hypertension in diabetic patients is a primary concern.

The aggressive reduction of blood pressure (BP) has been demonstrated to decrease the incidence of stroke in diabetics [51]. The UKPDS study showed that type 2 diabetics with hypertension at baseline were at two and a half times the risk for stroke than those without hypertension [52]. This study also demonstrated that tight BP control with a mean BP of 144/82 mmHg leads to a 44% reduction in stroke risk as compared with less stringent control (mean BP of 154/87) [53]. Hypertension has also been shown to augment the effect of hyperglycemia. Patients with a mean HbA1c ≥ 8.0% and systolic BP > 150 mmHg were at 13 times the risk for

Table 13.1 Overview of randomized controlled trials evaluating intensive vs. standard glycemic control and cardiovascular outcomes

	ACCORD	ADVANCE	VADT	UKPDS (post-trial)
Patient characteristics				
Number of subjects	10,251	11,140	1,791	3,277
Mean age (years)	62	66	60	63
Duration of diabetes (years)	10	8	11.5	17
Sex (% male)	39	42	97	SI: 60; M: 46
History of CVD (%)	35	32	40	0
BMI (kg/m²)	32	28	31	SI: 29; M: 46
Mean baseline HbA1c (%)	8.1	7.5	9.4	SI: 7.9; M: 8.4
Insulin use at baseline (%)	35	1.5	52	64
Protocol characteristics				
HbA1c target (%) (I vs. S)	<6.0 vs. 7.0–7.9	≤6.5 vs. local guidelines	<6.0 (action if >6.5) vs. planned separation of 1.5	Fasting plasma glucose <6 mmol/l
Glycemic control (I vs. S)	Multiple drugs in both groups	Multiple drugs with gliclazide vs. multiple drugs with no gliclazide	Multiple drugs in both groups (metformin, glimepiride, rosiglitazone, insulin)	Intensive therapy (SI; in overweight patients[c], M) vs. C (dietary restriction)
Risk factor management	Embedded BP and lipid trials	Embedded BP Trial	Intensive treatment in both groups	None
Study characteristics (I vs. S)				
Median follow-up (years)	3.5 (early termination)	5	5.6	8.8
Median HbA1c (%)	6.4 vs. 7.5	6.4 vs. 7.0	6.9 vs. 8.5	SI: 7.9 vs. 7.9; M: 8.1 vs. 8.1
On insulin[a] (%)	77 vs. 55	40 vs. 24	89 vs. 74	NA
On TZD[a] (%)	91 vs. 58	17 vs. 11	53 vs. 42	0
On statin[a] (%)	88 vs. 88	46 vs. 48	85 vs. 83	NA
On aspirin[a] (%)	7 vs. 76	57 vs. 55	88 vs. 86	NA
Mean blood pressure[a] (mmHg)				
Intensive glycemic control	126/67	136/74	127/68	NA
Standard glycemic control	127/68	138/74	125/69	NA
Participants with severe hypoglycemia[b] (%)				
Intensive glycemic control	16.2	2.7	21.2	NA
Standard glycemic control	5.1	1.5	9.9	NA

(continued)

Table 13.1 (continued)

	ACCORD	ADVANCE	VADT	UKPDS (post-trial)
Outcomes				
Primary outcome definition	Nonfatal MI, nonfatal stroke, CVD death	Micro and macrovascular (nonfatal MI, nonfatal stroke, CVD death) outcomes	Nonfatal MI, nonfatal stroke, CVD death, hospitalization for HF, revascularization	Any diabetes-related endpoint, diabetes-related death, death from any cause, MI, stroke, PVD, microvascular disease
HR for primary outcome (95% CI)	0.90 (0.78–1.04)	0.9 (0.82–0.98); macrovascular 0.94 (0.84–1.06)	0.88 (0.74–1.05)	SI: 0.91 (0.83–0.99); M: 0.79 (0.66–0.95)
HR for mortality findings (95% CI)	1.22 (1.01–1.46)	0.93 (0.83–1.06)	1.07 (0.81–1.42)	SI: 0.87 (0.79–0.96); M: 0.73 (0.590.89)

BMI Body mass index, *BP* blood pressure, *C* conventional therapy, *CVD* Cardiovascular disease, *HR* hazard ratio, *I* intensive glycemic control, *M* metformin, *NA* not available, *PVD* peripheral vascular disease, *S* standard glycemic control, *SI* sulfonylurea-insulin group, *TZD* thiazolidinedione

Adapted from Meier M, Hummel M. Cardiovascular disease and intensive glucose control in type 2 diabetes mellitus: moving practice toward evidence-based strategies. Vasc Health Risk Manag. 2009;5:859–71

[a]At the completion of the study
[b]One or more episodes
[c]Mean BMI 31 kg/m^2

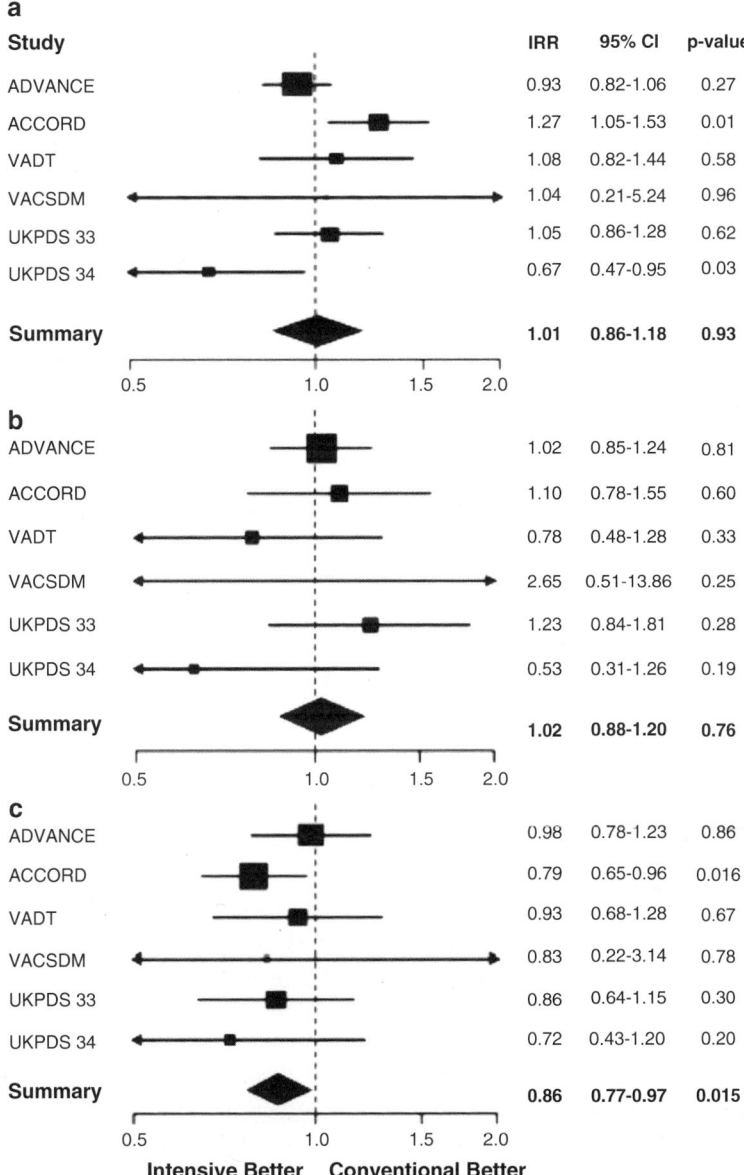

Fig. 13.2 Incidence rate ratios for (**a**) all-cause mortality, (**b**) nonfatal stroke, and (**c**) nonfatal myocardial infarction in patients randomized to intensive glucose or standard control. Intensive glucose management was not shown to be superior to conservative management in reducing the incidence of all-cause mortality or nonfatal stroke, but it has been shown to reduce the relative risk for nonfatal myocardial infarction by 14% (reprinted from Marso SP, Kennedy KF, House JA, et al. The effect of intensive glucose control on all-cause and cardiovascular mortality, myocardial infarction and stroke in persons with type 2 diabetes mellitus: a systemic review and meta-analysis. Diabetes Vasc Dis Res. 2010;7(2):119–30. With permission from SAGE Publications)

stroke as compared to those with HbA1c<6% and systolic BP<130 mmHg [54].

Thus, strict blood pressure targets in diabetics have been recommended. The American Heart Association (AHA) and the American Stroke Association (ASA) recommend blood pressure control in diabetic patients as one component of a multifactorial program to decrease cardiovascular risk (Class I Recommendation; Level of Evidence A) [48]. The Joint National Committee on Prevention, Detection, Evaluation, and Treatment of High Blood Pressure further recommends a goal of <130/80 in the diabetic population [55].

Several antihypertensive agents have been considered to reach blood pressure goals. The Heart Outcomes Prevention Evaluation (HOPE) study compared the addition of an ACE inhibitor (ACE-I) to the medical regimen in high-risk individuals, which included 3,577 patients with diabetes who experienced a prior cardiovascular event or had an additional cardiovascular risk factor. A significant 25% reduction in risk ($P=0.0004$) in the primary outcome of myocardial infarction, stroke, and cardiovascular mortality as well as a 33% reduction ($P=0.0074$) in stroke was achieved [56]. It remains unclear whether these dramatic findings are due to the effect of ACE-I administration or to the reduction in blood pressure.

The Losartan Intervention for Endpoint Reduction in Hypertension (LIFE) study compared the use of an angiotensinogen receptor blocker (ARB) with a β-adrenergic receptor blocker in diabetics with essential hypertension (160–200 mmHg/95–115 mmHg) and those with left ventricular hypertrophy [57]. A significant 24% reduction in major vascular events and a nonsignificant 21% reduction in stroke were observed in patients treated with an ARB compared to those treated with β-blockers. According to the AHA and ASA, the treatment of hypertension in diabetics with an ACE-I or an ARB is considered a beneficial method of managing hypertension (Class I Recommendation; Level of Evidence A) [48].

The effects of two antihypertensive treatments (amlodipine with perindopril or atenolol with thiazide) were evaluated in the Anglo-Scandinavian Cardiac Outcomes Trial (ASCOT) [58]. A blood pressure target of 130/80 was used in 5,137 diabetic patients, and the primary endpoint was the incidence of major cardiovascular events. This study underwent early termination due to reductions in mortality and stroke with the amlodipine/perindopril therapy. There was a significant decrease in the incidence of total cardiovascular events compared with that of the atenolol/thiazide regimen ($P=0.026$). Additionally, a 25% reduction in fatal and nonfatal strokes was observed in this population ($P=0.017$).

Dyslipidemia and Stroke in Diabetics

Diabetic patients with lipid dysregulation are characterized by elevated triglyceride and low-density lipid (LDL) cholesterol levels and decreased high-density lipid (HDL) cholesterol levels. The use of statins in diabetic subjects has been demonstrated to reduce the incidence of stroke, whereas the efficacy of fibrates in stroke prevention has been inconclusive.

Several studies have shown the benefit of statin therapy in the diabetic population. In the Medical Research Council/British Heart Foundation Heart Protection Study (HPS), 5,963 diabetic patients were randomly assigned to receive simvastatin (40 mg daily) versus placebo [59]. A 24% reduction in strokes (nonfatal or fatal stroke) was observed in the simvastatin group (95% confidence interval 6–39%; $P=0.01$). This effect was found to be independent of age, gender, lipid concentrations, glucose control, and presence of vascular disease. The Collaborative Atorvastatin Diabetes Study (CARDS) evaluated 2,838 diabetics with LDL cholesterol levels <160 mg/dl with no previous cardiovascular history; they were assigned to receive either atorvastatin (10 mg daily) or placebo [60]. This trial underwent early termination for a 48% reduction in stroke risk demonstrated in the atorvastatin group. A post hoc analysis of the Treating to New Targets (TNT) study analyzed the effect of decreasing LDL cholesterol on cardiovascular events in patients with coronary disease and diabetes with either high-dose or low-dose atorvastatin (80 mg daily vs. 10 mg daily, respectively) [61]. The higher dose group demonstrated a 40% reduction in time to cerebrovascular event ($P=0.037$). Thus, the AHA and ASA recommends the use of a statin to treat diabetic adults, especially in the presence of additional risk factors, to decrease the risk of an initial stroke (Class I Recommendation; Level of Evidence A) [48].

Low HDL cholesterol levels and increased triglyceride levels are independent risk factors for stroke. The use of fibrates has been demonstrated to improve these parameters [62]. The Department of Veterans Affairs High-Density Lipoprotein Intervention Trial (VA-HIT) assigned subjects to receive either gemfibrozil or placebo for 5.1 years [63]. Although gemfibrozil has not been associated with modification in stroke risk among nondiabetic subjects, it has been shown to cause a 40% reduction in stroke in diabetics ($P=0.046$). On the contrary, the Fenofibrate Intervention and Event Lowering in Diabetes (FIELD) study did not support these results [64]. 9,795 diabetics were studied to determine fenofibrate's effect on cardiovascular outcome. In 5 years, no effect on the incidence of stroke was observed in patients with fenofibrate therapy (4% vs. 3%; $P=NS$). These contradictory findings may be attributed to the higher proportion of patients in the placebo group compared to the fenofibrate group who started statin therapy during this trial, which may have masked a treatment benefit of the fibrate intervention. Additional studies are necessary to clarify the role of fibrates in preventing stroke in the diabetic population. The AHA and ASA states that monotherapy with a fibrate may be used to decrease the risk of stroke in diabetics (Class IIb Recommendation; Level of Evidence B) [48].

Antiplatelet Therapy and Stroke in Diabetics

Diabetes places patients at increased thrombotic risk, for it is associated with the presence of increased procoagulant factors (i.e., fibrinogen, von Willebrand factor, tissue factor, factor VII) and decreased antithrombotic factors (i.e., antithrombin III, protein C, and thrombomodulin) [26, 65]. Diabetic individuals are also characterized by increased platelet activation and aggregation as well as the promotion of antifibrinolytic factors. Therefore, antiplatelet and anticoagulation is critical in preventing stroke in the setting of diabetes [66].

The beneficial effect of aspirin therapy in minimizing stroke risk remains uncertain. Large randomized trials have shown that aspirin decreases the risk of stroke in the diabetic population [67]. A study by 163 Japanese institutions has analyzed 2,539 diabetic patients [68]. One group was given low-dose aspirin (81 or 100 mg/day) and the other was not treated with aspirin. Over 4.37 years, only a single fatal stroke occurred in the former group compared to five in the latter group. The study did not have sufficient power to determine aspirin's effect on stroke.

Many large trials have included subgroup analyses of diabetic patients. The Antithrombotic Trialists' Collaboration completed a meta-analysis of 287 randomized trials, which included 135,000 patients. The effects of antiplatelet therapy (predominantly aspirin) were compared with that of a control group [69]. In the subgroup of 5,126 diabetic patients, there was a nonsignificant 7% reduction in cardiovascular complications, including stroke.

Higher aspirin doses may be required in diabetic patients to achieve the same antiplatelet effects as nondiabetic individuals [70]. In diabetics, increased platelet hyperactivity has been demonstrated to respond poorly to aspirin [71]. These may represent explanations for why some reports have not shown a benefit of low-dose aspirin in diabetics. However, care providers must be mindful of the risk of gastrointestinal complications and bleeding that may occur with the use of higher doses of aspirin. According to the AHA and ASA, the aspirin therapy may be reasonable in patients at high cardiovascular risk (Class IIb Recommendation; Level of Evidence B) [48].

The use of clopidogrel versus aspirin has also been studied in the diabetic population. A post hoc analysis of the Clopidogrel vs. Aspirin in Patients at Risk of Ischaemic Events (CAPRIE) study has shown that clopidogrel decreases stroke risk as compared to aspirin [72]. The Management of Atherothrombosis with Clopidogrel in High-risk patients (MATCH) study showed no added benefit of combined therapy [73]. Aspirin was given to subjects who had experienced a previous stroke or TIA and were taking clopidogrel. No further reduction in stroke-related morbidity or mortality occurred; however, an increased risk of life-threatening bleeding was observed. The Clopidogrel for High Atherothrombotic Risk and Ischemic Stabilization, Management, and Avoidance (CHARISMA) study showed that dual antiplatelet therapy diminishes the risk of stroke by 21% in patients with cardiovascular disease or multiple risk factors [74]. Currently, there are insufficient data to support the use of dual therapy to prevent stroke in diabetic patients.

Carotid Disease and Biomarkers

High-grade carotid atherosclerosis is an important cause of TIA and stroke, accounting for 30–40% of ischemic cerebrovascular disease [75]. Carotid stenosis frequently occurs in the diabetic population and is considered to be another risk factor that augments diabetics' risk for cerebral infarction and death. Unlike hypertension or dyslipidemia, however, the presence of carotid disease is not as easy to ascertain without the presence of overt symptoms.

Carotid intima–media thickness (IMT) determined by ultrasound investigation is a surrogate marker for subclinical carotid disease, and it has been demonstrated to predict the future incidence of stroke [76]. It has been reported that 73% of type 2 diabetics possess carotid artery disease as well as increased carotid IMT [77]. This parameter is also significantly elevated in patients who later develop diabetes [78]. It has been shown that newly diagnosed type 2 diabetics often have carotid IMT that are significantly greater than that of nondiabetic controls [79]. Furthermore, type 1 diabetics also have significantly increased carotid IMT compared to that of nondiabetic controls, which suggests the early development of carotid atherosclerosis in this population [80].

In addition to ultrasound evaluation, increasing evidence has pointed to new serum biomarkers as determinants of carotid disease and predictors of vulnerable carotid plaques. In the last decade, a plethora of biomarkers has received recognition; they are listed in Table 13.2 [81]. Type 2 diabetes is regarded as a chronic low-grade inflammation, which accelerates the atherosclerotic process as compared to nondiabetics.

Table 13.2 Established biomarkers of carotid atherosclerosis in patients with type 2 diabetes

Category	Biomarkers
Inflammatory markers	CRP (and/or hsCRP) and fibrinogen
Adipokines	Adiponectin, leptin, and ghrelin
Cytokines	IL-6, -10 and -18
Growth factors	HGF
MMPs	MMP-9 and -8
Vascular calcification markers	Osteopontin and osteoprotegerin

CRP C-reactive protein, *hsCRP* high-sensitivity C-reactive protein, *MMP* matrix metalloproteinase
Adapted from Kadoglou NPE, Avgerinos ED, Liapis CD. An update on markers of carotid atherosclerosis in patients with type 2 diabetes. Biomark Med. 2010;4(4):601–9. With permission of Future Medicine Ltd.

Although the mechanism remains unclear, atherosclerosis and diabetes are believed to share a common inflammatory basis. Thus, the focus has been mostly on the systemic inflammatory markers and their relationship with carotid disease.

C-reactive protein (CRP) and fibrinogen are currently the most widely studied proinflammatory markers for carotid atherosclerosis. Despite the large number of studies investigating CRP's relationship with carotid disease, only a small number have examined the diabetic population exclusively. The predictive value of CRP has been better evaluated through high-sensitivity CRP (hsCRP). One study demonstrated a positive relationship of hsCRP with subclinical carotid disease as well as the occurrence of ischemic events in the diabetic population [82]. Likewise, fibrinogen has also been identified as a risk factor for cerebrovascular events. In patients with baseline asymptomatic carotid disease, it has been demonstrated that high fibrinogen levels were among the strongest indicators of cerebrovascular events [83]. Furthermore, patients with both high fibrinogen and CRP levels have exhibited additional risk for carotid atherosclerosis. Thus, these markers may be used to identify diabetic patients with advanced carotid stenosis at increased risk of thrombotic events; however, their clinical importance must be confirmed by future studies.

Adipokinins, cytokines, growth factors, metalloproteinases, and vascular calcification markers

Table 13.3 Recommendations for stroke risk modification in diabetes

Risk factor	Guideline	Recommendation/level of evidence[a]
Blood pressure	Blood pressure control in type 1 and type 2 diabetes should be a component of a comprehensive risk reduction plan Blood pressure goal <130/80, according to JNC 7[b] guidelines Antihypertensive of choice: ACE inhibitor[c] or ARB[d]	Class I/A
Hyperlipidemia	Treat diabetics with a statin (especially patients with additional risk factors) to lower the risk of initial stroke Fibrate monotherapy may be considered in diabetics to decrease stroke risk Adding a fibrate to statin therapy in diabetics is not effective for minimizing stroke risk	Class I/A Class IIb/B Class III/B
Platelet hyperactivity	The beneficial effect of aspirin to decrease stroke risk in diabetics has not been adequately demonstrated. However, aspirin therapy may be reasonable in patients at high cardiovascular risk	Class IIb/B

Based on data from Goldstein LB, Bushnell CD, Adams RJ, et al. On behalf of the American Heart Association Stroke Council on Cardiovascular Nursing Council on Epidemiology and Prevention Council for High Blood Pressure Research, Council on Peripheral Vascular Disease, and Interdisciplinary Council on Quality of Care and Outcomes Research. Guidelines for the primary prevention of stroke: a guideline for healthcare professionals from the American Heart Association/American Stroke Association. Stroke. 2011;42(5):517–84
[a]Based on American Heart Association Stroke Council Recommendations
[b]The Joint National Committee on Prevention, Detection, Evaluation, and Treatment of High Blood Pressure
[c]Angiotensin-converting enzyme inhibitor
[d]Angiotensin II receptor blocker

are other biomarkers that have garnered interest in predicting patients at increased cerebrovascular risk. The use of biomarkers may be a simple, cost-effective method for assessing carotid disease in diabetic subjects. However, the mechanism of action as well as the efficacy of these markers remains elusive. Further analysis and validation of these biomarkers may lead to appropriate and unique treatment strategies that may prevent the progression of carotid atherosclerosis and diminish cerebrovascular events in the rapidly increasing diabetic population.

Management of Cerebrovascular Disease in Diabetics

Several risk factors are implicated in predisposing patients with diabetes at greater risk for stroke. Table 13.3 summarizes the recent AHA/ASA guidelines. Besides these factors, the presence of tobacco use, atrial fibrillation, and metabolic syndrome contribute to making diabetic patients a high-risk group [66]. Therefore, healthcare providers must consider the patient as a whole rather than a collection of risk factors in order to minimize the risk for adverse cerebrovascular events.

The importance of multifactorial intervention is emphasized by findings of the Steno-2 study [84]. 160 diabetic patients were randomly assigned to two groups. The first group underwent aggressive risk management, which included strict glucose control, blood pressure control, smoking cessation, weight reduction, dietary modification, exercise, and aspirin therapy. The second group was managed with a conventional treatment regimen of risk factors. Patients receiving intensive therapy showed a 79% relative risk reduction in stroke over a mean follow up of 7.8 years. This benefit appeared to extend through another five and a half years of follow-up, during which time active intervention was not administered. These findings support the importance of comprehensive risk factor modification in managing diabetic patients.

Conclusions

Cerebrovascular disease is a well-recognized complication of diabetes. Strokes represent the most common cause of long-term morbidity and mortality in the diabetic population, with greater adverse neurological outcomes and morbidity following stroke in this group. High-risk factors, such as hypertension and hyperlipidemia, often present in diabetics and have been demonstrated to predispose patients to cerebrovascular disease. Although the AHA and ASA have made recommendations regarding specific goals of care, the management of diabetic individuals requires more than achieving specific glycemic targets or maintaining blood pressures below a certain threshold. Rather, appropriate management should also consider improving the lipid profile, administering antiplatelet agents, and encouraging life style changes through exercise and healthy diet. Thus, a multifactorial treatment regimen should be adopted and treatment strategies should be tailored to the individual rather than to any specific risk factor that may be present to ensure the best outcome. Further investigations regarding the pathophysiology of diabetes, the clinical outcome of risk factor modification, and the identification of surrogate markers for carotid disease are necessary to minimize the risk for debilitating cerebrovascular disease in this high-risk population.

References

1. Diabetes statistics. American Diabetes Association Web site. http://www.diabetes.org/diabetes-basics/diabetes-statistics/?loc=DropDownDB-stats. Updated 2011. Accessed 5 Nov 2011.
2. 2011 National Diabetes Fact Sheet. Centers for Disease Control and Prevention Web site. http://www.cdc.gov/diabetes/pubs/estimates11.htm#1. Published 5/23/11. Updated 2011. Accessed 15 Nov 2011.
3. Wild S, Roglic G, Green A, Sicree R, King H. Global prevalence of diabetes: estimates for the year 2000 and projections for 2030. Diabetes Care. 2004;27(5):1047–53.
4. Barrett-Conner E, Khaw K. Diabetes mellitus: an independent risk factor for stroke? Am J Epidemol. 1998;128:116–23.
5. Mukherjee D. Peripheral and cerebrovascular atherosclerotic disease in diabetes mellitus. Best Pract Res Clin Endocrinol Metab. 2009;23(3):335–45. doi:10.1016/j.beem.2008.10.015.
6. Rosamond WD, Folsom AR, Chambless LE, et al. Stroke incidence and survival among middle-aged adults: 9-year follow-up of the atherosclerosis risk in communities (ARIC) cohort. Stroke. 1999;30(4):736–43.
7. Screening for type 2 diabetes mellitus in adults: U.S. Preventative Services Task Force recommendation statement. Ann Intern Med. 2008;148:846–54.
8. Megherbi SE, Milan C, Minier D, et al. Association between diabetes and stroke subtype on survival and functional outcome 3 months after stroke: data from the European BIOMED Stroke Project. Stroke. 2003;34(3):688–94.doi:10.1161/01.STR.0000057975. 15221.40.
9. Andersen KK, Olsen TS. One-month to 10-year survival in the Copenhagen Stroke Study: interactions between stroke severity and other prognostic indicators. J Stroke Cerebrovasc Dis. 2011;20(2):117–23. doi:10.1016/j.jstrokecerebrovasdis.2009.10.009.
10. Harmsen P, Lappas G, Rosengren A, Wilhelmsen L. Long-term risk factors for stroke: twenty-eight years of follow-up of 7457 middle-aged men in Goteborg, Sweden. Stroke. 2006;37(7):1663–7. doi:10.1161/01. STR.0000226604.10877.fc.
11. Huber JD. Diabetes, cognitive function, and the blood-brain barrier. Curr Pharm Des. 2008;14(16): 1594–600.
12. Ergul A, Li W, Elgebaly MM, Bruno A, Fagan SC. Hyperglycemia, diabetes and stroke: focus on the cerebrovasculature.VasculPharmacol.2009;51(1):44– 9. doi:10.1016/j.vph.2009.02.004.
13. Carr ME. Diabetes mellitus: a hypercoagulable state. J Diabetes Complications. 2001;15(1):44–54.
14. Grant PJ. Diabetes mellitus as a prothrombotic condition. J Intern Med. 2007;262(2):157–72. doi:10.1111/j.1365-2796.2007.01824.x.
15. Brown CM, Marthol H, Zikeli U, Ziegler D, Hilz MJ. A simple deep breathing test reveals altered cerebral autoregulation in type 2 diabetic patients. Diabetologia. 2008;51(5):756–61. doi:10.1007/s00125-008-0958-3.
16. Quinn TJ, Dawson J, Walters MR. Sugar and stroke: cerebrovascular disease and blood glucose control. Cardiovasc Ther. 2010. doi:10.1111/j.1755-5922. 2010.00166.x.
17. Lithner F, Asplund K, Eriksson S, Hagg E, Strand T, Wester PO. Clinical characteristics in diabetic stroke patients. Diabetes Metab. 1988;14(1):15–9.
18. Woodward M, Zhang X, Barzi F, et al. The effects of diabetes on the risks of major cardiovascular diseases and death in the Asia-Pacific region. Diabetes Care. 2003;26(2):360–6.
19. Roehmboldt M, Palumbo P, Whisnant J, Elveback L. Transient ischemic attack and stroke in a community-based diabetic cohort. Mayo Clin Proc. 1983;58:56–8.
20. Abbott RD, Donahue RP, MacMahon SW, Reed DM, Yano K. Diabetes and the risk of stroke. The Honolulu Heart Program. JAMA. 1987;257(7):949–52.

21. Jorgensen H, Nakayama H, Raaschou HO, Olsen TS. Stroke in patients with diabetes. The Copenhagen Stroke Study. Stroke. 1994;25(10):1977–84.
22. Arboix A, Marti-Vilalta JL, Garcia JH. Clinical study of 227 patients with lacunar infarcts. Stroke. 1990;21(6):842–7.
23. Horowitz DR, Tuhrim S, Weinberger JM, Rudolph SH. Mechanisms in lacunar infarction. Stroke. 1992;23(3):325–7.
24. Iwase M, Yamamoto M, Yoshinari M, Ibayashi S, Fujishima M. Stroke topography in diabetic and non-diabetic patients by magnetic resonance imaging. Diabetes Res Clin Pract. 1998;42(2):109–16.
25. Vermeer SE, Den Heijer T, Koudstaal PJ, et al. Incidence and risk factors of silent brain infarcts in the population-based Rotterdam Scan Study. Stroke. 2003;34(2):392–6.
26. Air EL, Kissela BM. Diabetes, the metabolic syndrome, and ischemic stroke: epidemiology and possible mechanisms. Diabetes Care. 2007;30(12):3131–40. doi:10.2337/dc06-1537.
27. Weimar C, Kraywinkel K, Rodl J, et al. Etiology, duration, and prognosis of transient ischemic attacks: an analysis from the German Stroke Data Bank. Arch Neurol. 2002;59(10):1584–8.
28. Johnston C, Sidney S, Bernstein A, Gress D. A comparison of risk factors for recurrent TIA and stroke in patients diagnosed with TIA. Neurology. 2003;28:280–5.
29. Mankovsky BN, Ziegler D. Stroke in patients with diabetes mellitus. Diabetes Metab Res Rev. 2004;20(4):268–87. doi:10.1002/dmrr.490.
30. Whitmer RA. Type 2 diabetes and risk of cognitive impairment and dementia. Curr Neurol Neurosci Rep. 2007;7(5):373–80.
31. Yavuz BB, Ariogul S, Cankurtaran M, et al. Hippocampal atrophy correlates with the severity of cognitive decline. Int Psychogeriatr. 2007;19(4):767–77. doi:10.1017/S1041610206004303.
32. Sato T, Shimogaito N, Wu X, Kikuchi S, Yamagishi S, Takeuchi M. Toxic advanced glycation end products (TAGE) theory in Alzheimer's disease. Am J Alzheimers Dis Other Demen. 2006;21(3):197–208.
33. Luchsinger JA, Reitz C, Patel B, Tang MX, Manly JJ, Mayeux R. Relation of diabetes to mild cognitive impairment. Arch Neurol. 2007;64(4):570–5. doi:10.1001/archneur.64.4.570.
34. Cukierman T, Gerstein HC, Williamson JD. Cognitive decline and dementia in diabetes – systematic overview of prospective observational studies. Diabetologia. 2005;48(12):2460–9. doi:10.1007/s00125-005-0023-4.
35. Zhu X, Perry G, Smith MA. Insulin signaling, diabetes mellitus and risk of Alzheimer disease. J Alzheimers Dis. 2005;7(1):81–4.
36. Stead LG, Gilmore RM, Bellolio MF, et al. Hyperglycemia as an independent predictor of worse outcome in non-diabetic patients presenting with acute ischemic stroke. Neurocrit Care. 2009;10(2):181–6. doi:10.1007/s12028-008-9080-0.
37. Fuentes B, Ortega-Casarrubios MA, Sanjose B, et al. Persistent hyperglycemia >155 mg/dL in acute ischemic stroke patients: how well are we correcting it?: implications for outcome. Stroke. 2010;41(10):2362–5. doi:10.1161/STROKEAHA.110.591529.
38. Haratz S, Tanne D. Diabetes, hyperglycemia and the management of cerebrovascular disease. Curr Opin Neurol. 2011;24(1):81–8. doi:10.1097/WCO.0b013e3283418fed.
39. Parsons MW, Barber PA, Desmond PM, et al. Acute hyperglycemia adversely affects stroke outcome: a magnetic resonance imaging and spectroscopy study. Ann Neurol. 2002;52(1):20–8. doi:10.1002/ana.10241.
40. Clement S, Braithwaite SS, Magee MF, et al. Management of diabetes and hyperglycemia in hospitals. Diabetes Care. 2004;27(2):553–91.
41. Action to Control Cardiovascular Risk in Diabetes Study Group, Gerstein HC, Miller ME, et al. Effects of intensive glucose lowering in type 2 diabetes. N Engl J Med. 2008;358(24):2545–59. doi:10.1056/NEJMoa0802743.
42. ADVANCE Collaborative Group, Patel A, MacMahon S, et al. Intensive blood glucose control and vascular outcomes in patients with type 2 diabetes. N Engl J Med. 2008;358(24):2560–72. doi:10.1056/NEJMoa0802987.
43. Duckworth W, Abraira C, Moritz T, et al. Glucose control and vascular complications in veterans with type 2 diabetes. N Engl J Med. 2009;360(2):129–39. doi:10.1056/NEJMoa0808431.
44. Intensive blood-glucose control with sulphonylureas or insulin compared with conventional treatment and risk of complications in patients with type 2 diabetes (UKPDS 33). UK Prospective Diabetes Study (UKPDS) Group. Lancet. 1998;352(9131):837–53.
45. Holman RR, Paul SK, Bethel MA, Matthews DR, Neil HA. 10-year follow-up of intensive glucose control in type 2 diabetes. N Engl J Med. 2008;359(15):1577–89. doi:10.1056/NEJMoa0806470.
46. Meier M, Hummel M. Cardiovascular disease and intensive glucose control in type 2 diabetes mellitus: moving practice toward evidence-based strategies. Vasc Health Risk Manag. 2009;5:859–71.
47. Marso SP, Kennedy KF, House JA, McGuire DK. The effect of intensive glucose control on all-cause and cardiovascular mortality, myocardial infarction and stroke in persons with type 2 diabetes mellitus: a systematic review and meta-analysis. Diab Vasc Dis Res. 2010;7(2):119–30. doi:10.1177/1479164109353367.
48. Goldstein LB, Bushnell CD, Adams RJ, et al. Guidelines for the primary prevention of stroke: a guideline for healthcare professionals from the American Heart Association/American Stroke Association. Stroke. 2011;42(2):517–84. doi:10.1161/STR.0b013e3181fcb238.
49. Skyler JS, Bergenstal R, Bonow RO, et al. Intensive glycemic control and the prevention of cardiovascular events: implications of the ACCORD, ADVANCE, and VA diabetes trials: a position statement of the American Diabetes Association and a scientific statement of the American College of Cardiology

Foundation and the American Heart Association. Circulation. 2009;119(2):351–7. doi:10.1161/CIRCULATIONAHA.108.191305.
50. Kario K, Ishikawa J, Hoshide S, et al. Diabetic brain damage in hypertension: role of renin-angiotensin system. Hypertension. 2005;45(5):887–93. doi:10.1161/01.HYP.0000163460.07639.3f.
51. Tuomilehto J, Rastenyte D. Diabetes and glucose intolerance as risk factors for stroke. J Cardiovasc Risk. 1999;6(4):241–9.
52. Davis TM, Millns H, Stratton IM, Holman RR, Turner RC. Risk factors for stroke in type 2 diabetes mellitus: United Kingdom prospective diabetes study (UKPDS) 29. Arch Intern Med. 1999;159(10):1097–103.
53. Tight blood pressure control and risk of macrovascular and microvascular complications in type 2 diabetes: UKPDS 38. UK Prospective Diabetes Study Group. BMJ. 1998;317(7160):703–13.
54. Stratton IM, Cull CA, Adler AI, Matthews DR, Neil HA, Holman RR. Additive effects of glycaemia and blood pressure exposure on risk of complications in type 2 diabetes: a prospective observational study (UKPDS 75). Diabetologia. 2006;49(8):1761–9. doi:10.1007/s00125-006-0297-1.
55. Chobanian AV, Bakris GL, Black HR, et al. Seventh report of the joint national committee on prevention, detection, evaluation, and treatment of high blood pressure. Hypertension. 2003;42(6):1206–52. doi:10.1161/01.HYP.0000107251.49515.c2.
56. Effects of ramipril on cardiovascular and microvascular outcomes in people with diabetes mellitus: results of the HOPE study and MICRO-HOPE substudy. Heart Outcomes Prevention Evaluation Study Investigators. Lancet. 2000;355(9200):253–9.
57. Dahlof B, Devereux RB, Kjeldsen SE, et al. Cardiovascular morbidity and mortality in the losartan intervention for endpoint reduction in hypertension study (LIFE): a randomised trial against atenolol. Lancet. 2002;359(9311):995–1003. doi:10.1016/S0140-6736(02)08089-3.
58. Ostergren J, Poulter NR, Sever PS, et al. The Anglo-Scandinavian Cardiac Outcomes Trial: blood pressure-lowering limb: effects in patients with type II diabetes. J Hypertens. 2008;26(11):2103–11. doi:10.1097/HJH.0b013e328310e0d9.
59. Collins R, Armitage J, Parish S, Sleigh P, Peto R, Heart Protection Study Collaborative Group. MRC/BHF heart protection study of cholesterol-lowering with simvastatin in 5963 people with diabetes: a randomised placebo-controlled trial. Lancet. 2003; 361(9374):2005–16.
60. Colhoun HM, Betteridge DJ, Durrington PN, et al. Primary prevention of cardiovascular disease with atorvastatin in type 2 diabetes in the collaborative atorvastatin diabetes study (CARDS): multicentre randomised placebo-controlled trial. Lancet. 2004;364(9435):685–96. doi:10.1016/S0140-6736(04)16895-5.
61. Shepherd J, Barter P, Carmena R, et al. Effect of lowering LDL cholesterol substantially below currently recommended levels in patients with coronary heart disease and diabetes: the Treating to New Targets (TNT) study. Diabetes Care. 2006;29(6):1220–6. doi:10.2337/dc05-2465.
62. Rizos E, Mikhailidis DP. Are high density lipoprotein (HDL) and triglyceride levels relevant in stroke prevention? Cardiovasc Res. 2001;52(2):199–207.
63. Rubins HB, Robins SJ, Collins D, et al. Diabetes, plasma insulin, and cardiovascular disease: subgroup analysis from the department of veterans affairs high-density lipoprotein intervention trial (VA-HIT). Arch Intern Med. 2002;162(22):2597–604.
64. Keech A, Simes RJ, Barter P, et al. Effects of long-term fenofibrate therapy on cardiovascular events in 9795 people with type 2 diabetes mellitus (the FIELD study): randomised controlled trial. Lancet. 2005; 366(9500):1849–61. doi:10.1016/S0140-6736(05)67667-2.
65. Creager MA, Luscher TF, Cosentino F, Beckman JA. Diabetes and vascular disease: pathophysiology, clinical consequences, and medical therapy: Part I. Circulation. 2003;108(12):1527–32. doi:10.1161/01.CIR.0000091257.27563.32.
66. Hatzitolios AI, Didangelos TP, Zantidis AT, Tziomalos K, Giannakoulas GA, Karamitsos DT. Diabetes mellitus and cerebrovascular disease: which are the actual data? J Diabetes Complications. 2009;23(4):283–96. doi:10.1016/j.jdiacomp. 2008.01.004.
67. Colwell JA, American Diabetes Association. Aspirin therapy in diabetes. Diabetes Care. 2004;27 Suppl 1:S72–3.
68. Ogawa H, Nakayama M, Morimoto T, et al. Low-dose aspirin for primary prevention of atherosclerotic events in patients with type 2 diabetes: a randomized controlled trial. JAMA. 2008;300(18):2134–41. doi:10.1001/jama.2008.623.
69. Antithrombotic Trialists' Collaboration. Collaborative meta-analysis of randomised trials of antiplatelet therapy for prevention of death, myocardial infarction, and stroke in high risk patients. BMJ. 2002; 324(7329):71–86.
70. Evangelista V, Totani L, Rotondo S, et al. Prevention of cardiovascular disease in type-2 diabetes: how to improve the clinical efficacy of aspirin. Thromb Haemost. 2005;93(1):8–16. doi:10.1267/THRO05010008.
71. Sander D, Kearney MT. Reducing the risk of stroke in type 2 diabetes: pathophysiological and therapeutic perspectives. J Neurol. 2009;256(10):1603–19. doi:10.1007/s00415-009-5143-1.
72. Bhatt DL, Marso SP, Hirsch AT, Ringleb PA, Hacke W, Topol EJ. Amplified benefit of clopidogrel versus aspirin in patients with diabetes mellitus. Am J Cardiol. 2002;90(6):625–8.
73. Diener HC, Bogousslavsky J, Brass LM, et al. Aspirin and clopidogrel compared with clopidogrel alone after recent ischaemic stroke or transient ischaemic attack in high-risk patients (MATCH): randomised, double-blind, placebo-controlled trial. Lancet. 2004;364(9431):331–7. doi:10.1016/S0140-6736(04)16721-4.

74. Bhatt DL, Fox KA, Hacke W, et al. Clopidogrel and aspirin versus aspirin alone for the prevention of atherothrombotic events. N Engl J Med. 2006; 354(16):1706–17. doi:10.1056/NEJMoa060989.
75. Sacco RL, Ellenberg JH, Mohr JP, et al. Infarcts of undetermined cause: the NINCDS Stroke Data Bank. Ann Neurol. 1989;25(4):382–90. doi:10.1002/ana.410250410.
76. Chambless LE, Folsom AR, Davis V, et al. Risk factors for progression of common carotid atherosclerosis: the Atherosclerosis Risk in Communities Study, 1987-1998. Am J Epidemiol. 2002;155(1):38–47.
77. Henry RM, Kostense PJ, Spijkerman AM, et al. Arterial stiffness increases with deteriorating glucose tolerance status: the Hoorn Study. Circulation. 2003;107(16):2089–95. doi:10.1161/01.CIR.0000065222.34933.FC.
78. Hunt KJ, Williams K, Rivera D, et al. Elevated carotid artery intima-media thickness levels in individuals who subsequently develop type 2 diabetes. Arterioscler Thromb Vasc Biol. 2003;23(10):1845–50. doi:10.1161/01.ATV.0000093471.58663.ED.
79. Temelkova-Kurktschiev TS, Koehler C, Leonhardt W, et al. Increased intimal-medial thickness in newly detected type 2 diabetes: risk factors. Diabetes Care. 1999;22(2):333–8.
80. Nathan DM, Lachin J, Cleary P, et al. Intensive diabetes therapy and carotid intima-media thickness in type 1 diabetes mellitus. N Engl J Med. 2003;348(23):2294–303. doi:10.1056/NEJMoa022314.
81. Kadoglou NP, Avgerinos ED, Liapis CD. An update on markers of carotid atherosclerosis in patients with type 2 diabetes. Biomark Med. 2010;4(4):601–9. doi:10.2217/bmm.10.79.
82. Rizzo M, Corrado E, Coppola G, Muratori I, Novo G, Novo S. Markers of inflammation are strong predictors of subclinical and clinical atherosclerosis in women with hypertension. Coron Artery Dis. 2009;20(1):15–20. doi:10.1097/MCA.0b013e3283109065.
83. Corrado E, Rizzo M, Tantillo R, et al. Markers of inflammation and infection influence the outcome of patients with baseline asymptomatic carotid lesions: a 5-year follow-up study. Stroke. 2006;37(2):482–6. doi:10.1161/01.STR.0000198813.56398.14.
84. Gaede P, Vedel P, Larsen N, Jensen GV, Parving HH, Pedersen O. Multifactorial intervention and cardiovascular disease in patients with type 2 diabetes. N Engl J Med. 2003;348(5):383–93. doi:10.1056/NEJMoa021778.

Diabetic Considerations in Aortoiliac Disease

14

In-Kyong Kim and Rajeev Dayal

Keywords

Aortoiliac disease • Proximal disease • Diabetes • Infrarenal aorta • Iliac artery • Peripheral arterial disease

Definition of Aortoiliac Disease

Aortoiliac disease is an atherosclerotic process involving the abdominal aorta and the iliac arteries. It is an occlusive disease of the vascular inflow tract that leads to limited blood flow to the common femoral artery. This is in contrast to the outflow disease consisting of the arteries below the inguinal ligament. This classification is made not only to define the location of the disease, but also because the disease process and the treatment outcomes are distinctively different between the two regions.

Claudication

The symptoms of claudication attributable to aortoiliac occlusive disease are thigh or buttock pain

I.-K. Kim, M.D.
Department of General Surgery, Columbia University, New York Presbyterian Hospital, New York, NY, USA

R. Dayal, M.D. (✉)
Department of Surgery, North Shore University Hospital, 900 Northern Blvd., Great Neck, NY 11021, USA
e-mail: dayal.rajeev@gmail.com

with ambulation. In men, if the occlusion occurs in the bilateral iliac arteries and extends close to the origin of the hypogastric arteries, it leads to erectile dysfunction. Leriche syndrome encompasses the classic signs and symptoms of terminal aortoiliac disease and consists of thigh or buttock claudication, atrophy of the proximal leg muscles, impotence, and reduced femoral pulses. The symptoms of claudication are the result of lack of blood flow leading to regionally insufficient oxygenation, ischemic neuropathy involving the small unmyelinated A delta and C sensory fibers, and local intramuscular acidosis.

Chronic Limb Ischemia

Chronic limb ischemia describes the advanced symptoms of rest pain or tissue ischemia manifested usually by foot ulceration or gangrene. In the majority of patients with chronic aortoiliac disease, formation of collaterals from the infrainguinal segments to the popliteal artery allow for sufficient perfusion to avoid the symptoms of chronic limb ischemia. Therefore, the symptoms of these stages typically occur when there is an occlusion of two or more vascular beds, whether they are in sequence or in parallel circuit. Patients with diabetes often have distal, and especially infrapopliteal, disease, predisposing to these severe manifestations.

Asymptomatic Disease

Prior to progression to claudication and subsequently chronic limb ischemia, the process begins with vascular compromise without yet noticeable symptoms. The presence of asymptomatic disease is identified by the ankle–brachial index (ABI)<0.9. Detecting asymptomatic aortoiliac disease is often difficult, especially in individuals with diabetes and calcified vasculature that may confound proper ABI measurements.

Pathogenesis

Diverging theories exists to explain the process of atherosclerosis. The central theme, the order of which is debated, is injury to the arterial endothelial cells via varying proposed mechanisms, deposition of cholesterol molecules with accompanying inflammatory response via macrophages and T cells, and smooth muscle cell proliferation.

Mechanism of Vascular Injury in Diabetes

Endothelial cells maintain vascular homeostasis by providing a functional barrier and chemical medium that promote antiplatelet, anti-inflammatory, antiproliferative, and antioxidant properties [1]. The common channel that is believed to lead to atherogenesis is endothelial cell dysfunction. This occurs by means of decreased remodeling or repair after vascular injury secondary to reduction in the number of cells, defective mobilization from peripheral source, and impaired functional properties of vascular progenitor cells, including the endothelial progenitor cells (EPC) [2]. Several proposed mechanisms explain this phenomenon in diabetes

(1) glycated collagen releasing decreased amounts of nitric oxide, which is a stem cell growth factor and angiogenesis regulator [3, 4]; (2) formation of advanced glycation end products (AGE) and its interaction with receptor of AGE (RAGE) that enhance the release of proinflammatory oxidation products [5]; (3) decreased levels of stromal cell-derived factor (SDF)-1α that modulates EPC senescence and apoptosis [3].

In conjunction with the above chemical factors, there are mechanical factors that are associated with arterial disease. In vitro studies with glycated collagen show malalignment of cellular structures to sheer fluid stress [4]. Further, both diabetic and prediabetic patients with impaired fasting glucose are shown to have increased arterial wall stiffness as measured by pulse-wave velocity [6].

Diabetic Contributions to Aortoiliac Disease

There are important functional differences between proximal and distal diseases. Individuals with aortoiliac PAD have a higher volume of ischemic muscle mass with walking and have more symptoms of claudication [7]. Further, aortoiliac disease is associated with a higher mortality as compared with infrainguinal diseases independent of concominant risk factors and comorbidities [8]. As would be suspected, the risk factors differ depending on the disease distribution. Multivariate analysis of 132 affected segments (23 aortoiliac, 82 femoropopliteal, 27 tibial) by a group in Linz, Austria, found smoking to be a significant risk factor for the aortoiliac segment (Odds ratio 25.1 aortoiliac to 1.37 tibial) and diabetes to be a significant risk factor for the tibial segment (Odds ratio 4.60 aortoiliac to 43.1 tibial) [9]. Lower levels of HDL also were a statistically significant risk factor for the development of proximal disease. A study of patients with familial hypercholesterolemia also showed that age and increased levels of LDL were independent risk factors of aortoiliac disease. Diabetes was not an independent risk factor [10]. The studies suggest that aortoiliac disease is potentially more preventable than the tibial diseases in patients with diabetes via smoking session and cholesterol control.

Further, even though diabetes may not predispose to a greater incidence of proximal disease, there are evidences that it may change the manifestation of the disease. Exercise testing shows that within individuals with equivalent self-reported symptoms of claudication (as measured by reported distance prior to the onset of pain), individuals with diabetes have a significantly lower maximal walking distance on the treadmill (261 ± 257 and 339 ± 326 m, respectively; $P<0.05$ when adjusted for potential confounders) [11]. Potential association with this would be the decrease in aortic distensibility seen with increase in age and with worse glycemic control [12].

Epidemiology

Prevalence

Defining the prevalence of PAD in the diabetic population has been difficult due to the presence of peripheral neuropathy that dampen the outward symptoms and vascular calcification that confound the objective detection via ABI. The PAD Awareness, Risk, and Treatment: New Resources for Survival (PARTNERS) study estimates the prevalence of PAD in the diabetic population to be 29% [13], and Elhadd et al. estimates it to be 20% [14]. This is in contrast to the general population, where the prevalence is noted to be 4% [15]. However, when individuals with peripheral arterial disease are selected, the rate of proximal (aortoiliac) disease as measured by limb transcutaneous oxygen pressure is similar between the diabetic and the nondiabetic groups [11].

Progression of Disease

Regardless of the absolute prevalence, PAD imposes systemic and local effects during both symptomatic and asymptomatic stages of the disease. The morbidity and mortality associated with diabetic patients with PAD are staggering. In an 11-year follow-up study comparing diabetic patients with and without PAD (both symptomatic and asymptomatic as defined by $ABI<0.9$), the mortality equaled 58% and 16%, respectively ($P<0.001$) [16]. A health center at Catalonia, the only referral hospital in the region, studied specifically the impact of asymptomatic PAD. In the population of 329 registered type II diabetics, 242 were found to have PAD by $ABI<0.9$ criteria. The 10-year cumulative morbidity and mortality comparison between those without and with asymptomatic PAD was drastic: mortality 16.8% vs. 52.8% ($P<0.05$), rate of combined fatal and nonfatal MI 26.9% vs. 81.9% [17].

Diabetes also contributes to the faster progression of local disease. Nationwide age-adjusted amputation rate in diabetes is approximately 8 per 1,000 patient-years, with a prevalence of approximately 3%. Just the rate of amputation nearly parallels the overall prevalence of PAD in the general population (4% as mentioned previously).

Diagnosis

As can be inferred from the systemic and local implications of PAD in the diabetic population, a prompt diagnosis and aggressive treatment with the aim of secondary prevention is crucial. The American Diabetic Association recommends routine screening in all diabetic patients over age 50 by the use of ABI [18].

Physiologic and Hemodynamic Measurements

The most widely used definition of PAD is $ABI<0.9$. However, individuals with diabetes are significantly more prone to renal disease and medial calcification of the arterial system. This leads to vascular non-compressibility, and as a standard, $ABI>1.3$ is labeled as calcified vessels, and therefore nondiagnostic. Further, because the presence of calcification that may alter the compressibility to give an $ABI>1.3$, some advocate a higher cutoff value for ABI for the diagnosis of PAD in individuals with diabetes. Clairotte et al. examined 146 patients, 83 with diabetes, and assessed the presence of PAD as determined by duplex peak systolic velocity ratio>2. The oscillator ABI was utilized and compared with the duplex standard in the detection of PAD. The group found that the ABI cutoff of <0.9 was sufficient for diagnosing PAD in nondiabetic people. However, for those with diabetes, the cutoff values for the highest sensitivity and specificity were between 1.0 and 1.1, higher than the standard used for the general population [19].

The treadmill function test is also often utilized for the initial diagnosis. This consists of a comparison of the ankle pressure at rest with after a regimen of treadmill ambulation. Although this varies, an example of a regimen is walking at 3.5 km/h at a 12% incline until the symptoms of claudication followed by 3 min of recovery period. If the pressure at this point is decreased by more than 20%, the test is considered positive. Again, this test also requires compressible vessels for accuracy.

Imaging

All patients considered for a surgical or endovascular intervention need vascular imaging. Duplex ultrasound is a modality utilized often during the initial diagnosis. It does not expose the subject to harmful radiation and does not require any nephrotoxic contrast agents. However, duplex is of especially limited use in the aortoiliac segment secondary to view-obstructing bowel gas and large patient body habitus.

Many institutions utilize MRA enhanced with gadolinium. This modality has been shown to have a very high sensitivity and specificity, nearing 100% for both, especially in the proximal arterial disease [20]. The disadvantages of contrast-enhanced MRA (CEMRA) are the inability to accommodate those with metallic implants, causation of claustrophobia, and the potential of nephrogenic systemic fibrosis if performed on a person with GFR<30 mL/min (OR 6.671 after single exposure and 44.5 after multiple exposures) [21]. Additionally, MRA is known to overestimate the severity of the stenosis and requires the interpreter to have an experience with the degree of overestimation by the particular MRA utilized.

An interesting upcoming MRA technology may resolve a number of the above issues. Quiescent-interval single-shot (QISS) MRA is an unenhanced (therefore no contrast toxicity), non-substractive (therefore resistant to motion artifacts) technology that is significantly faster in obtaining the required images. The total imaging time from the infrarenal aorta down to the feet is 7 min. This technology acquires data using a modified single-shot 2-D balanced steady-state free precession pulse sequence. A recent study tested 25 individuals with contrast-enhanced MRA and the QISS MRA. Respective sensitivity and specificity of the two modalities determined by comparison to the gold-standard angiography was CEMRA 90.7%, 93.4% vs. QISS 96.2%, 96.1% [22].

Until the technology becomes widely and commercially available, most surgeon utilize the CEMRA, or in some centers, CT angiogram.

Biomarkers

A number of biomarkers have been studied for their association with PAD. If there is a concern for a prothrombotic state from patient or familial history, a hypercoagulability work-up is warranted and a fibrinogen level may be of value. Other nonspecific markers associated with atherosclerotic disease are CRP and homocysteine for those who develop PAD at an early age. Following are a few biomarkers that have been shown to specifically signify PAD in individuals with diabetes.

Ischemia-Modified Albumin

Ischemia-modified albumin, also called cobalt-binding albumin, is produced as a result of serum albumin flowing through ischemic tissues and is a marker of oxidative stress and ischemia. In a study of 290 participants with type II diabetes, the baseline ischemia-modified albumin levels were found to be significantly higher in those with PAD. Further, the levels had a positive correlation with HbA1c and homocysteine levels [23].

Plasma Osteoprotegerin

Plasma osteoprotegerin (OPG) is a glycoprotein from the tumor necrosis factor receptor superfamily and is typically involved in bone remodeling. The tissue concentrations of OPG in aorta and the hip bone are almost equal and approximately 500 times higher than in the plasma. It is implicated in vascular calcification inhibition, and thereby has become of interest in the field of vascular medicine. The most recent and one of the largest studies assessed 350 patients with type II diabetes for an association between OPG level and the presence of various cardiovascular diseases. Plasma OPG was significantly increased in patients with carotid and peripheral arterial disease compared to patients without ($P<0.001$, respectively); however, this was not the case for patients with myocardial ischemia versus those without ($P=0.71$) [24].

Treatment

Medical Therapy

General Cardiovascular Risk Reduction

As emphasized repeatedly, the presence of PAD indicates systemic atherosclerosis. Early treatments with the goal of controlling blood pressure, cholesterol, and glycemia have shown to have a significant impact in the progression of overall vascular diseases. In a large randomized control trial of 160 patients with type II diabetes, intensive therapy was compared with conventional therapy [25]. The intensive-therapy group had strict targets goals of HbA1c<6.5%, fasting serum total cholesterol <175 mg/dL, fasting serum triglyceride level <150 mg/dL, systolic BP<130, and diastolic <80 mmHg. All patients were treated with renin–angiotensin system blocker for microalbuminuria regardless of blood pressure and received low-dose aspirin therapy. Upon 6-year follow-up, the intensive-therapy group had lower mortality from cardiovascular causes (HR 0.43), lower cardiovascular events (HR 0.41), fewer incidence of progression to ESRD ($P=0.04$), and fewer retinal photocoagulation requirement (RR 0.45). The results clearly demonstrate the importance of tight glucose control, use of angiotensin receptor blockers, aspirin, and lipid-lowering agents.

However, intensive therapy has not been shown to delay the progression of peripheral arterial disease. In a recent study of 1,533 people with type II diabetes, patients were randomized to either the intensive-therapy group or routine-care group [26]. Participants were followed for 6 years; ABI and vibration and light touch sensations were measured throughout. At the end of the study, there was no statistically significant effect of intensive therapy on the prevalence of PAD or peripheral neuropathy as measured by above follow-up methods.

Treatment of PAD Symptoms
Lifestyle Modification

Although above intensive medical therapy regimen to improve systemic cardiovascular burden has not shown to decrease the progression of PAD, there are some lifestyle modifications that have been proven to improve the symptoms of PAD.

Supervised exercise has been shown to be significantly beneficial in delaying the progression of aortoiliac disease [7]. In the Claudication: Exercise Versus Endoluminal Revascularization (CLEVER) trial of 111 patients with known aortoiliac disease with moderate to severe claudication, the participants were randomly assigned to one of the three treatment arms: (1) optimal medical care (OMC) that includes cilastazol as well as exercise regimen recommendations; (2) supervised exercise (SE) of 26 weeks of exercise, three times a week, for 1 h at a time with a trainer that followed a given protocol; (3) stent revascularization (ST) of all hemodynamically significant stenosis (>50% by diameter) in the aorta and iliac arteries, with perioperative and postoperative antiplatelet medication at the discretion of the surgeon. At the 6-month follow-up, change in peak walking time (the primary end point) was greatest for the supervised exercise (SE) group, intermediate for the stent group (ST), and least with optical medical care (OMC) (mean change versus baseline, 5.8±4.6, 3.7±4.9, and 1.2±2.6 min, respectively; $P<0.001$ for the comparison of SE versus OMC, $P=0.02$ for ST versus OMC, and $P=0.04$ for SE versus ST). Similarly, the Edinburg trial compared exercise regimen plus aspirin against percutaneous balloon angiography (PTA) of the SFA or iliac arteries plus aspirin [27]. The study demonstrated that although PTA plus aspirin showed less extensive disease at the 2-year follow-up imaging, there was no functional difference between the two groups. Both of these studies point to the importance of supervised or regimented exercise.

Smoking session and diet change to lower cholesterol are also recommended. As discussed previously under pathogenesis, smoking, high LDL, and low HDL have been shown to be independent risk factors of aortoiliac disease. Therefore, although no randomized control can be done to assess these modifications, the lifestyle changes are recommended for secondary prevention of PAD.

Glycemic control is also emphasized. In the diabetic cohort from the Atherosclerosis Risk in Communities (ARIC) study, there was a positive, graded, and independent association between HbA1C and PAD risk for varying manifestations of the disease, including intermittent claudication to PAD-related hospitalization [28]. The results suggest that improvement in glycemic control in individuals with diabetes may substantially reduce the risk or progression of PAD.

Pharmacology

The only medication shown to improve the claudication symptoms of PAD is cilastazol (Pletal). This pharmacotherapy has been shown to be efficacious in the diabetic group as well [29]. Further, the usage of antiplatelets is well established.

As suggested by diet modification to improve cholesterol control, simvastatin is also shown to improve the symptoms of claudication. 40 mg/day of simvastatin for 6 months was tested against placebo in a randomized, placebo-controlled, double-blind study [30]. At the end of the study period, the mean pain-free walking distance had increased by 90-m more in the simvastatin group than in the placebo group ($P<0.05$), as well as statistically significant improvement in the total walking distance, and resting and post-exercise ABI. Of note, over 50% of the treatment and the placebo group had diabetes.

Prostaglandins, although not Food and Drug Administration (FDA) approved, have shown some efficacy in improving the symptoms of intermittent claudication. In specific, Iloprost is the only prostaglandin that has been shown to exert significant therapeutic effects in the diabetic population [31, 32]. The medication is given as intravenous infusion and has significant side effects of headache, flushing, and gastrointestinal symptoms with conflicting results and yet to be a widely approved treatment option.

Other medications that have been studied with conflicting evidence include levocarnitine, buflomedil, L-arginine, and ketanserin.

Operative Management

All patients with CLI should be treated by either open surgical or endovascular intervention. Typically, only severely limiting claudication not improved by medical therapy is treated operatively. However, for aortoiliac disease, as the outcomes of endovascular therapy are proven to be effective without significant morbidity and mortality, most claudicants are now treated via endovascular means without waiting for the outcomes of the medical treatment.

Collaterals

The presence of large collaterals plays a role in both open surgical and endovascular therapy. Especially in patients with chronic occlusive disease, significant collaterals may form (Fig. 14.1). Generally, large collaterals, such as lumbars, are avoided from coverage by covered stents. For the internal iliac arteries, coverage by either bare metal stents or covered stents can eventually lead to internal iliac thrombosis and occlusion. In order to avoid this occurrence and

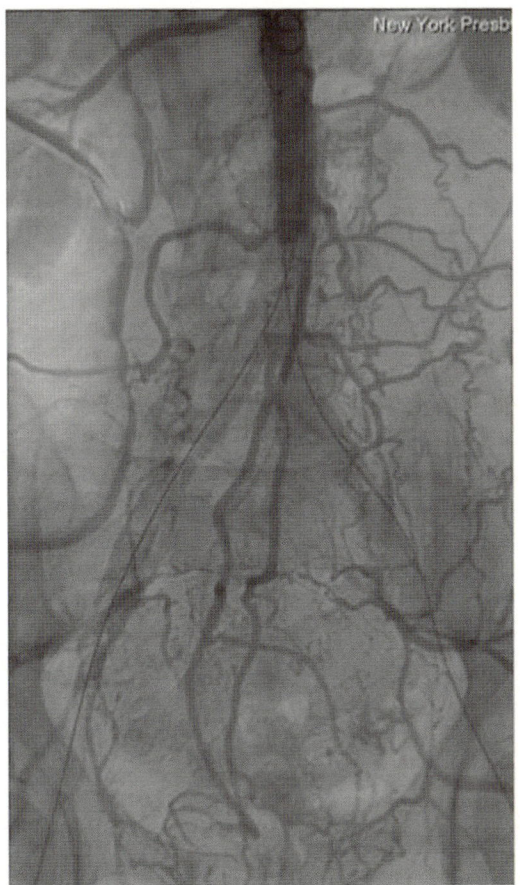

Fig. 14.1 A total occlusion of the aortoiliac segment. Significant collaterals via the systemic and visceral circulation can be seen

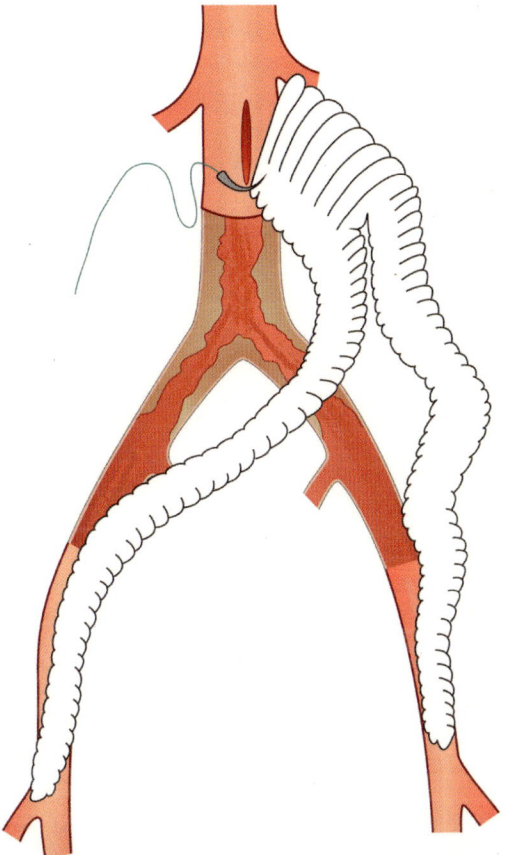

Fig. 14.2 End-to-side anastomosis. The distal aorta and the common iliac arteries are patent and allows for antegrade flow into the hypogastric arteries. To preserve this flow, end-to-side anastomosis is performed (courtesy of Stephen Cassidy)

the resulting symptoms of buttock claudication, coverage of internal iliac arteries by any type of stents is avoided.

When treating via open surgery, the patency of the distal aorta or the common iliac arteries dictates the type of anastomosis. If this distal segment is patent, end-to-side anastomosis is favored (Fig. 14.2). If the segment is occluded, an end-to-end proximal anastomosis allows for an improved anatomical alignment, decreased erosion into the duodenum, and construction to be closer to the renal arteries (Fig. 14.3). Further discussion on the anastomosis will be included in the surgical portion of this chapter.

Endovascular Intervention
Endovascular Outcomes

The disease of the aortoiliac segment is distinct from other lower extremity segments in that the outcome of endovascular therapy is similar to open surgery with decreased morbidity and mortality [33]. Endovascular intervention, therefore, is considered first-line therapy (Fig. 14.4).

There were initial concerns that the results may not hold true for the diabetic population. A study at Yale University that included 142 PTA intervention (94 in iliac arteries, 46 in femoropopliteal segment) showed absence of diabetes, as assessed via chi-square testing, was a patient factor that favored a superior outcome as assessed

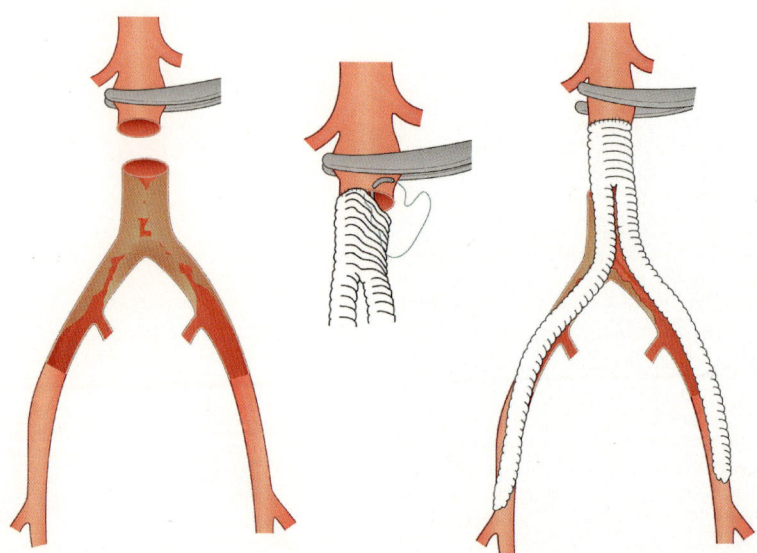

Fig. 14.3 End-to-end anastomosis. The distal aorta and the common iliac arteries are occluded. The hypogastric arteries are perfused by retrograde flow from the external iliac arteries. Therefore, no antegrade flow needs to be preserved. In such circumstances, end-to-end proximal anastomosis is preferred to allow for an improved anatomical construction (courtesy of Stephen Cassidy)

by resolution or improvement of symptoms [34]. Further, data from PTA of the femoropopliteal region at the British Royal Infirmary showed that the cumulative patency of PTA in individuals with diabetes was 37.2% vs. 53.1% in nondiabetic patients, although it did not reach statistical significance on logrank testing [35].

However, there is now evidence that, for aortoiliac disease, endovascular intervention is equally as effective as open surgery even in individuals with diabetes. A consecutive series of 159 iliac PTA performed in conjunction with infrainguinal arterial bypass in 126 patients was reviewed [36]. In this series, 99 patients (78.6%) had diabetes. Average follow-up was 20.2 months. Graft patency was determined by clinical pulse examination, Doppler examination, as well as selective color-flow duplex exam. Overall perioperative morbidity was 4.8% (myocardial infarction, acute renal failure, pneumonia), complications 8.7% (hematoma, wound infection, wound dehiscence), and 30-day mortality 1% in those with diabetes and 0% nondiabetics. There was no significant difference in any of the above rates between the diabetic and the nondiabetic cohort. Further, the graft patency between the two cohorts remained similar. A total of 159 iliac PTA were performed (92 common iliac artery (CIA) and 67 external iliac artery (EIA)). The mean pressure gradient prior to PTA was 41.0 ± 28.2 mmHg (range 11–106 mmHg). The mean pressure gradient after PTA completion was 1.6 ± 2.6 mmHg (range 0–4.7 mmHg). There was no significant difference in gradients between diabetic and nondiabetic patients ($P=NS$). With the evidence taken together, the current standard of care for symptomatic aortoiliac disease in diabetic or nondiabetic patients is endovascular therapy.

Endovascular Techniques

As reported above, PTA alone has positive outcomes in aortoiliac disease in diabetic patients. PTA is known to work well for short segment CIA stenosis or occlusion. However, if there is significant vessel recoil, residual stenosis, flow-limiting dissection, or persistent gradient, then the usage of stenting is well established. Additional evidence from the Palmaz group indicate that primary stent placement is also safe and involving >50% diameter) and freedom from occlusion for the TransAtlantic Inter-Society Consensus (TASC) B lesions. However, for TASC C and D lesions, covered stents had a significantly higher freedom from binary restenosis (HR 0.136). This suggests the superiority of covered stents for the more severe lesion types in the proximal arteries.

Diabetic Considerations for Endovascular Complications

The most notable complication of endovascular therapy in the diabetic patient population is contrast-induced nephropathy. The debate on the methods to lower the incidence of this complication is still ongoing. The only proven factor currently is hydration. Evidence for the type of intravenous fluid, although some exists in favor of bicarbonate solution, is not well established. The role of N-acetylcysteine is also still controversial.

Surgical Intervention

As discussed previously, iliac artery PTA and stenting have excellent outcomes nearing that of aortofemoral bypass. Therefore, surgical interventions are now considered second- or third-line therapy in the treatment of aortoiliac occlusive lesions.

Surgical Bypass Results in Diabetics

Although the efficacy of surgical bypass in the diabetic population has not been of debate, the controversy has centered on the potential need for a combined proximal as well as infrainguinal bypass. Some surgeons believe that, as diabetes affects distal arteries often, patients with diabetes should undergo a distal bypass at the time of the proximal bypass to avoid the increased morbidity and mortality of undergoing multiple operations.

Most recent data appear to refute this suggestion. Between 1990 and 1999, a total of 504 inflow arterial reconstructions were performed (diabetic = 301, 59.7%; nondiabetic = 203, 40.3%) [39]. Procedures included aortofemoral (370, 73%), axilofemoral (56, 11%), and the rest femorofemoral bypass. Throughout the follow-up time period, there was no statistical difference in

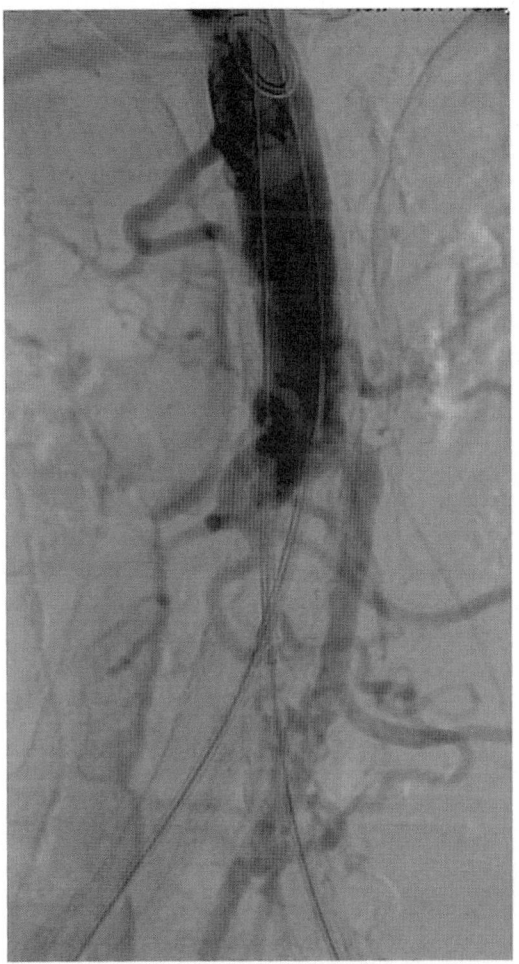

Fig. 14.4 Endovascular management of complete aortoiliac occlusion. Two balloon-expandable stents are placed into the aorta below the level of inferior mesenteric artery

efficacious with a clinical success rate above 98% and primary patency reaching 90% at 2 years [37] (Fig. 14.5).

Also of interest is the efficacy of covered versus bare-metal expandable stents in the treatment of aortoiliac disease. The Covered Versus Balloon Expandable Stent Trial (COBEST), a prospective, multicenter, randomized control trial, was recently performed involving 168 iliac arteries in 125 patients [38]. The patients were randomized into the covered balloon-expandable stent group or the bare-metal stent group. Patients were followed at 1, 6, 12, and 18 months. The study showed that the two stents had similar rate of freedom from binary restenosis (stenosis

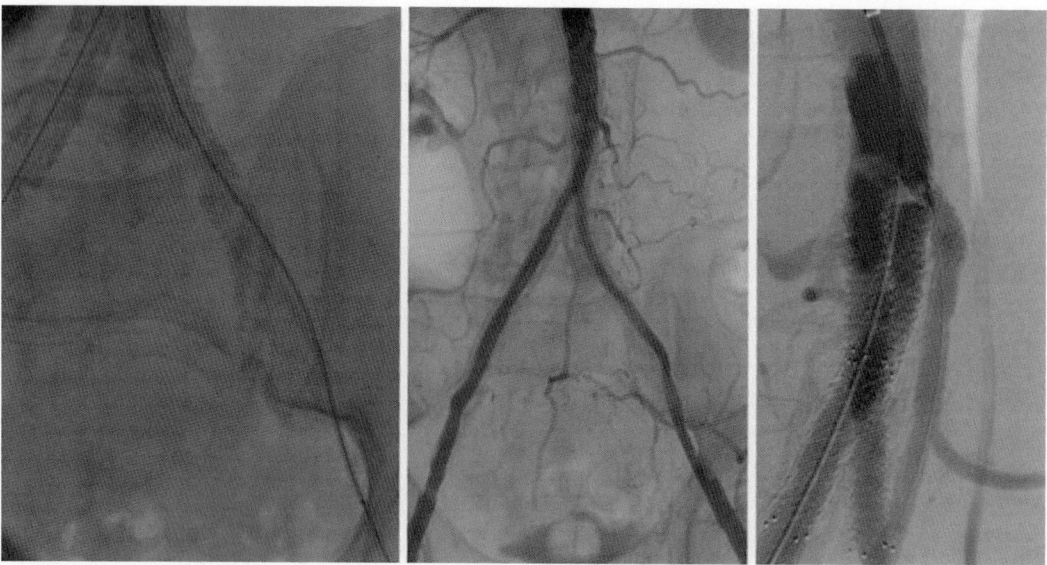

Fig. 14.5 8 mm Viabahn stent grafts (Gore, Flagstaff, Arizona) placed into bilateral CIA and EIA. The completion angiogram showed occlusion of the inferior mesenteric artery requiring additional stent placement

cumulative patency or limb salvage rate between the bypasses performed in the diabetic and the nondiabetic patients (graft patency = diabetic 100% at 5 years, nondiabetic 88%; Limb salvage = diabetic 91% at 5 years, non-diabetic 80%). Further, the presence of diabetes was not an independent risk factor for the need for multiple revascularization procedures. Therefore, the study concluded that there was no rationale for simultaneous inflow and outflow procedures.

Aortoiliac Endarterectomy

Aortoiliac endarterectomy is currently rarely performed owing to the superior outcomes of endovascular treatments and aortofemoral bypass for those requiring open treatment. Therefore, this procedure has become of historical interest only. For those who continue to possess the proper training and technique for aortoiliac endarterectomy, it may be of benefit in the diabetic population, because it avoids the use of prosthetic material, and the infection rate is practically nonexistent.

Aortofemoral Bypass

Aortofemoral bypass is the open surgical treatment of choice for those cases in which endovascular therapy is not amenable. As discussed previously, there are some instances when end-to-end versus end-to-side proximal anastomosis would be preferred; however, there is no strong evidence to support one technique over another under circumstances in which either method is technically able to be performed.

In addition to the instances described previously, there is one more circumstance in which end-to-end anastomosis is preferred. This pertains to a calcified infrarenal aorta. This is of special concern for patients with diabetes as the disease has been traditionally associated with medial arterial calcification. A recent controlled study of 260 subjects from the Rochester Diabetic Neuropathy Study with matched cohort from the Rochester Diabetic Neuropathy Study—Healthy Subject cohort ($n = 221$) took a radiograph of the lower extremities and found the presence of arterial calcification to be four times as prevalent as in the diabetic group [40]. If the calcification is present at the infrarenal aorta, then the tandem partial-occluding clamping utilized during the end-to-side anastomosis is difficult to perform, and an end-to-end method is recommended. To obtain the proximal anastomotic site on the aorta, dissection should be carried out to or just above the left renal vein. Calcification is often less severe at this proximal point just below the renal arteries. The clamp should be applied at this point. Once the aorta is transected, endarterectomy should be performed to create a 1- to 2-cm cuff that is free of calcification. This supplies a cuff made of aortic adventitia and external elastic lamina. According to Brewster's experience reported in Haimovici's Vascular Surgery, this cuff is adequate for graft anastomosis without additional complications of bleeding, suture line disruption, or pseudoaneurysm formation at the anastomotic site [41]. If the aorta just distal to the renals is calcified and occluded, proximal clamp can be applied above the renal arteries. In this case, it is very important to dissect and loop the renals, then clamp the renals prior to clamping the aorta. Once the clamp is secure, the aorta should be transected 3–4 cm below the renals. A circumferential endarterectomy should be performed by passing a large fogarty balloon through the occlusion into the suprarenal aorta and pulling the plug out. This quick flush technique will remove the debris and allow for the suprarenal clamp to be now moved below the renals. The renal clamps are then removed. This would then allow for a sufficient cuff for the anastomosis. The infrarenal cuff can be shortened, if needed, at this point. This sequence is of utmost importance to prevent renal dysfunction that may result from this procedure.

Regardless of the proximal anastomotic technique, it is important to establish an adequate outflow prior to the distal anastomosis. If the superficial femoral artery (SFA) is diseased, then the profunda can be utilized, since it is often spared even in patients with diabetes. In virtually all cases, the distal anastomosis should be hooded over the origin of the profunda femoris.

The graft selection, Dacron or polytetrafluoroethylene (PTFE), is at the discretion of the surgeon. There is no strong evidence to favor one material to another. A randomized control study was performed to compare the two graft materials in 85 patients undergoing femoropopliteal bypass, and the results were equivocal [42]. Early limb salvage rates for Dacron and PTFE were 100 and 97.7% ($P>0.05$). Early (30-day) complications (bleeding 2.38 and 2.32%; wound infection 11.9 and 11.63%) occurred in both groups with similar frequency ($P>0.05$). There is a general belief that Dacron may cause less needle hold bleeding and thereby cause decreased bleeding difficulties at the proximal anastomosis. There are no strong data currently to support this conjecture.

For either Dacron or PTFE, it is crucial to not oversize the graft. Oversizing can lead to sluggish flow in graft limbs and increased deposition of laminar pseudointima. This can eventually lead to occlusion of the graft. Therefore, the recommended size is 16×8 mm, with the smaller size of 14×7 mm when appropriate, such as in some female patients [41].

Extra-Anatomic Bypass

There are instances in which extra-anatomic bypass is performed. Femorofemoral bypass can be utilized for uni-iliac disease without any stenosis in the contralateral iliac artery. This procedure is technically simpler than the aortofemoral bypass and has good long-term results. Therefore, this procedure provides a surgical option for those patients who are not amenable to endovascular procedures but are too high risk (comorbidities, prior abdominal surgeries, anatomic configuration) or elderly to safely undergo an anatomic procedure. There is controversy; however, concerning the progression of disease in the aorta to the donor iliac artery, however, this can be readily treated with an iliac stent. Most definitive treatment, if any concern, would be to perform a bilateral reconstruction with a bifurcated prosthetic graft. With this in mind, femorofemoral bypass can also be used in cases of unilateral obstruction after a previous aortofemoral bypass [43].

Axillofemoral bypass is an option for an infected abdominal field as it can avoid the region of native infection. Of important note, this is not useful for an infected groin, as the operation still requires the distal anastomosis to be performed at the groin region. For both of these extra-anatomic bypasses, the patency is dependent on the runoff status of the distal vessels.

Postoperative Considerations for Diabetics

Two of the early complications are of particular concern for the diabetic population. First is the concern of distal atheroemboli, or "trash foot." As discussed earlier, the arterial system in the diabetic population is significantly more likely to be calcified. Therefore, prevention of distal emboli or "trash foot" hinges on meticulous intraoperative management. Aortic clamping should be applied judiciously, and every measure should be taken as described above to avoid clamping a significantly calcified segment.

The second, and a preventable complication, is wound infection. It is well known that diabetic patients are at greater risk of infectious complications. It is also well known that tight glycemic control during the perioperative period can significantly lower the infectious complication rate. Therefore, the insulin drip should be carefully titrated while the patient is under NPO status and should be transitioned to standard long-acting insulin or oral glycemic agent as appropriate.

As shown in the previous sections, the long-term complications of graft occlusion appear to be similar between the diabetic and the nondiabetic population. Regardless of circumstances, the most important concept in avoiding the complications attributable to diabetes is glycemic control.

References

1. De Caterina R. Endothelial dysfunctions: common denominators in vascular disease. Curr Opin Lipidol. 2000;11(1):9–23.
2. Madonna R, De Caterina R. Cellular and molecular mechanisms of vascular injury in diabetes – part II: cellular mechanisms and therapeutic targets. Vascul Pharmacol. 2011;54(3–6):75–9.
3. Gallagher KA, Liu ZJ, Xiao M, et al. Diabetic impairments in NO-mediated endothelial progenitor cell mobilization and homing are reversed by hyperoxia and SDF-1 alpha. J Clin Invest. 2007;117(5):1249–59.
4. Kemeny SF, Figueroa DS, Andrews AM, Barbee KA, Clyne AM. Glycated collagen alters endothelial cell actin alignment and nitric oxide release in response to fluid shear stress. J Biomech. 2011;44(10):1927–35.
5. Barlovic DP, Soro-Paavonen A, Jandeleit-Dahm KA. RAGE biology, atherosclerosis and diabetes. Clin Sci (Lond). 2011;121(2):43–55.
6. Shin JY, Lee HR, Lee DC. Increased arterial stiffness in healthy subjects with high-normal glucose levels and in subjects with pre-diabetes. Cardiovasc Diabetol. 2011;10:30.
7. Murphy TP, Cutlip DE, Regensteiner JG, et al. Supervised exercise versus primary stenting for claudication resulting from aortoiliac peripheral artery disease: six-month outcomes from the Claudication: Exercise Versus Endoluminal Revascularization (CLEVER) study. Circulation. 2012;125(1):130–9.
8. Aboyans V, Desormais I, Lacroix P, Salazar J, Criqui MH, Laskar M. The general prognosis of patients with peripheral arterial disease differs according to the disease localization. J Am Coll Cardiol. 2010;55(9):898–903.
9. Haltmayer M, Mueller T, Horvath W, Luft C, Poelz W, Haidinger D. Impact of atherosclerotic risk factors on the anatomical distribution of peripheral arterial disease. Int Angiol. 2001;20(3):200–7.
10. Yagi K, Hifumi S, Nohara A, et al. Difference in the risk factors for coronary, renal and other peripheral arteriosclerosis in heterozygous familial hypercholesterolemia. Circ J. 2004;68(7):623–7.
11. Mahe G, Ouedraogo N, Leftheriotis G, Vielle B, Picquet J, Abraham P. Exercise treadmill testing in patients with claudication, with and without diabetes. Diabet Med. 2011;28(3):356–62.
12. Stacey RB, Bertoni AG, Eng J, Bluemke DA, Hundley WG, Herrington D. Modification of the effect of glycemic status on aortic distensibility by age in the multi-ethnic study of atherosclerosis. Hypertension. 2010;55(1):26–32.
13. Hirsch AT, Criqui MH, Treat-Jacobson D, et al. Peripheral arterial disease detection, awareness, and treatment in primary care. JAMA. 2001;286(11):1317–24.
14. Elhadd TA, Jung RT, Newton RW, Stonebridge PA, Belch JJ. Incidence of asymptomatic peripheral arterial occlusive disease in diabetic patients attending a hospital clinic. Adv Exp Med Biol. 1997;428:45–8.
15. Selvin E, Erlinger TP. Prevalence of and risk factors for peripheral arterial disease in the United States: results from the National Health and Nutrition Examination Survey, 1999-2000. Circulation. 2004;110(6):738–43.
16. Kallio M, Forsblom C, Groop PH, Groop L, Lepantalo M. Development of new peripheral arterial occlusive disease in patients with type 2 diabetes during a mean follow-up of 11 years. Diabetes Care. 2003;26(4):1241–5.
17. Bundo M, Munoz L, Perez C, et al. Asymptomatic peripheral arterial disease in type 2 diabetes patients: a 10-year follow-up study of the utility of the ankle brachial index as a prognostic marker of cardiovascular disease. Ann Vasc Surg. 2010;24(8):985–93.
18. American Diabetes Association. Peripheral arterial disease in people with diabetes. Diabetes Care. 2003;26(12):3333–41.
19. Clairotte C, Retout S, Potier L, Roussel R, Escoubet B. Automated ankle-brachial pressure index measure-

ment by clinical staff for peripheral arterial disease diagnosis in nondiabetic and diabetic patients. Diabetes Care. 2009;32(7):1231–6.
20. Holland GA, Dougherty L, Carpenter JP, et al. Breath-hold ultrafast three-dimensional gadolinium-enhanced MR angiography of the aorta and the renal and other visceral abdominal arteries. AJR Am J Roentgenol. 1996;166(4):971–81.
21. Othersen JB, Maize JC, Woolson RF, Budisavljevic MN. Nephrogenic systemic fibrosis after exposure to gadolinium in patients with renal failure. Nephrol Dial Transplant. 2007;22(11):3179–85.
22. Hodnett PA, Ward EV, Davarpanah AH, et al. Peripheral arterial disease in a symptomatic diabetic population: prospective comparison of rapid unenhanced MR angiography (MRA) with contrast-enhanced MRA. AJR Am J Roentgenol. 2011; 197(6):1466–73.
23. Ma SG, Wei CL, Hong B, Yu WN. Ischemia-modified albumin in type 2 diabetic patients with and without peripheral arterial disease. Clinics (Sao Paulo). 2011;66(10):1677–80.
24. Poulsen MK, Nybo M, Dahl J, et al. Plasma osteoprotegerin is related to carotid and peripheral arterial disease, but not to myocardial ischemia in type 2 diabetes mellitus. Cardiovasc Diabetol. 2011;10:76.
25. Gaede P, Lund-Andersen H, Parving HH, Pedersen O. Effect of a multifactorial intervention on mortality in type 2 diabetes. N Engl J Med. 2008;358(6):580–91.
26. Charles M, Ejskjaer N, Witte DR, Borch-Johnsen K, Lauritzen T, Sandbaek A. Prevalence of neuropathy and peripheral arterial disease and the impact of treatment in people with screen-detected type 2 diabetes: the ADDITION-Denmark study. Diabetes Care. 2011;34(10):2244–9.
27. Whyman MR, Fowkes FG, Kerracher EM, et al. Is intermittent claudication improved by percutaneous transluminal angioplasty? A randomized controlled trial. J Vasc Surg. 1997;26(4):551–7.
28. Selvin E, Wattanakit K, Steffes MW, Coresh J, Sharrett AR. HbA1c and peripheral arterial disease in diabetes: the Atherosclerosis Risk in Communities study. Diabetes Care. 2006;29(4):877–82.
29. Rosales RL, Santos MM, Mercado-Asis LB. Cilostazol: a pilot study on safety and clinical efficacy in neuropathies of diabetes mellitus type 2 (ASCEND). Angiology. 2011;62(8):625–35.
30. Mondillo S, Ballo P, Barbati R, et al. Effects of simvastatin on walking performance and symptoms of intermittent claudication in hypercholesterolemic patients with peripheral vascular disease. Am J Med. 2003;114(5):359–64.
31. Piaggesi A, Vallini V, Iacopi E, et al. Iloprost in the management of peripheral arterial disease in patients with diabetes mellitus. Minerva Cardioangiol. 2011; 59(1):101–8.
32. Altstaedt HO, Berzewski B, Breddin HK, et al. Treatment of patients with peripheral arterial occlusive disease Fontaine stage IV with intravenous iloprost and PGE1: a randomized open controlled study. Prostaglandins Leukot Essent Fatty Acids. 1993; 49(2):573–8.
33. Kashyap VS, Pavkov ML, Bena JF, et al. The management of severe aortoiliac occlusive disease: endovascular therapy rivals open reconstruction. J Vasc Surg. 2008;48(6):1451–7, 1457.e1–3.
34. Cambria RP, Faust G, Gusberg R, Tilson MD, Zucker KA, Modlin IM. Percutaneous angioplasty for peripheral arterial occlusive disease. Correlates of clinical success. Arch Surg. 1987;122(3):283–7.
35. Jeans WD, Cole SE, Horrocks M, Baird RN. Angioplasty gives good results in critical lower limb ischaemia. A 5-year follow-up in patients with known ankle pressure and diabetic status having femoropopliteal dilations. Br J Radiol. 1994;67(794):123–8.
36. Faries PL, Brophy D, LoGerfo FW, et al. Combined iliac angioplasty and infrainguinal revascularization surgery are effective in diabetic patients with multilevel arterial disease. Ann Vasc Surg. 2001;15(1):67–72.
37. Murphy KD, Encarnacion CE, Le VA, Palmaz JC. Iliac artery stent placement with the Palmaz stent: follow-up study. J Vasc Interv Radiol. 1995;6(3):321–9.
38. Mwipatayi BP, Thomas S, Wong J, et al. A comparison of covered vs bare expandable stents for the treatment of aortoiliac occlusive disease. J Vasc Surg. 2011;54(6):1561–70, e1561.
39. Faries PL, LoGerfo FW, Hook SC, et al. The impact of diabetes on arterial reconstructions for multilevel arterial occlusive disease. Am J Surg. 2001;181(3):251–5.
40. Moon JS, Clark VM, Beabout JW, Swee RG, Dyck PJ. A controlled study of medial arterial calcification of legs: implications for diabetic polyneuropathy. Arch Neurol. 2011;68(10):1290–4.
41. Ascher E, Haimovici H. Haimovici's vascular surgery. 5th ed. Malden, MA: Blackwell; 2004.
42. Davidovic L, Jakovljevic N, Radak D, et al. Dacron or ePTFE graft for above-knee femoropopliteal bypass reconstruction. A bi-centre randomised study. Vasa. 2010;39(1):77–84.
43. Testini M, Todisco C, Greco L, Impedovo G, Fullone M, Regina G. Femoro-femoral graft after unilateral obstruction of aorto-bifemoral bypass. Minerva Cardioangiol. 1998;46(1–2):15–9.

Abdominal Aortic Aneurysms in Patients with Diabetes

William F. Johnston and Gilbert R. Upchurch Jr.

Keywords
Diabetes mellitus • Abdominal aortic aneurysm • Risk factors • Complications • Protective factors

Introduction

Abdominal aortic aneurysms (AAAs) are common and are increased in patients with atherosclerotic risk factors. Aneurysms are defined as a 50% dilation of a blood vessel. The diameter of the normal abdominal aorta is approximately 2 cm (range = 1.9–2.3 cm in men, 1.7–1.9 cm in women); therefore, an AAA has been conventionally defined as an aortic diameter greater than 3 cm [1].

AAAs result in over 15,000 deaths annually with an increased incidence in elderly men. AAAs are discovered in 3.6–7.2% of older men and 0.3–1.3% of older women [2–6]. While aneurysms do occur elsewhere in the aorta, the abdominal aorta is the most prevalent site for aneurysm formation with approximately 80–90% of aortic aneurysms occurring here. Through population studies, female gender and African-American race are independently associated with a decreased incidence of AAAs [2, 5]. Importantly, diabetes is also independently correlated with a lower incidence of AAA, indicating that diabetes, female sex, and African-American race are all protective of AAA disease.

The pathogenesis of AAAs remains largely unknown and is therefore an intense area of research. Despite significant advancements in understanding the etiology of AAAs, surgical management remains the only effective treatment, as there are no currently available medical or pharmacologic therapies for the treatment or prevention of aneurysm growth. Prospective evaluation of AAAs shows that most aneurysms expand over time; however, growth is usually slow, averaging 0.3 cm/year of expansion [7]. With persistent growth, the question traditionally in AAA treatment becomes when, not if, to repair a patient's AAA.

Surgical management is a delicate balance between the risks of surgery and the risks of aortic rupture. Operative mortality, while improving slowly by decade, remains greater than 40% [8], while overall mortality for AAA rupture is 75–90% [9]. Aortic aneurysm diameter is most

W.F. Johnston, M.D. • G.R. Upchurch Jr., M.D. (✉)
Division of Vascular and Endovascular Surgery,
Department of Surgery, University of Virginia,
PO Box 800679, Charlottesville, VA 22908-0679, USA
e-mail: wfj3u@virginia.edu; gru6n@virginia.edu

Table 15.1 Estimated annual risk of AAA rupture based on aneurysm maximal diameter

Estimated annual rupture risk

AAA diameter (cm)	Annual rupture risk (%/year)
<4	0
4–5	0.5–5
5–6	3–15
6–7	10–20
7–8	20–40
>8	30–50

Adapted from Brewster DC, Cronenwett JL, Hallett Jr JW, Johnston KW, Krupski WC, Matsumara JS. Guidlines for the treatment of abdominal aortic aneurysms. Report of a subcommittee of the Joint Council of the American Association for Vascular Surgery and Society for Vascular Surgery. J Vasc Surg. 2003;37:1106–17 [79]. With permission from Elsevier

closely associated with rupture risk. Annual rupture risk of AAAs based on aortic diameter from the Joint Council of the American Association for Vascular Surgery and Society for Vascular Surgery is found in Table 15.1.

The risk of aortic rupture dramatically increases from 5 to 6 cm. Therefore, patients with AAAs greater than 5.5 cm should be evaluated for repair. The UK Small Aneurysm Trial demonstrated that surgery for aneurysms less than 5.5 cm in men does not confer a survival advantage [10]. Since AAAs are more prevalent among men, many trials have limited their study cohorts to male patients only. When female patients are included and compared with men, women with AAAs measuring 5.0–5.9 cm have a four-time higher risk of rupture (3.9% women versus 1.0% men with AAA 5.0–5.9 cm) [11]. Importantly, women who experienced aortic rupture all had AAAs less than 5.5 cm. Therefore, the threshold for surgical evaluation in women should likely be lower than for men; 5.0 cm has been the recommended indication for surgical intervention in women with AAAs.

This chapter reviews the epidemiology of diabetes and AAAs, the pathologic effects of diabetes on AAA formation and growth, preoperative comorbidities in diabetics with AAAs, operative repair of AAAs in patients with diabetes, and postoperative management in diabetics following open or endovascular AAA repair (EVAR).

Diabetes Is Protective Against AAA Formation

The Veterans Affairs Aneurysm Detection and Management (ADAM) trial documented risk factors for AAAs: smoking, male sex, family history, increasing age, and atherosclerotic disease [2]. Other studies have shown an association between AAAs and hypercholesterolemia, hypertension, and coronary artery disease [12–14]. Therefore, AAAs and atherosclerosis share many of the same risk factors, and for years, atherosclerosis was thought to be the primary contributing factor for AAA pathogenesis [15]. Further evidence of the link between AAAs and atherosclerosis includes autopsy studies of human aortas demonstrating that sites with atherosclerotic plaque deposition had localized aortic dilation, wall thinning, and loss of elastic lamina [16].

Although many risk factors are shared with atherosclerotic disease (smoking, hypertension, hyperlipidemia), diabetes stands alone as a traditional cardiovascular risk factor that does not contribute to aortic aneurysms. In fact, the ADAM trial found that diabetes (along with African-American race and female sex) is protective against AAA formation [2]. Multivariate analyses show that diabetics have nearly half the odds ratio for having an AAA greater than or equal to 4.0 cm (odds ratio = 0.52; 95% confidence interval = 0.45–0.61). Similar results have been found by Blanchard et al. who showed that diabetes is associated with an odds ratio of 0.15 (95% confidence interval = 0.03–0.79) for having an AAA greater than or equal to 4.0 cm [17]. Since the presence of diabetes has been shown to be protective for AAA formation, but contributes to atherosclerotic disease, the link between atherosclerosis and AAA formation has been questioned. While AAAs were once thought to be secondary to atherosclerotic disease, alternative pathways are now considered more critical to AAA formation, including inflammatory mediators and genetic differences.

Diabetes is a complex multifactorial disease that includes hyperglycemia, insulin resistance or decreased insulin production, and microvascular

Fig. 15.1 The Law of Laplace applied to the aorta. In diabetic aortas, increased wall thickness results in decreased wall stress (shown in *checkered arrows*)

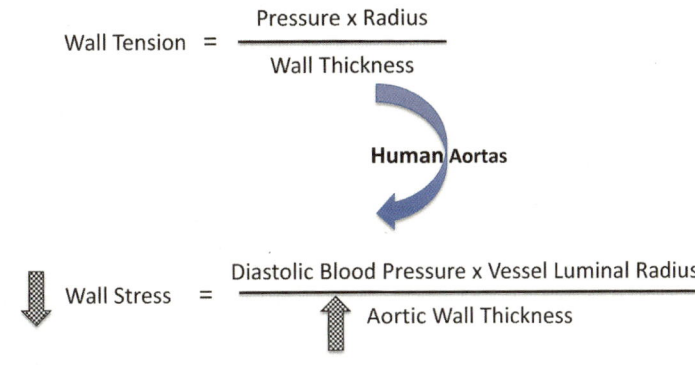

complications. Of these factors, hyperglycemia appears to be the most significant contributing factor for AAA protection. There is an inverse relationship between serum fasting glucose concentration and aortic diameter in patients with and without diabetes [18]. Furthermore, hyperglycemia without concomitant diabetes reduces AAA diameter in a murine model [19]. Hyperglycemic mice have decreased AAA mural neovascularity and less macrophage infiltration of the aortic wall, both of which have been positively correlated with AAA diameter. As expected, the addition of insulin therapy in hyperglycemic mice decreased serum glucose levels in a dose responsive fashion. However, the addition of insulin therapy correlated with larger aneurysm formation. Insulin-mediated reductions in hyperglycemia partially negate the protective effects of diabetes on AAA progression in the murine elastase model, suggesting that the elevated serum glucose concentration provides a protective environment against aneurysm formation.

In the UK Small Aneurysm Trial with over 2,600 patients, diabetics had a slower AAA growth rate [20]. Aneurysm growth rate was diminished by 30% in diabetics (1.8 mm/year in diabetics versus 2.6 mm/year in control patients). In a similar study comparing aortic growth in diabetics versus controls with 30–45 mm AAAs, diabetics had approximately half of the rate of progression of AAA diameter. Mean annual increase in aortic diameter in diabetics was 0.63 mm/year compared to control patients with mean increase of 1.20 mm/year [21]. Despite the differences in actual growth rates between the two previous studies, the trend that diabetes is associated with a decreased progression of AAA growth in humans persists.

Pathologic Differences that Decrease AAA Growth in Diabetics

Increased Aortic Wall Thickness

Aortic diameter is clearly linked with AAA rupture risk, with larger diameter aneurysms having an increased risk of rupture. This relates to the Law of Laplace, which demonstrates the relationship between wall tension, vessel diameter, and wall thickness. Wall tension is directly associated with the risk of AAA rupture [22]. From the Law of Laplace, vessels with a larger diameter, higher pressure, and thinner walls have increased wall tension. This concept has been applied to human aortas to determine wall stress changes over time (Fig. 15.1).

Wall thickening appears to play an important role in the protective mechanism of diabetes against AAA formation and progression. Astrand et al used ultrasound to measure and compare aortic wall thickness of diabetics with normal-sized aortas to nondiabetics with similar aortic diameters. Aortic wall thickness in non-AAA diabetics is 22% greater than in control, nondiabetic patients ($P<0.001$) [23]. This translates to a 20% overall decrease in aortic wall stress ($P<0.001$). To further strengthen the relationship, the duration of diabetes is positively correlated with increasing aortic wall thickness. Patients with a longer duration of diabetes

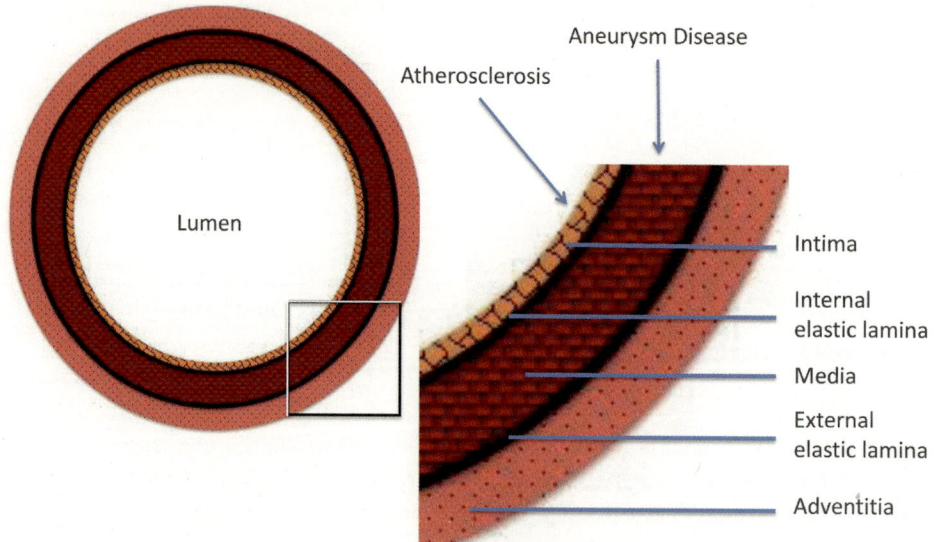

Fig. 15.2 Anatomic overview of an arterial vessel. Atherosclerotic disease occurs mostly in the intimal layer, while abdominal aortic aneurysms result from destruction of the medial layer

have increased wall thickness when compared to patients with diabetes for a shorter duration. This increased wall thickness results in increased vessel wall strength and decreased compliance. In patients with type 1 diabetes, the aorta has been shown to have reduced compliance [24]. The aorta is even less distensible with increased duration of diabetes or the presence of microvascular complications (microalbuminuria, retinopathy, neuropathy). Thus, long-standing diabetes likely has an effect on the aortic wall and surrounding microenvironment.

Decreased Matrix Metalloproteinases

The microenvironment surrounding the aorta in diabetics is likely different from nondiabetics and may partially explain the protective effect of diabetes. Matrix metalloproteinases (MMPs) are enzymes that are frequently elevated in the aortic wall and surrounding tissue in AAAs. MMPs are a family of structurally related proteolytic enzymes that function to degrade extracellular matrix in many normal biological and pathological processes [25]. MMPs appear to play an important role in aortic remodeling in diabetic patients and in AAA formation.

Patients with AAAs suffer from significant degeneration of the tunica media layer of the aortic wall. This contrasts with atherosclerosis, in which the pathology is mostly confined to the tunica intima of the vessel wall. The tunica media is the muscular, middle layer of an artery composed of vascular smooth muscle cells surrounded by the internal and external elastic lamina (Fig. 15.2). In AAAs, there is widespread destruction of elastic lamellae in the tunica media and decreased smooth muscle cells [26]. MMPs are thought to play a pivotal role in the medial destruction seen in AAAs, as they have the ability to degrade all structural and interstitial proteins in the aortic wall. There are a variety of MMPs, but MMP2 and 9 have been found to be upregulated in human AAA tissue [26]. Both MMP2 and 9 are also increased in murine models of aortic aneurysms that are used to study the pathogenesis of AAAs [27, 28]. These MMPs are produced by cells that are endogenous to the aorta and function to degrade collagen, gelatin, elastin, and laminin [29].

MMP2 is primarily produced by mesenchymal cells, including smooth muscle cells and fibroblasts [30]. While MMP2 activity is not upregulated in large human AAA specimens [31],

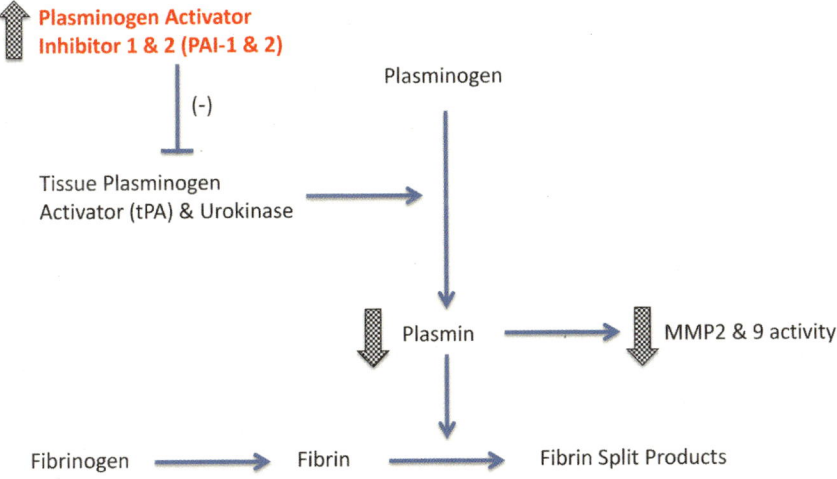

Fig. 15.3 Mechanism of plasminogen activator inhibitor-1 (PAI-1) leading to decreased activation of plasmin. Diabetic patients have elevated PAI-1 that blocks the activation of plasminogen to plasmin and therefore leads to lower MMP2 and 9 levels (shown by *checkered arrows*)

MMP2 is significantly elevated in smaller AAAs (4.0–5.5 cm in diameter) [32], suggesting MMP2 may play a key early role in the pathogenesis of AAAs. Importantly, MMP2 is decreased in large arteries in diabetic patients [33], and may contribute to the decreased wall destruction and increased wall thickness that reduce AAA development. Multiple MMPs are required to work in concert to cause aortic aneurysms. In a murine model of AAAs, neither mice deficient in the expression of MMP2 nor MMP9 alone (MMP2 and MMP9 knockouts) developed aneurysms [34]. However, when MMP9 producing macrophages were reinfused into the MMP9 knockout mice, aneurysms developed. In contrast, reinfusion of MMP9 producing macrophages into MMP2 knockouts did not result in AAA formation. This suggests that MMP2 and MMP9 work together and are both required for AAA formation.

MMP9 is markedly increased in AAA and has been localized to aneurysm infiltrating macrophages [31]. In vivo analyses show that these MMP9 producing macrophages are primarily located in the medial layer where overt damage is present. MMP9 levels are more elevated in AAA than in aortic tissue with atherosclerotic disease. To further strengthen the relationship between MMP9 and inflammatory conditions leading to AAAs, MMP9 is upregulated by inflammatory cytokines, including interleukin-1β, interluekin-6, and tumor necrosis factor-α (TNF-α). MMP9 is the most prominent MMP in AAA and may be associated with vessel damage seen in AAA. Importantly, hyperglycemia reduces MMP9 activity in an AAA model, correlating with a relative preservation of elastin fibers in the medial layer of the aortic wall and a decrease in macrophage infiltration [19, 35].

Increased Plasminogen Activator Inhibitor-1

MMPs are secreted in zymogen form and require activation by plasmin to become active proteases. Plasmin is also secreted in zymogen form and requires activation with plasminogen activators, such as tissue plasminogen activator (tPA) and urokinase-type plasminogen activator (uPA). Plasminogen activator levels are elevated in smooth muscle cells from human AAA samples [36]. Plasminogen activator inhibitor-1 (PAI-1) inhibits tPA and uPA, thereby linking this protease inhibitor with AAA formation and MMP production (Fig. 15.3). Increases in PAI-1 decrease plasmin activation of MMPs. Elimination of PAI-1 leads to dramatic increases in AAA formation as there is less inhibition of MMP activation [37]. In hyperglycemic murine models, plasma PAI-1 levels are significantly increased in diabetic aortas and in diabetic AAA tissue, which may contribute to attenuate AAA formation [35]. Hyperglycemia increases PAI-1 expression, which mediates inhibition of plasmin leading to decreased MMP activation. In summary, this results in decreased elastin degradation and aortic wall degradation.

The molecular mechanisms that result in decreased incidence and delayed progression of AAA disease among diabetics continue to be under investigation. Results from this research will lead to a better understanding of the complex etiology of aneurysm formation.

Preoperative Comorbidities in Patients with AAAs and Diabetes

Despite the protective effects of diabetes on AAA development and growth, many diabetics develop AAAs that must undergo repair. As the incidence of diabetes is rapidly increasing, the surgical team is required to be increasingly aware of diabetic management. The incidence of diabetes in the USA has increased 57% over the past two decades from 6.0% in 1988 to 9.4% in 2008 [38]. This is largely secondary to increases in type 2 diabetes and metabolic syndrome. The approach to operative care in diabetics must include consideration of the comorbidities frequently associated with diabetes.

Increased Coronary Artery Disease

Diabetes is a risk factor for coronary artery disease (CAD) and increases the risk of death from CAD. The relative risk for death from CAD is 1.8 in diabetic men and 2.5 in diabetic women [39]. Importantly, diabetes reverses the protective effects of female gender on CAD. Diabetes is one of the Eagle clinical predictors of postoperative cardiac events in patients undergoing vascular surgery, along with age >70 years, angina, history of ventricular ectopy, and Q waves [40]. The Eagle Criteria have been shown to be more sensitive than cardiac stress imaging for predicting perioperative adverse cardiac events [41]. Patients with diabetes and concomitant CAD may not have the classic angina symptoms, as myocardial ischemia is silent in greater than one in five asymptomatic diabetic patients [42]. Therefore, a low threshold for diagnostic and therapeutic coronary angiography should be maintained in diabetics undergoing major vascular surgery.

Diabetes confers an increased risk for perioperative myocardial infarction in patients undergoing AAA repair. In a review of 570 AAA repairs, Kertai et al. documented that although the incidence of diabetes among patients with AAAs is infrequent (6.3% of patients), diabetics are twice as likely to suffer perioperative mortality or myocardial infarction following AAA repair (16.7% in diabetics versus 8.7% in nondiabetics, odds ratio=2.2) [43]. This risk may be reduced with medical therapy. In the highest risk patient (defined as having three or more of the following: ischemic heart disease, history of congestive heart failure, history of cerebrovascular disease, insulin-dependent diabetes, and/or renal insufficiency), the combination of statins and beta-blockers has been associated with a sevenfold reduction in perioperative mortality and nonfatal myocardial infarction [43].

Diabetic Nephropathy

Diabetic nephropathy is characterized by proteinuria and/or an impaired glomerular filtration rate. It is the leading cause of kidney disease in the developed world and accounts for almost half of patients with end stage renal disease (ESRD) in the USA [44]. Approximately 40% of people with diabetes develop diabetic nephropathy. Even though the prevalence of diabetic kidney disease has remained stable, the incidence of diabetic nephropathy is increasing secondary to the increase in diabetes in the USA. The prevalence of diabetic nephropathy increases with age and

Table 15.2 Risk factors for all-cause mortality after major vascular surgery

Independent predictors for all-cause mortality	Multivariate Odds Ratio (95% confidence interval)	P-Value
Postoperative dialysis (temporary or persistent)	3.45 (1.99–5.96)	<0.001
COPD	1.53 (1.29–1.81)	<0.001
Smoking	1.32 (1.13–1.53)	<0.001
Kidney injury	1.24 (1.06–1.45)	0.007
Diabetes mellitus	**1.18 (1.00–1.43)**	**0.048**
Age (per 1 year increase)	1.04 (1.03–1.05)	<0.001
Baseline kidney function		
CrCl (per 1 mL/min increase)	0.993 (0.990–0.996)	<0.001
Estimated GFR (per 1 mL/min/1.73 m² increase)	0.994 (0.991–0.998)	<0.001
Statin use	0.60 (0.48–0.75)	<0.001

COPD chronic obstructive pulmonary disease, *CrCl* creatinine clearance, *GFR* glomerular filtration rate
Adapted from Welten GMJM, Chonchol M, Schouten O, et al. Statin use is associated with early recovery of kidney injury after vascular surgery and improved long-term outcome. Nephrol Dial Transplant. 2008; 23:3867–73

affects approximately 50% of people with diabetes older than 65 years old [38]. Since many of the patients who are evaluated for AAA repair are greater than 65 years old, renal dysfunction must be investigated preoperatively, and all attempts should be made to avoid nephrotoxic agents unless necessary.

Concomitant Arterial Occlusive Disease

Diabetic patients are at increased risk for atherosclerotic disease, which must be considered during the workup for a diabetic patient who is to undergo AAA repair. Diabetes is significantly more common in patients with aorto-iliac occlusive disease (AIOD) than with AAAs (36% of patients with AIOD vs. 6% of patients with AAAs) [45]. Diabetes also increases the odds ratio nearly threefold for patients to undergo femoral artery bypass for peripheral arterial disease compared to healthier controls [46]. In diabetic patients, arterial occlusive disease is often asymptomatic and unknown to the patient [47]. This may potentially translate to an increased incidence of AIOD and peripheral occlusive disease, which may not be previously diagnosed. Therefore, diabetic patients being worked up for AAA repair should be evaluated for carotid, femoral, iliac, and renal artery occlusive lesions that may impact repair.

Repair of AAA

The effect of diabetes on AAA repair is controversial [48–50]. According to Hua et al., diabetics do not have significantly increased mortality or morbidity following open or endovascular repair of AAA [48]. However, an analysis of over 1,900 patients from Rotterdam documented that diabetes confers a mild increase in risk for mortality following all major vascular operations [49] (Table 15.2). This is similar to other factors that have been shown to be protective for AAA formation and progression as both female sex and African-American race have been shown to be related to increased mortality rates following open AAA repair [50]. Both Hua et al. and the Rotterdam study agree that the protective effects of diabetes do not persist once AAA repair is indicated.

Examining patients undergoing major vascular surgery, diabetes is linked with an increased risk of perioperative death or cardiovascular complication [51]. However, when confounding comorbidities, such as renal insufficiency, are accounted for, diabetes alone does not appear to increase the rates of perioperative death or cardiovascular complications following aortic reconstruction. Patients with diabetes are most likely to have severe comorbidities, including congestive heart failure, renal insufficiency, renal failure requiring dialysis, and proteinuria. Each of these comorbid conditions is a risk factor for poor outcomes following vascular surgery.

AAA repair is commonly performed though two approaches: open surgical and endovascular catheter-based repair. There have been multiple large, randomized studies to compare endovascular repair with an open approach. The most recent of these studies is the Open Versus Endovascular Repair (OVER) study from the Veterans Affairs Hospital System. EVAR was associated with decreased 30-day mortality, decreased hospital and ICU stay, decreased blood loss, and reduced transfusion requirement [52]. At 2 years, aneurysm-related mortality occurred equally between endovascular and open repair. Endovascular repair was shown to be a less morbid operation with similar outcomes to open repair.

Although EVAR is considered first line therapy for prevention of aortic rupture, open AAA repair should be considered when the aneurysm cannot be repaired endovascularly, including patients with inadequate proximal or distal landing zones, difficult vascular access, mycotic aneurysms, or patient preference. Contemporary open repair can be performed with low overall morbidity and mortality. In a recent review of over 400 patients who underwent open AAA repair between 2003 and 2009, 30-day survival was over 95%, with 1- and 5-year survival of 90% and 65%, respectively [53]. Nineteen percent of patients had decreased postoperative renal function, 17% experienced cardiac complications, and 11% had pulmonary complications. Chronic renal insufficiency (CRI) and chronic obstructive pulmonary disease (COPD) were independently associated with decreased 30-day, 1-year, and 5-year survival. Compared to patients without CRI, patients with CRI had a 30-day survival of 92.0% versus 98.3% and a 5-year survival of 51% versus 73% [53]. The importance of renal function on patient survival extends beyond the effects of CRI. Patients who had postoperative kidney injury (even if the injury appeared to later resolve) were associated with a significantly decreased 5-year survival (41% vs. 72%). The significance of postoperative kidney injury is not limited to patients undergoing open AAA repair, but has also been shown in patients undergoing any major abdominal surgery. Postoperative acute kidney injury, even with small changes in the serum creatinine level, is an independent long-term risk for death [54].

With a clear correlation between renal insufficiency (both chronic and postoperative) and long-term outcomes, strategies aimed at minimizing kidney injury during AAA repair may improve patient outcomes. This is especially important in diabetics, given the increased risk of nephropathy. Known risk factors for developing kidney injury after major vascular surgery are shown in Table 15.3. Patients with diabetes have almost half the odds of recovering full renal function if acute kidney injury occurs following major vascular surgery [49].

Statin usage has been associated with a fourfold reduction in perioperative mortality in patients undergoing major vascular surgery [55]. Although statin usage has not been shown to prevent acute kidney injury following major vascular surgery, it is associated with early complete recovery of kidney function. Statin usage nearly doubles the odds ratio of complete kidney function recovery [49].

Special Consideration for Open Repair

During open repair, the surgeon must cross-clamp the aorta above the aneurysm to anastomose normal caliber aorta with graft. The cross-clamp may be placed infrarenal, suprarenal, supramesenteric, or supraceliac, based on relative position to the visceral vessels. Suprarenal (and supramesenteric/supraceliac) aortic clamping prevents renal perfusion and is associated with an increased risk of postoperative kidney injury (Table 15.3). Therefore, attempts should be made to limit suprarenal clamp time. If suprarenal clamping is required, renal

Table 15.3 Risk factors for developing kidney injury after major vascular surgery

Independent predictors for AKI	Multivariate Odds Ratio (95% confidence interval)	P-Value
Suprarenal aortic cross-clamping	4.07 (2.76–6.00)	<0.001
Hypertension	1.48 (1.15–1.89)	0.002
Baseline kidney function		
CrCl (per 1 mL/min increase)	1.010 (1.006–1.014)	<0.001
Estimated GFR (per 1 mL/min/1.73 m^2 increase)	1.008 (1.004–1.013)	<0.001
Age (per 1 year increase)	1.03 (1.02–1.04)	<0.001

AKI acute kidney injury, *CrCl* creatinine clearance, *GFR* glomerular filtration rate
Adapted from Welten GMJM, Chonchol M, Schouten O, et al. Statin use is associated with early recovery of kidney injury after vascular surgery and improved long-term outcome. Nephrol Dial Transplant. 2008;23:3867–73. With permission from Oxford University Press

hypothermia with continuous cold perfusion of the kidneys with normal saline may reduce postoperative renal complications [56]. Additionally, renal revascularization during AAA repair may improve postoperative renal function [57].

Special Considerations for EVAR

EVAR has gained tremendous popularity and is a safe, durable, and effective method to reduce the risk of aneurysm rupture. The proximal end of the stent graft must conform to the shape of the aorta in order to prevent migration of the stent, exclude blood flow in the aneurysm sac, and secure hemostatic stent implantation. If the proximal landing zone is too short, the stent will not have sufficient overlap with the aorta to assume the same shape. Proximal endoleaks can result in continued aneurysm growth and increased risk of rupture. The proximal landing zone of the endovascular stent may be infrarenal or suprarenal, based on its relation to the ostia of the renal arteries. Suprarenal fixation stents have uncovered proximal ends with barbs for stent fixation. The placement of proximal fixation does not appear to affect postprocedural renal dysfunction or long-term renal function [58, 59].

Close proximity of the aneurysm to the renal and visceral vessel origins is the most common factor precluding EVAR. Current options for treating juxtarenal AAAs with EVAR include fenestrated stents, renal artery stenting with endograft encroachment, and renal artery "snorkel" stent placement. Fenestrated endovascular stents have fabric fenestrations in the wall of the stent that may be coupled with stents to provide visceral branch perfusion while providing a secure proximal seal (Fig. 15.4). Fenestrated stents are safe, but have a nearly 40% reintervention

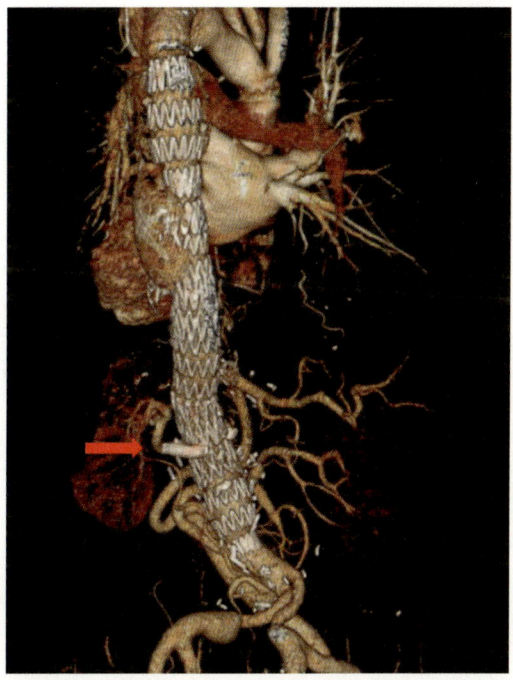

Fig. 15.4 Three-dimensional reconstruction of CT angiography illustrating fenestrated EVAR. Fenestration shown (*arrow*) with stent placed in the left renal artery

rate due to graft-related complications, commonly involving renal artery stent fracture/stenosis or endoleaks [60]. Endovascular manipulation of renal arteries may result in embolism of atheromatous debris distally causing renal infarction. Presently, fenestrated EVAR grafts are available only in designated trial centers in the USA, but are widely available throughout Europe and Australia.

Renal artery encroachment involves usual deployment of the EVAR graft with special attention paid to the proximal end of the graft. A renal stent graft is inserted through the proximal portion of the uncovered stent. This allows the endograft to sit just below the renal artery origin or even partially cover the ostia while maintaining renal perfusion through the renal artery stent. The renal artery "snorkel" technique likewise involves renal artery stenting. In this procedure, the renal artery is typically accessed from above via the brachial artery prior to EVAR deployment. A stent graft is placed in the renal artery with the proximal portion of the stent remaining in the aorta. The EVAR is then deployed with the goal that the renal stent will sit beside the EVAR. Endoleaks are common following both the encroachment method and the snorkel method, but most have few long-term effects [61]. Currently, juxtarenal AAAs can be safely repaired endovascularly, but the treatment is not straightforward and requires creativity to solve this complex issue.

Endovascular repair is frequently performed through femoral or iliac artery access. The vessel lumen should have a diameter of 6–8 mm to accommodate the sheath and device delivery system. Manufacturers are developing newer systems that are lower profile, but care must be taken in patients with severe femoral or iliac artery disease. These lesions are more prevalent in patients with diabetes [46, 47] and may therefore preclude an endovascular approach or necessitate a conduit directly to the aorta or common iliac artery.

Compared to open repair, EVAR requires exposure to intravenous contrast. Angiography is needed to define the vascular anatomy for stent placement and to evaluate stent positioning following deployment. Angiography requires the use of potentially nephrotoxic contrast agents. Patients with preexisting renal insufficiency (a frequent comorbidity of diabetes) have a decreased ability to recover from contrast exposure [62]. EVAR also requires lifelong follow-up with more frequent imaging since the long-term effects of EVAR are unknown. Follow-up imaging often consists of computed tomography angiography (CTA) to evaluate for aneurysm diameter, endoleaks, and stent migration. Exposure to iodinated contrast with CTA carries a risk of contrast-induced nephropathy.

Intravascular infusion of radiopaque contrast is the third leading cause of hospital-acquired acute renal failure [63]. Diabetes, especially when coupled with coexisting renal insufficiency, is a risk factor for contrast nephropathy. Parfrey et al. demonstrated that diabetic patients with coexisting renal insufficiency have a twofold increase in their relative risk of developing acute renal failure following contrast infusion when compared to nondiabetic patients with renal insufficiency (8.8% for diabetic patients with preexisting renal insufficiency vs. 4.5% for nondiabetic patients with preexisting renal insufficiency) [64]. Diabetics with normal renal function do not appear to have increased risk of contrast-induced acute renal failure [64], but careful consideration should be given to these patients as risks of lifelong frequent contrast exposure have not been evaluated.

Carbon dioxide (CO_2) digital subtraction angiography may be employed for AAA diagnosis and repair with less effect on renal function. Intravenous CO_2 is eliminated by one pass through the pulmonary circulation and is the only intravenous contrast agent that is non-allergenic and non-nephrotoxic [65]. Image quality can be decreased with bowel gas or motion, and obtaining clear, quality diagnostic images is more labor intense. However, CO_2 angiography may be effectively used for EVAR placement and endoleak detection [66]. A renal-protective approach for EVAR placement in azotemic patients is using CO_2 digital subtraction angiography to guide

EVAR placement with supplemental iodinated contrast for confirmation if needed. CO_2 angiography is also safe and effective for EVAR of ruptured AAA with no postoperative decreases in renal function [67].

Postoperative Considerations

Diabetes increases hospital length of stay for patients undergoing AAA repair. This increased length of stay (LOS) is even more apparent in insulin-dependent diabetics. Diabetics requiring insulin for glucose management had a 26% increased LOS, while diabetic patients managed by oral hypoglycemic medications had a 10% increased LOS [51]. This is likely secondary to the comorbidities associated with diabetes, including renal insufficiency and decreased immune function.

Prevention of Contrast-Induced Nephropathy

With contrast nephropathy being prevalent, many drugs have been evaluated to decrease or prevent contrast-induced nephropathy, including sodium bicarbonate, *N*-acetylcysteine, fenoldopam, dopamine, statins, furosemide, mannitol, and theophylline. Of these, intravenous sodium bicarbonate, *N*-acetylcysteine, and theophylline have been shown to have some potential for risk reduction [68]. Use of these agents is controversial and has mixed results. Meler et al. found that preprocedural hydration with sodium bicarbonate was superior to normal saline and reduced the rate of contrast-induced nephropathy (odds ration 0.52, $P=0.003$). However, From et al. documented that the use of sodium bicarbonate was independently associated with increased contrast induced nephropathy in their retrospective review of over 7,900 patients [69]. *N*-acetylcysteine has been shown to reduce the risk of contrast nephropathy by 72% [70]. Theophylline has likewise been associated with reduced risk for contrast-induced nephropathy (relative risk=0.49) [68].

At our institution, intravenous sodium bicarbonate hydration and *N*-acetylcysteine are frequently used based on the strategy that both might provide the diabetic patient potential benefit with minimal risk.

The easiest way to decrease contrast-induced nephropathy is to avoid the use of iodinated contrast by employing alternative methods for aneurysm surveillance. For follow-up on diabetic patients after open or EVAR, ultrasound may be considered as a diagnostic modality for screening for endoleaks, aneurysm sac enlargement, and stent/graft position [71, 72]. An example of endoleak detection by ultrasound is shown in Fig. 15.5. If CT imaging is desired, a noncontrast study can show stent placement and change in aneurysm sac diameter to suggest potential endoleaks.

Wound Healing in Patients with Diabetes

Diabetes is frequently associated with wound complications secondary to poor wound healing. The etiology of poor wound healing in diabetics is multifactorial, including decreased or impaired growth factors, angiogenesis, macrophage function, collagen formation, quantity of granulation tissue, fibroblast proliferation, and remodeling by MMPs [73]. As a result, diabetes is an independent risk factor for wound complications following abdominal surgery [74]. This likely contributes to the nearly threefold increase in surgical wound infections seen in diabetics following vascular surgery [75]. In a retrospective review of over 1,500 patients, postoperative glucose levels were the most important risk factor for a surgical site infection following general surgical operations [76]. The increased risk of postoperative wound infections with hyperglycemia extends to both diabetic and nondiabetic patients. Vascular surgery patients alone are at increased risk of surgical site infections regardless of their serum glucose levels (10.3% of vascular surgery patients developed wound complications versus 7.4% of all patients). However, when combining vascular

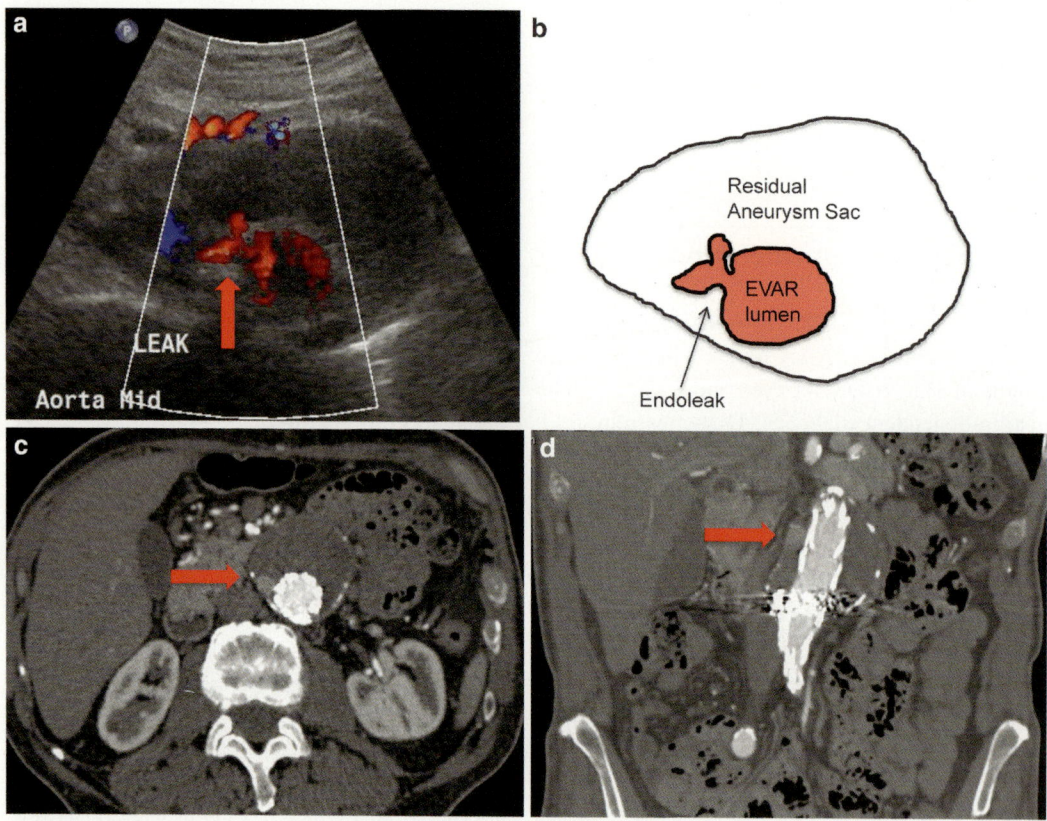

Fig. 15.5 Ultrasound surveillance of EVAR with endoleak detected. Ultrasound demonstrates high flow endoleak (*arrow*) (**a** and **b**). This was followed by CT angiography that confirms contrast outside of the graft (*arrow*) in the axial (**c**) and coronal (**d**) planes

surgery patients with postoperative serum glucose of greater than 220 mg/dL, surgical site infection rate nearly doubles (20.0%) [76].

Postoperative Glucose Management

To decrease the rate of wound infections, hyperglycemia must be avoided. All type 1 and 2 diabetic patients should be managed with insulin and dextrose solution for glycemic control. Oral anti-glycemic medications should not be used following major surgery as stress responses to surgery alter patients' normal serum glucose levels. The American College of Cardiology and American Heart Association guidelines recommend maintaining blood glucose concentrations less than 150 mg/dL following vascular procedures [77]. In our institution, all patients following open AAA repair are placed in the intensive care unit (ICU) postoperatively and their serum glucose levels are checked hourly. Insulin infusions are frequently used to maintain glucose < 150 mg/dL. On the surgical floor units, blood glucose is typically controlled with sliding scale insulin. A recent randomized study has shown that a better regimen for blood glucose control on floor units is a basal–bolus insulin regimen [78]. The basal–bolus regimen included glargine as the long acting basal insulin with glulisine given before meals as a rapid acting agent. The basal–bolus regimen significantly improved glycemic control and reduced postoperative complications, including wound infection.

Conclusions

Patients with diabetes are protected from AAA development and have slower rates of AAA growth. This is associated with an increased aortic wall thickness, decreased MMP production, and increased PAI-1 levels. The protective effects of diabetes disappear once AAA repair is indicated. The treatment team must be cognizant of the concomitant complications of diabetes, including increased rates of coronary artery disease, renal insufficiency, atherosclerotic disease, and decreased would healing. The risks of open AAA repair in diabetic patients (large incision, aortic cross-clamping) must be weighed against the risks of endovascular repair (frequent reintervention, increased use of contrast agents during surveillance). All attempts should be made to minimize these risks. Adapting postoperative care and follow-up to the individual needs of the diabetic patient may result in improved long-term outcomes.

References

1. Lederle FA, Johnson GR, Wilson SE, et al. Relationship of age, gender, race, and body size to infrarenal aortic diameter. J Vasc Surg. 1997;26:595–601.
2. Lederle FA, Johnson GR, Wilson SE, et al. The aneurysm detection and management study screening program: validation cohort and final results. Arch Intern Med. 2000;160:1425–30.
3. Norman PE, Jamrozik K, Lawrence-Brown MM, et al. Population based randomised controlled trial on impact of screening on mortality from abdominal aortic aneurysm. BMJ. 2004;329:1259.
4. Scott RAP, Bridgewater SG, Ashton HA. Randomized clinical trial of screening for abdominal aortic aneurysm in women. Br J Surg. 2002;89:283–5.
5. Lederle FA, Johnson GR, Wilson SE. Abdominal aortic aneurysm in women. J Vasc Surg. 2001;34:122–6.
6. Lederle FA, Larson JC, Margolis KL, et al. Abdominal aortic aneurysm events in the women's health initiative: cohort study. BMJ. 2008;337:a1724.
7. Guirguis EM, Barber GG. The natural history of abdominal aortic aneurysms. Am J Surg. 1991;162:481–3.
8. Bown MJ, Sutton AJ, Bell PRF, Sayers RD. A meta-analysis of 50 years of ruptured abdominal aortic aneurysm repair. Br J Surg. 2002;89:714–30.
9. Semmens JB, Norman PE, Lawrence-Brown MMD, Holman CDAJ. Influence of gender on outcome from ruptured abdominal aortic aneurysm. Br J Surg. 2000;87:191–4.
10. Powell JT. Final 12-year follow-up of surgery versus surveillance in the UK Small Aneurysm Trial. Br J Surg. 2007;94:702–8.
11. Brown PM, Zelt DT, Sobolev B. The risk of rupture in untreated aneurysms: the impact of size, gender, and expansion rate. J Vasc Surg. 2003;37:280–4.
12. Pleumeekers HJ, Hoes AW, van der Does E, et al. Aneurysms of the abdominal aorta in older adults. The Rotterdam Study. Am J Epidemiol. 1995;142:1291–9.
13. Alcorn HG, Wolfson Jr SK, Sutton-Tyrrell K, Kuller LH, O'Leary D. Risk factors for abdominal aortic aneurysms in older adults enrolled in the cardiovascular health study. Arterioscler Thromb Vasc Biol. 1996;16:963–70.
14. Singh K, BØnaa KH, Jacobsen BK, BjØrk L, Solberg S. Prevalence of and risk factors for abdominal aortic aneurysms in a population-based study. Am J Epidemiol. 2001;154:236–44.
15. Lee AJ, Fowkes FGR, Carson MN, Leng GC, Allan PL. Smoking, atherosclerosis and risk of abdominal aortic aneurysm. Eur Heart J. 1997;18:671–6.
16. Xu C, Zarins CK, Glagov S. Aneurysmal and occlusive atherosclerosis of the human abdominal aorta. J Vasc Surg. 2001;33:91–6.
17. Blanchard JF, Armenian HK, Friesen PP. Risk factors for abdominal aortic aneurysm: results of a case-control study. Am J Epidemiol. 2000;151:575–83.
18. Le MT, Jamrozik K, Davis TM, Norman PE. Negative association between infra-renal aortic diameter and glycaemia: the Health in Men Study. Eur J Vasc Endovasc Surg. 2007;33:599–604.
19. Miyama N, Dua MM, Yeung JJ, et al. Hyperglycemia limits experimental aortic aneurysm progression. J Vasc Surg. 2010;52:975–83.
20. Brady AR, Thompson SG, Fowkes FGR, Greenhalgh RM, Powell JT. Abdominal aortic aneurysm expansion: risk factors and time intervals for surveillance. Circulation. 2004;110:16–21.
21. Golledge J, Karan M, Moran CS, et al. Reduced expansion rate of abdominal aortic aneurysms in patients with diabetes may be related to aberrant monocyte-matrix interactions. Eur Heart J. 2008;29:665–72.
22. Fillinger MF, Marra SP, Raghavan ML, Kennedy FE. Prediction of rupture risk in abdominal aortic aneurysm during observation: wall stress versus diameter. J Vasc Surg. 2003;37:724–32.
23. Astrand H, Ryden-Ahlgren A, Sundkvist G, Sandgren T, Lanne T. Reduced aortic wall stress in diabetes mellitus. Eur J Vasc Endovasc Surg. 2007;33:592–8.
24. Giannattasio C, Failla M, Piperno A, et al. Early impairment of large artery structure and function in Type I diabetes mellitus. Diabetologia. 1999;42:987–94.
25. Nagase H, Woessner JF. Matrix metalloproteinases. J Biol Chem. 1999;274:21491–4.
26. Thompson RW, Parks WC. Role of matrix metalloproteinases in abdominal aortic aneurysms. Ann N Y Acad Sci. 1996;800:157–74.

27. Eagleton MJ, Ballard N, Lynch E, Srivastava SD, Upchurch Jr GR, Stanley JC. Early increased MT1-MMP expression and late MMP-2 and MMP-9 activity during angiotensin II induced aneurysm formation. J Surg Res. 2006;135:345–51.
28. Ailawadi G, Eliason JL, Roelofs KJ, et al. Gender differences in experimental aortic aneurysm formation. Arterioscler Thromb Vasc Biol. 2004;24:2116–22.
29. Visse R, Nagase H. Matrix metalloproteinases and tissue inhibitors of metalloproteinases. Circ Res. 2003;92:827–39.
30. Davis V, Persidskaia R, Baca-Regen L, et al. Matrix metalloproteinase-2 production and its binding to the matrix are increased in abdominal aortic aneurysms. Arterioscler Thromb Vasc Biol. 1998;18:1625–33.
31. Thompson RW, Holmes DR, Mertens RA, et al. Production and localization of 92-kilodalton gelatinase in abdominal aortic aneurysms. An elastolytic metalloproteinase expressed by aneurysm-infiltrating macrophages. J Clin Invest. 1995;96:318–26.
32. Freestone T, Turner RJ, Coady A, Higman DJ, Greenhalgh RM, Powell JT. Inflammation and matrix metalloproteinases in the enlarging abdominal aortic aneurysm. Arterioscler Thromb Vasc Biol. 1995;15:1145–51.
33. Portik-Dobos V, Anstadt MP, Hutchinson J, Bannan M, Ergul A. Evidence for a matrix metalloproteinase induction/activation system in arterial vasculature and decreased synthesis and activity in diabetes. Diabetes. 2002;51:3063–8.
34. Longo GM, Xiong W, Greiner TC, Zhao Y, Fiotti N, Baxter BT. Matrix metalloproteinases 2 and 9 work in concert to produce aortic aneurysms. J Clin Invest. 2002;110:625–32.
35. Dua MM, Miyama N, Azuma J, et al. Hyperglycemia modulates plasminogen activator inhibitor-1 expression and aortic diameter in experimental aortic aneurysm disease. Surgery. 2010;148:429–35.
36. Louwrens HD, Kwaan HC, Pearce WH, Yao JST, Verrusio E. Plasminogen activator and plasminogen activator inhibitor expression by normal and aneurysmal human aortic smooth muscle cells in culture. Eur J Vasc Endovasc Surg. 1995;10:289–93.
37. DiMusto PD, Lu G, Ghosh A, Roelofs KJ, Su G, Zhao Y, Lau CL, Sadiq O, McEvoy B, Laser A, Diaz JA, Wakefield TW, Henke PK, Eliason JL, Upchurch GR, Jr. Increased pai-1 in females compared with males is protective for abdominal aortic aneurysm formation in a rodent model. Am J Physiol Heart Circ Physiol. 2012;302:H1378–86.
38. de Boer IH, Rue TC, Hall YN, Heagerty PJ, Weiss NS, Himmelfarb J. Temporal trends in the prevalence of diabetic kidney disease in the United States. JAMA. 2011;305:2532–9.
39. Lee WL, Cheung AM, Cape D, Zinman B. Impact of diabetes on coronary artery disease in women and men: a meta-analysis of prospective studies. Diabetes Care. 2000;23:962–8.
40. Eagle KA, Coley CM, Newell JB, et al. Combining clinical and thallium data optimizes preoperative assessment of cardiac risk before major vascular surgery. Ann Intern Med. 1989;110:859–66.
41. Back MR, Schmacht DC, Bowser AN, et al. Critical appraisal of cardiac risk stratification before elective vascular surgery. Vasc Endovascular Surg. 2003;37: 387–97.
42. Wackers FJ, Young LH, Inzucchi SE, et al. Detection of silent myocardial ischemia in asymptomatic diabetic subjects: the DIAD study. Diabetes Care. 2004;27:1954–61.
43. Kertai MD, Boersma E, Westerhout CM, et al. A combination of statins and beta-blockers is independently associated with a reduction in the incidence of perioperative mortality and nonfatal myocardial infarction in patients undergoing abdominal aortic aneurysm surgery. Eur J Vasc Endovasc Surg. 2004;28:343–52.
44. USRDS. 2011 USRDS Annual Date Report: atlas of chronic kidney disease and end-stage renal disease in the United States. Bethesda, MD: US Renal Data System; 2011.
45. Shteinberg D, Halak M, Shapiro S, et al. Abdominal aortic aneurysm and aortic occlusive disease: a comparison of risk factors and inflammatory response. Eur J Vasc Endovasc Surg. 2000;20:462–5.
46. LaMorte WW, Scott TE, Menzoian JO. Racial differences in the incidence of femoral bypass and abdominal aortic aneurysmectomy in Massachusetts: relationship to cardiovascular risk factors. J Vasc Surg. 1995;21:422–31.
47. Hooi JD, Stoffers HE, Kester AD, et al. Risk factors and cardiovascular diseases associated with asymptomatic peripheral arterial occlusive disease. The Limburg PAOD Study. Peripheral Arterial Occlusive Disease. Scand J Prim Health Care. 1998;16:177–82.
48. Hua HT, Cambria RP, Chuang SK, et al. Early outcomes of endovascular versus open abdominal aortic aneurysm repair in the National Surgical Quality Improvement Program-Private Sector (NSQIP-PS). J Vasc Surg. 2005;41:382–9.
49. Welten GMJM, Chonchol M, Schouten O, et al. Statin use is associated with early recovery of kidney injury after vascular surgery and improved long-term outcome. Nephrol Dial Transplant. 2008;23:3867–73.
50. Dardik A, Lin JW, Gordon TA, Williams GM, Perler BA. Results of elective abdominal aortic aneurysm repair in the 1990s: a population-based analysis of 2335 cases. J Vasc Surg. 1999;30:985–95.
51. Axelrod DA, Upchurch Jr GR, DeMonner S, et al. Perioperative cardiovascular risk stratification of patients with diabetes who undergo elective major vascular surgery. J Vasc Surg. 2002;35:894–901.
52. Lederle FA, Freischlag JA, Kyriakides TC, et al. Outcomes following endovascular vs open repair of abdominal aortic aneurysm: a randomized trial. JAMA. 2009;302:1535–42.
53. Nathan DP, Brinster CJ, Jackson BM, et al. Predictors of decreased short- and long-term survival following open abdominal aortic aneurysm repair. J Vasc Surg. 2011;54:1237–43.

54. Bihorac A, Yavas S, Subbiah S, et al. Long-term risk of mortality and acute kidney injury during hospitalization after major surgery. Ann Surg. 2009;249:851–8.
55. Poldermans D, Bax JJ, Kertai MD, et al. Statins are associated with a reduced incidence of perioperative mortality in patients undergoing major noncardiac vascular surgery. Circulation. 2003;107:1848–51.
56. Yeung KK, Jongkind V, Coveliers HME, Tangelder GJ, Wisselink W. Routine continuous cold perfusion of the kidneys during elective juxtarenal aortic aneurysm repair. Eur J Vasc Endovasc Surg. 2008;35: 446–51.
57. Nathan DP, Brinster CJ, Woo EY, Carpenter JP, Fairman RM, Jackson BM. Predictors of early and late mortality following open extent IV thoracoabdominal aortic aneurysm repair in a large contemporary single-center experience. J Vasc Surg. 2011;53:299–306.
58. Mehta M, Cayne N, Veith FJ, et al. Relationship of proximal fixation to renal dysfunction in patients undergoing endovascular aneurysm repair. J Cardiovasc Surg (Torino). 2004;45:367–74.
59. Lau LL, Hakaim AG, Oldenburg WA, et al. Effect of suprarenal versus infrarenal aortic endograft fixation on renal function and renal artery patency: a comparative study with intermediate follow-up. J Vasc Surg. 2003;37:1162–8.
60. Tambyraja AL, Fishwick NG, Bown MJ, Nasim A, McCarthy MJ, Sayers RD. Fenestrated aortic endografts for juxtarenal aortic aneurysm: medium term outcomes. Eur J Vasc Endovasc Surg. 2011;42:54–8.
61. Hiramoto JS, Chang CK, Reilly LM, Schneider DB, Rapp JH, Chuter TA. Outcome of renal stenting for renal artery coverage during endovascular aortic aneurysm repair. J Vasc Surg. 2009;49:1100–6.
62. Haddad F, Greenberg RK, Walker E, et al. Fenestrated endovascular grafting: the renal side of the story. J Vasc Surg. 2005;41:181–90.
63. Waybill MM, Waybill PN. Contrast media-induced nephrotoxicity: identification of patients at risk and algorithms for prevention. J Vasc Interv Radiol. 2001;12:3–9.
64. Parfrey PS, Griffiths SM, Barrett BJ, et al. Contrast material-induced renal failure in patients with diabetes mellitus, renal insufficiency, or both. A prospective controlled study. N Engl J Med. 1989;320:143–9.
65. Hawkins IF, Cho KJ, Caridi JG. Carbon dioxide in angiography to reduce the risk of contrast-induced nephropathy. Radiol Clin North Am. 2009;47:813–25, v–vi.
66. Chao A, Major K, Kumar SR, et al. Carbon dioxide digital subtraction angiography-assisted endovascular aortic aneurysm repair in the azotemic patient. J Vasc Surg. 2007;45:451–8.
67. Knipp BS, Escobar GA, English S, Upchurch Jr GR, Criado E. Endovascular repair of ruptured aortic aneurysms using carbon dioxide contrast angiography. Ann Vasc Surg. 2010;24:845–50.
68. Kelly AM, Dwamena B, Cronin P, Bernstein SJ, Carlos RC. Meta-analysis: effectiveness of drugs for preventing contrast-induced nephropathy. Ann Intern Med. 2008;148:284–94.
69. From AM, Bartholmai BJ, Williams AW, Cha SS, Pflueger A, McDonald FS. Sodium bicarbonate is associated with an increased incidence of contrast nephropathy: a retrospective cohort study of 7977 patients at mayo clinic. Clin J Am Soc Nephrol. 2008;3:10–8.
70. Baker CSR, Wragg A, Kumar S, De Palma R, Baker LRI, Knight CJ. A rapid protocol for the prevention of contrast-induced renal dysfunction: the RAPPID study. J Am Coll Cardiol. 2003;41:2114–8.
71. Nagre SB, Taylor SM, Passman MA, et al. Evaluating outcomes of endoleak discrepancies between computed tomography scan and ultrasound imaging after endovascular abdominal aneurysm repair. Ann Vasc Surg. 2011;25:94–100.
72. Schmieder GC, Stout CL, Stokes GK, Parent FN, Panneton JM. Endoleak after endovascular aneurysm repair: duplex ultrasound imaging is better than computed tomography at determining the need for intervention. J Vasc Surg. 2009;50:1012–7. Discussion 7–8.
73. Brem H, Tomic-Canic M. Cellular and molecular basis of wound healing in diabetes. J Clin Invest. 2007;117:1219–22.
74. Sorensen LT, Hemmingsen U, Kallehave F, et al. Risk factors for tissue and wound complications in gastrointestinal surgery. Ann Surg. 2005;241:654–8.
75. Richet HM, Chidiac C, Prat A, et al. Analysis of risk factors for surgical wound infections following vascular surgery. Am J Med. 1991;91:S170–2.
76. Ata A, Lee J, Bestle SL, Desemone J, Stain SC. Postoperative hyperglycemia and surgical site infection in general surgery patients. Arch Surg. 2010;145:858–64.
77. Fleisher LA, Beckman JA, Brown KA, et al. ACC/AHA 2007 guidelines on perioperative cardiovascular evaluation and care for noncardiac surgery: a report of the American College of Cardiology/American Heart Association Task Force on Practice Guidelines (Writing Committee to Revise the 2002 Guidelines on Perioperative Cardiovascular Evaluation for Noncardiac Surgery) developed in collaboration with the American Society of Echocardiography, American Society of Nuclear Cardiology, Heart Rhythm Society, Society of Cardiovascular Anesthesiologists, Society for Cardiovascular Angiography and Interventions, Society for Vascular Medicine and Biology, and Society for Vascular Surgery. J Am Coll Cardiol. 2007;50:e159–242.
78. Umpierrez GE, Smiley D, Jacobs S, et al. Randomized study of basal-bolus insulin therapy in the inpatient management of patients with type 2 diabetes undergoing general surgery (RABBIT 2 surgery). Diabetes Care. 2011;34:256–61.
79. Brewster DC, Cronenwett JL, Hallett Jr JW, Johnston KW, Krupski WC, Matsumara JS. Guidlines for the treatment of abdominal aortic aneurysms. Report of a subcommittee of the Joint Council of the American Association for Vascular Surgery and Society for Vascular Surgery. J Vasc Surg. 2003;37:1106–17.

Evolving Technology in the Treatment of Peripheral Vascular Disease

16

Francesco A. Aiello and Nicholas J. Morrissey

Keywords

Drug eluting stents • Drug eluting balloons • Paclitaxel (taxol) • Sirolimus (rapamune) • Everolimus • Zotarolimus • Biological treatment • Peripheral arterial disease • Lower extremity angioplasty

Introduction

Endovascular technology continues to evolve at a fascinating rate, facilitating the advent of new devices and challenging existing principles. The idea of using drug eluting stents (DES) and balloons (DEB) has been around for decades but the actual accumulation of quality data is relatively recent. The theory behind this technology was the prevention or limitation of restenosis and occlusion due to neointimal hyperplasia. The enthusiasm for drug technology comes from its success in the coronary literature but it became clear early on that this success could not easily translate to the peripheral circulation. Ultimately, newer technologies need to result in improved patency and of course superior clinical outcomes. These technologies have continued to develop over the last 10–20 years with newer pharmacology-based devices demonstrating the potential to change the paradigm of lower extremity revascularization.

Drug Eluting Stents for Lower Extremity Arterial Disease

DES were first studied in the human coronary system, which demonstrated a sustained suppression of neointimal hyperplasia at both 6 and 12 months, revolutionizing the treatment of coronary artery disease in actual clinical practice [1, 2]. The benefits were further substantiated in subsequent studies using multiple different compounds, which helped push the technology into the peripheral circulation [3]. The first study to explore the use of DES in the superficial femoral artery was the Sirolimus Coasted Cordis Self-expandable Stent (SIROCCO) trial [4]. The premise was based on previous studies looking at

F.A. Aiello, M.D. (✉)
Division of Vascular and Endovascular Surgery,
University of Massachusetts Medical School,
55 Lake Avenue North, Worcester, MA 01655
e-mail: francesco.aiello@umassmemorial.org

N.J. Morrissey
Division of Vascular Surgery and Endovascular Interventions, Columbia University College of Physicians and Surgeons, New York Presbyterian Hospital, New York, NY, USA

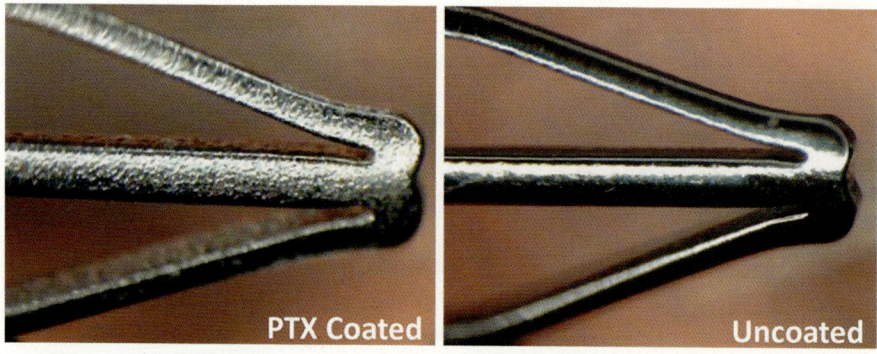

Fig. 16.1 The Zilver PTX stent (permission for use granted by Cook Medical Incorporated, Bloomington, IN)

the effects of sirolimus (Rapamune) on smooth muscle cell (SMC) proliferation and migration. The immunosuppressive effects showed benefit in renal transplant patients with a comparable safety profile but it was the effect on SMC that sparked an interest among vascular interventionists [5]. In vitro and in vivo models studying the effects beyond immunosuppression proved that rapamycin, primarily through inhibiting cell cycle-dependent kinases and phosphorylation, could significantly inhibit SMC migration and cause cell cycle arrest in late G1 phase [6]. DNA synthesis and cell growth inhibition could be seen in human and rat vascular SMCs at concentrations as low as 1 ng/ml [7]. Rapamycin could, as a result of these properties, cause a decrease in inflammation, cell proliferation, and migration in very low concentrations possibly altering the safety profile [5]. The SIROCCO trial was the first to test these hypotheses in the peripheral circulation.

Studies to investigate sirolimus eluting stents in the peripheral circulation were begun in the Europe. The SIROCCO trial investigated a sirolimus eluting self-expanding Smart stent (Cordis Endovascular (Bridgewater, NJ) in superficial femoral artery (SFA) disease to determine if these devices would cause lower rates of restenosis and stent failure. The initial study, SIROCCO I, looking at a small cohort of patients showed no significant difference in mean in-stent diameter stenosis, 22.6% vs. 30.9%, but proved the feasibility and safety of sirolimus in the peripheral circulation [4]. The SIROCCO group, combining SIROCCO I and SIROCCO II, randomized 93 patients to bare metal stents or sirolimus eluting stents. While there was a trend towards improved patency in the drug eluting stents, no significant improvement was seen in ankle–brachial index (ABI), in-stent restenosis, target vessel revascularization (TVR) or target lesion revascularization (TLR) for up to 2 years [8]. In addition, there was a significant rate of stent fracture, 18% at 6 months, which may contribute to restenosis and treatment failure. Drug delivery, including dose delivery and duration of release, play a significant role in optimizing effect of treatment. The DES group did have more severe lesion calcification, 57% vs. 35%, $p=0.03$. This may have affected drug delivery and overall performance [9, 10]. Also, the DES used in this study required a copolymer, which has been associated with hypersensitivity and inflammatory reactions [10, 11]. This study highlights the fact that the peripheral circulation may behave quite differently than the coronary vessels. The SFA and popliteal arteries are subject to numerous forces due to ambulation, muscle contractions, and positional changes that these forces may alter the efficacy of stents.

The Zilver PTX study represents the largest randomized controlled study of any SFA intervention to date [12]. The Zilver PTX stent consists of the nitinol Zilver stent with a non-polymer-based paclitaxel coating (Fig. 16.1). There were 479 patients enrolled and event-free survival (EFS) as well as patency, stent fractures and clinical outcomes were analyzed. The EFS was significantly greater in the DES group compared to the PTA group, 12 months 90.4% vs. 82.6%, $p=0.004$. The primary patency was also significantly improved in the initial analysis of all comers in the DES group, 83.1% vs. 32.8%, as well as the optimal percutaneous transluminal angioplasty (PTA) group, 83.1% vs. 65.3%. The subgroup analysis comprising acute PTA failures who underwent subsequent randomization to bare metal stent or DES also revealed improved primary patency, 83.1% vs. 73.4%. Zilver PTX trial may have revealed better EFS and primary patency but the secondary clinical outcomes, although improved up to 12 months post procedure, were not significantly different between treatment modalities. These similar clinical results between the two groups were only achieved with an almost twofold higher reintervention rate in the PTA group, 17.5% vs. 9.5%; $p=0.01$). The Provisional group, consisting of those PTA patients who underwent acute failure, also had a greater than 60% reduction in restenosis rate. A recent 12-month follow-up to this study looking at 787 patients and 900 lesions with 1,722 Zilver PTX stents deployed continued to yield very high EFS, 89%, as well as primary patency, 86.2%, and freedom from TLR, 90.5%. (The limitations of using TLR as an endpoint in this setting are discussed in Chap. 9) [13]. These results differ from the previously reported studies looking at DES. The important difference in preparation of the Zilver stents is the polymer-free paclitaxel coating. As mentioned previously, these polymers have been associated with thrombotic reactions in other studies and both the SIROCCO and the superficial femoral artery treatment with drug-eluting stents (STRIDES) trials employed this mechanism of stent preparation, possibly attributing to the clinical results observed. A Food and Drug Administration (FDA) advisory panel has recently recommended the Zilver PTX stent for approval in peripheral circulation intervention. This should represent the first drug-coated stent approved for lower extremity use in the USA.

The development of new drug regimens, preparations, and delivery is a continuously evolving process. Lammer et al. recently published the first clinical trial looking at everolimus-eluting stent implantation for peripheral arterial occlusive disease, SFA Treatment with Drug-Eluting Stents Study (STRIDES) Trial [14]. These DES provided a greater concentration of drug delivery, improved sustained release and an increased flexibility. Primary patency was 94% at 6 months but fell to 68% at 12 months despite a stent fracture rate less than 2%. The overall success of DES seems to be far greater during the first 6 months but as seen in this study as well as others, there tends to be a significant drop in patency after this time. Pharmacokinetics and the systemic effects of these drugs are not completely understood in the peripheral circulation. Everolimus was shown to have a dose-dependent peak systemic effect which was constant at 24 h then underwent linear dose release over time [15]. This has led to the research and development of diffusion models which could help determine the release pattern and, therefore, alterations in coating thickness and diffusion coefficients providing a more sustained drug effect [16]. Also, the concomitant use of medical therapy is being studied and may play a more critical in clinical improvement [17]. Economic consideration must be paid since DES are significantly more expensive than their bare metal stent (BMS) counterpart. Although this comparison can at best be approximated given differing costs, reimbursement, patient selection and surveillance it has been estimated that there is a 40% increase in cost per 100 patients, treatment and 12 month surveillance, and as much as 93% increase when compared to open bypass for that same population [18]. This will play a significant role in the decision making process as we try to rein in medical expenditures and better disperse healthcare.

These advancements are also leading to more distal lesion treatment with DES. As already discussed, DES was originally proven to be beneficial in the coronary circulation and the hypothesis was that this would be replicated in the similar sized tibial vessels [19]. There have been several single-center cohort, pilot and nonrandomized single arm registries that have shown clinically significant improvements at up to 3 years [20, 21]. Bosiers et al. recently published the Drug Eluting Stents in the Critically Ischemic Lower Leg (DESTINY) trial, a prospective, randomized clinical trial comparing DES to BMS for treatment of tibial lesions in patients with critical limb ischemia (CLI) [19]. The 12 month primary patency was significantly improved in the DES group, 85% vs. 54%; $p=0.0001$, as was the freedom from TLR, 92% vs. 65%; $p=0.005$. The improvement in primary patency, however, was dependent on stent location. Proximal lesions were found to have a statistically significant improvement, 85 vs. 58%; $p=0.0002$, while there was a trend towards improvement in the distal lesion, this did not reach statistical significance, 87% vs. 43%; $p=0.08$, most likely due to the small sample size. It is also important to note that there was a <50% follow up in this study group, reflective of the severity of underlying pathology in this patient population. There are several studies currently underway looking at DES for popliteal and infrapopliteal lesions of varying severity and lesion length, which will certainly help shed light on their future role in distal peripheral lesions [20]. While primary stenting in infrapopliteal arteries has never been viewed as first line therapy, the results with DES could dramatically change the standard approach for the treatment of infrapopliteal arteries. Since tibial arteries are generally treated in cases of limb threatening ischemia, the improved patency seen with DES recently can have a major impact on limb salvage. Combining this with the knowledge that limb salvage patients are generally sicker than claudicants, the physiologic gain from drastically improving patency and limb salvage with minimally invasive technology will be dramatic.

Drug Eluting Balloons

Several agents have been conceived as options for DEB with some proven unsuccessful in animal models, methotrexate and azathioprine, others requiring prolonged contact or a better carrier, sacrolimus, and new agents, zotarolimus, still undergoing clinical evaluation [22–24]. The most studied, successful and published anti-proliferative agent used to treat vascular disease is paclitaxel (Taxol). Paclitaxel is extrapolated from the Pacific yew (*Taxus brevifolia*) and although first discovered in the 1960s, it was not isolated as the active substrate until 1971; a result of the National Cancer Institute program to discover and develop anticancer medications [25]. It remained relatively underutilized until 1979 when its exact mechanism of action and clinical application was further recognized and its medical potential recognized [26]. Paclitaxel is a lipophilic taxane which allows for rapid intracellular uptake and dose-dependent irreversible effect on microtubules, with antiproliferative properties seen at nanomolar concentrations [27]. Unlike its *Vinca* alkaloid counterparts, which prevent the polymerization of tubulin and microtubule stabilization, paclitaxel stabilizes microtubules and essentially renders them dysfunctional when bound. This alters spindle fibers and cell division but a host of cellular functions, including signal transduction and gene activation [28]. Paclitaxel is also able to inhibit angioplasty-induced smooth muscle cell migration by binding to the hydrophobic sites of the artery while leaving endothelial cell growth unaffected [29]. These multimodal effects on dividing cells allow Taxol to be very antiproliferative drug with multiple capabilities in preventing neointimal hyperplasia in treated vessels.

The biochemical and cellular interactions of paclitaxel are extensive as are its antineoplastic properties, but the effect on arterial smooth muscle and neointimal proliferation are most important to vascular interventionalists. Prevention and treatment of neointimal proliferation and restenosis have largely been unsuccessful and contribute to both short- and long-term endovascular failure. This may be attributed to the incomplete understanding of neointimal hyperplasia as well as the suboptimal effects of other antiproliferative, antimetabolic, and antimitotic agents used in experimental animal models, which do not always translate to clinical results in humans [22]. In vitro studies by Axel et al. utilizing human arterial smooth muscle cells and in vivo studies in rabbit models found paclitaxel to have a very potent and dose-dependent inhibitory effect on both proliferation and migration, yielding significantly reduced wall thickness and degree of stenosis. The extended antiproliferative effects were observed long after the administration of paclitaxel, and its effect on smooth muscle cells was several folds greater than that on some tumor cell lines [28].

Solubility and Application

The initial studies looking at paclitaxel dissolved the drug in normal saline and other aqueous media and clinical application required intricate delivery systems, which could also induce vascular injury [28, 30]. Scheller et al. made a significant discovery when paclitaxel was dissolved in hydrophilic contrast medium, iopromide (Ultravist™), increasing the concentration 20-fold [31, 32]. Paccocath™ denotes standard angioplasty balloons coated with contrast medium and paclitaxel, 3 µg/mm². Contrast media not only acts as a solvent but its adherence to the vessel wall could also serve as a matrix. This combined effect contributes to the sustained efficacy seen with shorter incubation times and equivalent arterial tissue paclitaxel concentrations despite treatments ranges of 10–120 s [32, 33]. The drug coating, drug loading, can be performed in three different manners: micropipetting, spray coating, and dip coating [29]. The most commonly employed technique is micropipetting where the folded balloon is turned while micropipette application of the drug with extra attention to the folds of the balloon. The spray technique is the application of the drug on an unfolded balloon. This allows for more even distribution but there is an unknown drug loss with the refolding. The last and probably least controlled application is the dip coating technique. This entails the immersion of the balloon into solution but it is very difficult to control the application and distribution, this was the preparation of the first clinical trials [29, 30].

The lipophilic nature of taxanes promotes a rapid uptake and crossing of the cell membrane but it is also hydrophilic and requires a spacer to permit high surface area of contact and high bioavailability on the target side [9]. Therefore, drug coating is as important as the balloon technology and medium used to ensure application and even distribution to the vessel wall. The concentration of paclitaxel most is usually 1–3 µg/mm² with dispersing or dipping being the most common coating application. As previously mentioned, the contrast agent iopromide (Ultravist™) was the initial spacer. Recently, the organic substrate urea was found to be as effective in animal models both in vessel wall uptake, 20–30%, and effectiveness [34]. This may prove to overcome some of the limitations seen with iopromide-coated balloons but further clinical trials are needed.

Initial Clinical Studies in Animals and Humans

The effects on vascular smooth muscle cells have been documented since the late 1980s with in vitro confirmation on human smooth muscle and animal models shortly thereafter [28, 35]. The clinical application in trials was bolstered by the modification of drug delivery. Scheller et al, utilizing porcine model of coronary overstretch, found a significant reduction in neointimal proliferation, 63% reduction of neointimal area, with the effects lasting for days despite a short insufflation time [30]. About 80% of the drug was released during the inflation with only 6% lost during the delivery. These findings were followed by the first human trial confirming significant improvements in late lumen loss (LLL) and restenosis at 6 months as well as improved clinical results at 24 months [36]. The application in coronary studies were impressive but peripheral arteries are very different from the coronary circulation, both anatomically and physiologically, and a direct correlation cannot be assumed [11].

Albrecht et al. performed the first study of paclitaxel-coated balloons in swine peripheral vessels, observing a significant dose-dependent reduction in stenosis and late lumen loss [37]. This study observed a statistically significant reduction in stenosis and late lumen loss of both the balloon-coated treatment group as well as an admixture of contrast and paclitaxel. The reduction was dose dependent and although results were derived from angiographic studies, no histological analysis was performed. Milewski et al. was able to detect significant reduction in neointimal proliferation compared to control balloon angioplasty with histologic analysis confirming safety and biocompatibility comparable to controls on porcine ilio-femoral vasculature [38]. Recent animal studies exploring other antiproliferative agents have shown that zotarolimus (mTOR inhibitor)-coated balloons are also safe and effective with therapeutic levels maintained within the arterial wall over time with reduced neointimal proliferation and area stenosis [24]. This encourages the development and study of other potentially beneficial agents yet to be utilized.

Clinical Peripheral Vascular Studies

The first randomized human study of DEB was the Local Taxane with Short Exposure for Reduction of Restenosis in Distal Arteries (THUNDER) trial [39]. 154 patients were randomly assigned to undergo treatment with uncoated balloons, paclitaxel-coated balloons, Paccocath™ balloons, or paclitaxel added to contrast medium. The primary endpoint, late lumen loss at 6 months, was significantly reduced for the paclitaxel-coated balloon treatment group compared to both the control and paclitaxel in medium group (0.4 ± 1.2 mm vs. 1.7 ± 1.8 vs. 2.2 ± 1.6, $p<0.001$). There was no difference between the control group and the group receiving paclitaxel in the contrast medium. These results were consistent even when comparing nonstented patient groups. TVR was also significantly lower at both 12 and 24 months in the paclitaxel-coated balloon group compared with the control group or the group treated with paclitaxel in the contrast medium. These results were in contrast to animal studies of both coronary and peripheral treatments when looking at the paclitaxel in contrast medium. The study investigators attributed this finding to the differences in circulation, vessel diameter, and capillary supply to adjacent muscle [39].

The Femoral Paclitaxel (FemPac) trial randomly assigned 87 patients with femoropopliteal disease to undergo treatment with uncoated or paclitaxel-coated balloons [40]. The 6-month follow-up study revealed significantly less late lumen loss and TLR, which was maintained at 18 months. Both the THUNDER and the FemPac studies observed significant improvement in LLL and TLR without any increase adverse events related to balloon coating.

Newer studies such as the LEVANT I trial (presented by Dierk Scheinert at Transcatheter Cardiovascular Therapeutics (TCT) annual meeting 2010) using the Moxy™ balloon also found a significant reduction in LLL at 6 months but failed to prove a difference it TLR during that same time period. This finding may be explained by the lower coating dose (2 $\mu g/mm^2$) of the Moxy™ balloon. Interestingly, there was a lower rate of clinical events, and treatment with the drug-coated balloon may lead to shorter duration of antiplatelet therapy. Further clinical endpoints and will be pursued by researchers in LEVANT II. Balloon technology continues to evolve and newer studies are currently either underway or in the process of recruiting patients. The Advance™ 18PTX™ balloon catheter trial for SFA and popliteal vessels has completed the enrollment and results are pending. The PACIFIER study, also looking at SFA disease, is recruiting patients. The DEFINITIVE™ AR trial will attempt a novel approach and utilize plaque excision, SilverHawk or TurboHawk (EV3, Inc., Plymouth, MN), followed by treatment with a Cotavance™ Paccocath balloon (Medrad, Inc., Pittsburgh, PA) for treatment of lower extremity lesions with an additional registry for patients with severe calcification [10]. The enrollment of patients with severe SFA calcification will help create a more applicable clinical scenario encountered by most clinicians.

There is a paucity of data regarding below the knee interventions with DEB's. The first registry (Leipzig, Germany) using the IN.PACT™ Amphirion balloon revealed a reduction in 3 month restenosis (69% vs. 31%) but randomized clinical trials are currently underway [10, 41]. The Paclitaxel Coated Balloons for Prevention of

Restenosis in Small Arteries Below the Knee Compared to Angioplasty Using Uncoated Balloons (PICCOLO) is a randomized, double-blind trial (in respect of the primary end point) of treatment of stenotic lesions. INPACT-DEEP trial will examine approximately 357 patients with BTK critical limb ischemia comparing PTA balloon to IN.PACT™ Amphirion drug-coated balloon with a 5-year follow-up period. These trials will help shed some light on potentially game changing tibial treatment options.

Limitations, Advantages, and Potential Pitfalls

Thunder and FEMPAC showed promising results and have helped spark an increased interest in DEB's. It should be noted that despite their significantly improved results, patients with severe calcification were not enrolled. Severely calcified SFA disease is seen in approximately 15% of interventions and the barrier created by such lesions may affect the homogeny and dosage of drug distribution [9, 10]. Both studies also treated a small number of patients with in-stent restenosis, thereby not permitting an assessment of this patient population [42]. These are issues that will most likely be addressed by newer studies as outlined previously. Tibial lesions are also more prone to have severe calcification, wall irregularities, and longer segment occlusion. The longer distance for target lesion treatment, insufficient protection of the DEB by catheters and sheaths, and the inability to always predilate the lesions can all contribute to significant drug loss in transit. Newer devices, including longer working lengths and smaller profiles as well as a multimodality approach, i.e. atherectomy, allow for more successful interventions and the addition of DEB's to our armamentarium in the future [43].

DEBs offer several potential advantages over DES in treatment of peripheral lesions. DEB possess a larger surface area and can provide a homogenous distribution while DES generally only come in contact with 15% of the vessel [11, 44]. DEBs can carry a larger amount of antiproliferative compounds delivered at the very early stages of intimal injury, may be used in areas not otherwise favorable to stents and avoids the use of a polymer, which may be associated with a hypersensitivity and inflammatory reaction [10, 11]. The use of DEBs does not limit the option of utilizing other interventions, stents, or atherectomy, and there is also a potential to reduce antiplatelet therapy [41].

Paclitaxel has shown promise in clinical trials but possible detrimental effects have yet to be fully assessed. The majority of the drug is lost to systemic circulation with less than 20–30% found within the arterial wall. The uptake has not been fully studied in heavily calcified vessels and could result in greater systemic loss than expected. The concentration used for treatment is usually less than 1–2% of the dose used for cancer treatments with typical side effects rarely seen [34, 37]. However, when excessive doses were administered intentionally, there was a higher rate of thrombotic stent occlusion [34]. This may be explained by the reduced expression of thrombomodulin and augmented release of tissue factor when tumor necrosis factor-alpha is in the presence of paclitaxel, leading to a prothrombotic state [45]. The true clinical significance remains to be known but it does reveal some potential side effects to DEBs.

Biological Treatments

Treatment of stents or potentially grafts with biological substances to encourage healing on the stent surface has been studied with the OrbusNeich R Stent™. This stent is coated with monoclonal antibodies specific for vascular endothelial cells. The cells attach to the antibody-coated surface and allow early healing of the surface. Results in the coronary circulation demonstrate a target lesion revascularization rate of 0.05% and a subacute thrombosis rate of 0.37%. Thus the OrbusNeich R stent gives excellent prevention of coronary restenosis while having a significantly lower rate of subacute thrombosis, a complication which is challenging the utility and safety of drug eluting stents in the coronary circulation [46].

Conclusion

The management of peripheral vascular disease is evolving rapidly and newer technologies must include the full utilization of mechanical, biological, and chemical advancement to help ensure optimal peripheral interventions in the vascular patient. Understanding the physiology of drug–vessel interactions has permitted the evolution of pharmacologic technology to involve shorter exposure times with perhaps equivalent results. The approval of these newer technologies is on the horizon and each new study brings us one step closer to successful interventions in the least invasive manner possible, ultimately, creating a methodology of minimal mechanical impact and maximal pharmacologic effect.

References

1. Sousa JE, Costa MA, Abizaid A, et al. Lack of neointimal proliferation after implantation of sirolimus-coated stents in human coronary arteries. A quantitative coronary angiography and three-dimensional intravascular ultrasound study. Circulation. 2001;103:192–5.
2. Sousa JE, Costa MA, Abizaid AC, et al. Sustained suppression of neointimal proliferation by sirolimus-eluting stents: one-year angiographic and intravascular ultrasound follow-up. Circulation. 2001;104:2007–11.
3. Serruys PW, Kutryk MJB, Ong ATL. Coronary-artery stents. N Engl J Med. 2006;354:483–95.
4. Duda SH, Pusich B, Richter G, et al. Sirolimus-eluting stents for the treatment of obstructive superficial femoral artery disease: six-month results. Circulation. 2002;106:1505–9.
5. Groth CG, Backman L, Morales JM, et al. Sirolimus (rapamycin)-based therapy in human renal transplantation: similar efficacy and different toxicity compared with cyclosporine. Sirolimus European renal transplant study group. Transplantation. 1999;67:1036–42.
6. Poon M, Marx SO, Gallo R, et al. Rapamycin inhibits vascular smooth muscle cell migration. J Clin Invest. 1996;98:2277–83.
7. Marx SO, Jayaraman T, Go LO, Marks AR. Rapamycin-FKBP inhibits cell cycle regulators of proliferation in vascular smooth muscle cells. Circ Res. 1995;76:412–7.
8. Duda SH, Bosiers M, Lammer J, et al. Drug-eluting and bare nitinol stents for the treatment of atherosclerotic lesions in the superficial femoral artery: long-term results from the SIROCCO trial. J Endovasc Ther. 2006;13:701–10.
9. Zeller T, Schmitmeier S, Tepe G, Rastan A. Drug-coated balloons in the lower limb. J Cardiovasc Surg. 2011;52:235–43.
10. Tepe G, Schmitmeier S, Zeller T. Drug-coated balloons in the peripheral arterial disease. EuroIntervention. 2011;7:K70–6.
11. Schnorr B, Speck U, Scheller B. Review of clinical data with Paccocath™-coated balloon catheters. Minerva Cardioangiol. 2011;59:431–45.
12. Dake MD, Ansel GM, Jaff MR, et al. Paclitaxel-eluting stents show superiority to balloon angioplasty and bare metal stents in femoropopliteal disease: twelve-month Zilver PTX randomized study results. Circ Cardiovasc Interv. 2011;4:495–504.
13. Dake MD, Scheinert D, Tepe G, et al. Nitinol stents with polymer-free paclitaxel coating for lesions in the superficial femoral and popliteal arteries above the knee: twelve-month safety and effectiveness results from the Zilver PTX single-arm clinical study. J Endovasc Ther. 2011;18:613–23.
14. Lammer J, Bosiers M, Zeller T, et al. First clinical trial of nitinol self-expanding everolimus-eluting stent implantation for peripheral arterial occlusive disease. J Vasc Surg. 2011;54:394–401.
15. Lammer J, Scheinert D, Vermassen F, et al. Pharmacokinetic analysis after implantation of everolimus-eluting stent self-expanding stents in the peripheral vasculature. J Vasc Surg. 2012;55:400–5.
16. Zhao HQ, Jayasinghe D, Hossainy S, Schwartz LB. A theoretical model to characterize the drug release behavior of drug-eluting stents with durable polymer matrix coating. J Biomed Mater Res A. 2012;100:120–4.
17. Tepe G, Schmehl J, Heller S, et al. Drug eluting stents versus PTA with GP IIb/IIIa blockade below the knee in patients with current ulcers-The BELOW study. J Cardiovasc Surg. 2010;51:203–12.
18. Bosiers M, Deloose K, Keirse K, et al. Are drug-eluting stents the future of SFA treatment? J Cardiovasc Surg. 2010;51:115–9.
19. Bosiers M, Scheinert D, Peeters P, et al. Randomized comparison of everolimus-eluting versus bare-metal stents in patients with critical limb ischemia and infrapopliteal arterial occlusive disease. J Vasc Surg. 2012;55:390–9.
20. Chan YC, Cheng SW. Drug-eluting stents and balloons in peripheral arterial disease: evidence so far. Int J Clin Pract. 2011;65:664–8.
21. Bosiers M, Cagiannos C, Deloose K, et al. Drug-eluting stents in the management of peripheral arterial disease. Vasc Health Risk Manag. 2008;4:553–9.

22. Schwartz RS, Holmes DR, Topol EJ. The restenosis paradigm revisited: an alternative proposal for cellular mechanisms. J Am Coll Cardiol. 1992;20:1284–93.
23. Gray WA, Granada JF. Drug-coated balloons for the prevention of vascular restenosis. Circulation. 2010;121:2627–80.
24. Granada JF, Milewski K, Zhao H, et al. Vascular response to zotarolimus-coated balloons in the injured superficial femoral arteries of the familial hypercholesterolemic swine. Circ Cardiovasc Interv. 2011;4:447–55.
25. Wani MC, Taylor HL, Wall ME, Coggan P, McPhail AT. Plant antitumor agents. VI. The isolation and structure of taxol, a novel antileukemic and antitumor agent from Taxus brevifolia. J Am Chem Soc. 1971;93:2325–7.
26. Rowinsky EK, Donehower RC. Paclitaxel (Taxol). N Engl J Med. 1995;332:1004–14.
27. Crossin KL, Carney DH. Microtubule stabilization by taxol inhibits initiation of DNA synthesis by thrombin and by epidermal growth factor. Cell. 1981;27(2 Pt 1):341–50.
28. Axel DI, Kunert W, Goggelmann C, et al. Paclitaxel inhibits arterial smooth muscle cell proliferation and migration in vitro and in vivo using local drug delivery. Circulation. 1997;96:636–45.
29. Cortese B, Bertoletti A. Paclitaxel coated balloons for coronary artery interventions: a comprehensive review of preclinical and clinical data. Int J Cardiol. 2011.
30. Scheller B, Speck U, Abramjuk C, et al. Paclitaxel balloon coating, a novel method for prevention and therapy of restenosis. Circulation. 2004;110:810–4.
31. Scheller B, Speck U, Romeike B, et al. Contrast media as carriers for local drug delivery. Successful inhibition of neointimal proliferation in the porcine coronary model. Eur Heart J. 2003;24:1462–7.
32. Scheller B, Speck U, Schmitt A, et al. Addition of paclitaxel to contrast media prevents restenosis after coronary stent implantation. J Am Coll Cardiol. 2003;42:1415–20.
33. Cremers B, Speck U, Kaufels N, et al. Drug-eluting balloon: very short-term exposure and overlapping. Thromb Haemost. 2009;101:201–6.
34. Kelsch B, Schneller B, Biederman M, et al. Dose response to paclitaxel-coated balloon catheters in the porcine coronary overstretch and stent implantation model. Invest Radiol. 2011;46:255–63.
35. Schiff PB, Fant J, Horwitz SB. Promotion of microtubule assembly in vitro by taxol. Nature. 1979;277:665–7.
36. Scheller B, Hehrlein C, Bocksch W, et al. Treatment of coronary in-stent restenosis with paclitaxel-coated balloon catheters. N Engl J Med. 2006;355:2113–24.
37. Albrecht T, Speck U, Baier C, et al. Reduction of stenosis due to intimal hyperplasia after stent supported angioplasty of peripheral arteries by local administration of paclitaxel in swine. Invest Radiol. 2007;42:579–85.
38. Milewski K, Tellez A, Abodi MS, et al. Paclitaxel-iopromide coated balloon followed by "bail-out" bare metal stent in porcine iliofemoral arteries: first report on biological effects in peripheral circulation. EuroIntervention. 2011;7:362–8.
39. Tepe G, Zeller T, Albrecht T, et al. Local delivery of paclitaxel to inhibit restenosis during angioplasty of the leg. N Engl J Med. 2008;358:689–99.
40. Werk M, Langner S, Reinkensmeier B, et al. Inhibition of restenosis in femoropopliteal arteries. Paclitaxel-coated versus uncoated balloons: femoral paclitaxel randomized pilot trial. Circulation. 2008;118:1358–65.
41. Scheller B. Opportunities and limitations of drug-coated balloons in interventional therapies. Herz. 2011;36:232–40.
42. Manzi M, Cester G, Palena M. Paclitaxel-coated balloon angioplasty for lower extremity revascularization: a new way to fight in-stent restenosis. J Cardiovasc Surg. 2010;51:567–71.
43. Schwarzwalder U, Zeller T. Below-the-knee revascularization. Advanced techniques. J Cardiovasc Surg. 2009;50:627–34.
44. Tepe G, Schmitmeier S, Schnorr B, et al. Advances in drug-coated balloons. J Cardiovasc Surg. 2010;51:125–43.
45. Wood SC, Tang X, Tesfamariam B. Paclitaxel potentiates inflammatory cytokine-induced prothrombotic molecules in endothelial cells. J Cardiovasc Surg. 2010;55:276–85.
46. Nakazawa G, Granada JF, Alviar CL, et al. Anti-CD34 antibodies immobilized on the surface of sirolimus-eluting stents enhance stent endothelialization. JACC Cardiovasc Interv. 2010;3:68–75.

Index

A

Abdominal aortic aneurysms (AAAs)
  aortic aneurysm diameter, 211–212
  aortic rupture, 212
  vs. diabetic AAA, 212–213
    decreased matrix metalloproteinases, 214–215
    increased aortic wall thickness, 213–214
    increased plasminogen activator inhibitor-1, 215–216
  endovascular AAA repair, 218
    carbon dioxide digital subtraction angiography, 220–221
    computed tomography angiography, 220
    femoral or iliac artery access, 220
    fenestrated endovascular stents, 219–220
    intravascular infusion, radiopaque, 220
    vs. open repair, 220
    proximal endoleaks, 219
    renal artery encroachment, 220
    suprarenal fixation stents, 219
  incidence, 211
  open repair
    chronic renal insufficiency, 218
    comorbid conditions, 217–218
    kidney injury after, 218, 219
    mortality, 217
    suprarenal clamping, 218–219
  pathogenesis of, 211
  postoperative considerations
    contrast-induced nephropathy prevention, 221
    glucose management, 222
    increased length of stay, 221
    poor wound healing, 221–222
  preoperative comorbidities in
    concomitant arterial occlusive disease, 217
    diabetic nephropathy, 216–217
    increased coronary artery disease, 216
Abnormal biothesiometer readings, 40
Above-knee amputation, 174
Action to Control Cardiovascular Risk in Diabetes (ACCORD) trial, 35, 184
Aldose reductase inhibitors, 48
α-lipoic acid (ALA), 48
Aminoglycosides, 98

Aminoguanidine, 48
Amputation, 163. *See also* Lower extremity amputation
Angioplasty, 121–122
Anglo-Scandinavian Cardiac Outcomes Trial (ASCOT), 188
Ankle-brachial index (ABI), 4, 104
Antiplatelet therapy, 124
Aortoiliac disease
  asymptomatic disease, 198
  chronic limb ischemia, 197–198
  claudication, 197
  definition, 197
  diabetes
    exercise testing, 199
    proximal disease, 198–199
    vascular injury mechanism, 198
  diagnosis
    biomarkers, 200–201
    imaging, 200
    physiologic and hemodynamic measurements, 199–200
  epidemiology, 199
  operative management
    aortofemoral bypass, 206–207
    aortoiliac endarterectomy, 206
    collaterals, 202–203
    endovascular intervention, 202–205
    extra-anatomic bypass, 207
    postoperative considerations, 208
    surgical bypass, 205–206
  prevalence, 199
  progression of, 199
  treatment
    diet modification, 202
    general cardiovascular risk reduction, 201
    lifestyle modifications, 201–202
Aorto-iliac occlusive disease (AIOD), 217
Arterial duplex scanning, 1091–110
Arterial imaging
  arterial duplex scanning, 1091–110
  arteriography (*see* Arteriography)
  noninvasive (*see* Noninvasive arterial studies (NIAS))

Arterial insufficiency, 72
Arteriography
   computed tomographic angiography
      contrast induced nephropathy, 111–112
      CT scanners, 110
      3D reconstruction, 111
      image acquisition, 110–111
      lower extremity vasculature, 111
      occlusive lesions, 111
      pros and cons of, 115
      reconstruction-based artifacts, 111
   contrast arteriography
      CO_2 injection, 114–115
      contrast agent, 113–114
      digital subtraction arteriography, 113
      metformin, 114
      nephrotoxicity, 114
      pros and cons of, 115
      toxic side effects, 114
   magnetic resonance angiography, 112–113, 115
Arteriovenous shunting, 57
Asymmetrical neuropathies
   autonomic neuropathy, 44
   cardiovascular autonomic neuropathy, 44
   CIDP, 43
   cranial mononeuropathy, 43
   diabetic amyotrophy, 43
   gastrointestinal, 44
   genitourinary, 44–45
   nerve entrapment syndromes, 43
   orthostatic hypotension, 44
   proximal asymmetric mononeuropathy, 43
   sudomotor dysfunction, 45
   truncal radiculopathy, 43
Atherectomy, 123
Atherosclerosis
   acute vascular occlusion, 14, 15
   advanced glycation endproducts, 18
   angiogenesis, 22–23
   arteries layers, 14
   atherosclerotic plaques, 14
   endothelial cells, 16
   endothelial progenitor cells, 23, 24
   endothelin-1, 22
   hexosamine pathway, 18
   hypercoagulability, 22, 23
   hyperglycemia, 16
   hyperlipidemia, 21–22
   injury response, 22
   insulin resistance, 19–21
   lower extremity lesions, 14
   mitochondria, 16–17
   monocytes, 16
   PKC pathway, 18
   platelet aggregation, 22
   polyol pathway, 18–19
   reactive oxygen species, 17–18
   type I DM, 13
   type II DM, 13
   vascular smooth muscle cells, 14, 16

Atherosclerosis Risk in Communities (ARIC) study, 202
Autonomic neuropathy, 44

B
Bare metal stents, 122
Below-knee amputation, 172–174

C
Cardiovascular autonomic neuropathy (CAN), 44
Carotid endarterectomy (CEA), 14
Carotid intima–media thickness (IMT), 190
Cephalosporins, 95
Cerebrovascular disease
   carotid disease and biomarkers, 190–191
   diabetes
      cognitive decline, 182–183
      cognitive impairment and dementia, 183
      dyslipidemia and stroke, 188–189
      hemorrhagic strokes, 182
      hyperglycemia and stroke, 183–184
      hypertension and stroke, 184, 187–188
      ischemic strokes, 182
      lacunar strokes, 182
      management of, 191
      transient ischemic attacks, 182
   pathophysiology of, 181–182
Charcot's foot, 68
Chopart's amputation, 171–173
Chronic hyperglycemia, 40
Chronic inflammatory demyelinating polyradiculopathy (CIDP), 43
Claudication: Exercise Versus Endoluminal Revascularization (CLEVER) trial, 5, 134, 201
Clindamycin, 95, 97, 98
Clopidogrel for High Atherothrombotic Risk and Ischemic Stabilization, Management, and Avoidance (CHARISMA) study, 190
Clopidogrel vs. Aspirin in Patients at Risk of Ischaemic Events (CAPRIE) study, 189
Common femoral artery (CFA), 120
Computed tomographic angiography (CTA)
   contrast induced nephropathy, 111–112
   CT scanners, 110
   3D reconstruction, 111
   image acquisition, 110–111
   lower extremity vasculature, 111
   occlusive lesions, 111
   pros and cons of, 115
   reconstruction-based artifacts, 111
Contrast arteriography
   CO_2 injection, 114–115
   contrast agent, 113–114
   digital subtraction arteriography, 113
   metformin, 114
   nephrotoxicity, 114
   pros and cons of, 115
   toxic side effects, 114

Index

Contrast induced nephropathy (CIN)
   arteriography, 111–112
   contrast arteriography, 114
Coronary artery bypass grafting (CABG), 13
Coronary artery disease (CAD), 13
Covered stents, 122–123
Cranial mononeuropathy, 43
C-reactive protein (CRP), 190
Critical limb ischemia (CLI)
   infrainguinal occlusive disease (*see* Infrainguinal occlusive disease)prevalence of, 1, 119
   revascularization strategy in, 135
Cryoplasty, 123

D

Dacron, 207
Daptomycin, 97
Diabetes Control and Complication Trial (DCCT), 40
Diabetes mellitus
   abdominal aortic aneurysms (*see* Abdominal aortic aneurysms (AAAs))amputation, 163 (*see also* Lower extremity amputation)aortoiliac disease (*see* Aortoiliac disease)atherosclerosis (*see* Atherosclerosis)cerebrovascular disease
      cognitive decline, 182–183
      cognitive impairment and dementia, 183
      dyslipidemia and stroke, 188–189
      hemorrhagic strokes, 182
      hyperglycemia and stroke, 183–184
      hypertension and stroke, 184, 187–188
      ischemic strokes, 182
      lacunar strokes, 182
      management of, 191
      transient ischemic attacks, 182
   clinical findings, 2
   complications, 27
   management goals in
      hospitalized patients, 36
      nonhospitalized patients, 34–35
   micro-and macrovascular complications, 33
   peripheral arterial disease
      co-prevalence, 1
      diabetes control, 28–29
      diagnosis, 29–30
      diagnosis of, 4
      epidemiology of, 2–3
      guidelines and outcome metrics, 6–8
      limb salvage approach, 9–10
      major amputation, 8–9
      morbidity and mortality, 28
      pathophysiology of, 3–4
      pedal sepsis, 8
      prediabetes, 29
      reduced revascularization, 28
      risk factors, 27
      surgical bypass and endovascular therapy, 5–6
      T2DM treatment (*see* Type 2 diabetes mellitus)wound care and debridement, 8
   therapy and outcomes
      intensive care unit, 133–134
      non-ICU patient, 34
   type 1 and type 2 diabetes, 27
   vasculopathy, 1
Diabetic amyotrophy, 43
Diabetic foot
   clinical effects, 53
   infections
      antibiotics, 95–98
      cellulitis, 98, 100
      clinical syndromes and microbiology, 94
      follow-up, 99
      osteomyelitis, 99–100
      pathogenesis, 93–94
      patient evaluation, 94–95
      risk factors for, 94
      therapy duration, 100
      ulcer, 98–100
   microvasculature changes
      capillary perfusion, 56–57
      clinical significance, 60–61
      endothelial dependent vasodilation, 57
      function, 54, 55
      functional changes, 56
      nerve–axon reflex, 58
      oxidative stress, 58–59
      structural changes, 54–56
      structure, 53
      vascular permeability, 58–59
   ulceration (*see* Diabetic foot ulceration)
Diabetic foot ulceration
   arterial disease impact
      anaerobic infections, 71
      cardiovascular disease, 71
      diabetic occlusive lesions, 68
      infection, 70–71
      renal complications, 71–72
      toe-brachial index, 68
   epidemiologic studies, 64
   HRQOL, 64, 65
   limb-threatening ischemia, 64
   lower extremity disease, 63
   management
      bioengineered alternative tissues, 85–87
      infection control, 80–81
      negative pressure wound therapy, 83–84
      off-loading techniques, 84
      revascularization, 85
      surgical debridement techniques, 80
      wound closure, 81–93
   metabolic control, 87
   patient assessment
      history, 72
      imaging techniques, 77–78
      neurologic examination, 75–77
      physical examination, 73
      ulcer evaluation, 73–74
      vascular examination, 74–75
   pedal soft-tissue deficits, 64

Diabetic foot ulceration (*continued*)
   prevention, 87–88
   reconstructive ladder, 87
   walking biomechanics
      bunions, 66
      diabetic foot, 66
      gait, 65
      musculoskeletal deformities, 68–69
      neuropathy, 66–68
      pathophysiologic mechanisms, 66
      sensory input, 65
Diabetic neuropathy (DN)
   classification
      asymmetrical DN (*see* Asymmetrical neuropathies)symmetrical DN (*see* Symmetrical neuropathies)diagnosis, 46–47
   encephalopathies
      hypoglycemia, 45–46
      nerve–axon reflex vasodilation, 45
   epidemiology, 39–40
   pathophysiology
      chronic hyperglycemia, 40
      nonenzymatic glycation, 40–41
      oxidative stress, 41
      PKC, 41
      polyol pathway abnormalities, 40
   treatment
      antiarrhythmics, 48
      anticonvulsants, 47
      NMDA, 47–48
      opioids, 47
      pathogenic mechanisms, 48–49
      topical therapy, 48
      tricyclic antidepressants, 47
Digital pressures, 104
Distal sensory and sensory-motor neuropathy, 42
Drug eluting balloons (DEB)
   advantages, 233
   biological treatment, 233–234
   clinical peripheral vascular studies
      Advance™ 18PTX™ balloon catheter trial, 232
      DEFINITIVE™ AR trial, 232
      FemPac trial, 232
      IN.PACT™ Amphirion drug-coated balloon, 232–233
      LEVANT I trial, 232
      PACIFIER study, 232
      THUNDER trial, 232
   limitations, 233
   paclitaxel, 230
      antiproliferative effects, 230–231
      biochemical and cellular interactions, 230
      clinical charcteristics, 230
      clinical studies, 231–232
      neointimal hyperplasia, 230
      solubility and application, 231
Drug eluting stents (DES), 124
   biological treatment, 233–234
   DESTINY trial, 229–230
   distal lesion treatment, 229
   drug delivery, 228
   economic consideration, 229
   percutaneous transluminal angioplasty, 229
   popliteal and infrapopliteal lesions, 230
   popliteal arteries, 228
   proximal lesion, 230
   SIROCCO trial, 227–228
   SMC proliferation and migration, 227–228
   STRIDES trial, 229
   superficial femoral artery, 227
   Zilver PTX stent, 228–229
Drug Eluting Stents in the Critically Ischemic Lower Leg (DESTINY) trial, 229–230
Drug-eluting technology, 124
Dyslipidemia, 188–189

E

Encephalopathies
   hypoglycemia, 45–46
   nerve–axon reflex vasodilation, 45
   Endovascular therapy. *See also* Peripheral endovascular interventionangioplasty, 121–122
   arterial circulation assessment, 119–120
   atherectomy, 123
   bare metal stents, 122
   covered stents, 122–123
   crossing lesions, 120–121
   cryoplasty, 123
   diagnostic angiography, 120, 121
   drug-eluting technology, 124
   endovascular AAA repair, 218
      carbondioxide digital subtraction angiography, 220–221
      computed tomography angiography, 220
      femoral or iliac artery access, 220
      fenestrated endovascular stents, 219–220
      intravascular infusion, radiopaque, 220
      vs. open repair, 220
      proximal endoleaks, 219
      renal artery encroachment, 220
      suprarenal fixation stents, 219
   follow-up and surveillance, 125
   peri-procedural management, 124–125
End-stage renal disease (ESRD), 71–72
Erectile dysfunction (ED), 44–45

F

Femoral Paclitaxel (FemPac) trial, 231
Fenofibrate Intervention and Event Lowering in Diabetes (FIELD) study, 189
Foot ulcers
   diabetes (*see* Diabetic foot ulceration)infections, 98–100

G

Glucagon-like peptide-1 (GLP-1), 33
Glucose transporters (GLUTs), 58
Glycation inhibitors, 48

Index

H
Heart Outcomes Prevention Evaluation (HOPE) study, 188
Hexokinase, 40
Hip disarticulation, 175
Hydrostatic capillary pressure, 54
Hyperglycemia
  atherosclerosis, 16
  diabetic neuropathy, 40
  stroke, 183–184
Hypertension, 184, 187–188

I
Impaired fasting glycemia (IFG), 40
Infrainguinal occlusive disease
  bypass technique
    anesthesia, 139–140
    circumferential calcification, 141
    clinical outcomes, 143–145
    early graft failure, 142
    functional assessment, 141–142
    intraoperative angiography, 142
    minimal touch technique, 140
    postoperative care, 142–143
    preoperative vein mapping, 140
    proximal anastomosis, 141
    saphenofemoral junction exposure, 140
    tourniquet, 141
    valve lysis, 140–141
    vein graft orientation, 140
    vein graft tunneling, 141
    venous conduit quality, 140
  revascularization
    angiosome concept, 137–138
    conduit considerations, 135–137
    distal origin grafts, SFA, 137, 138
    lower extremity, CFA, 137
    patient selection for, 134–135
    pedal and tarsal arteries, 138–139
    preoperative imaging studies, 137
Insulin, 32
Intermittent claudication (IC), 134
Intravenous immunoglobulins, 49
Intrinsic minus foot, 68
Iopromide, 231
Ischemia-modified albumin, 200–201
Ischemic diabetic foot ulcers, 70
Ischemic strokes, 182

K
Knee disarticulation, 174

L
Lacunar strokes, 182
Large fiber neuropathy, 42–43
Linezolid, 97
Lisfranc amputation, 171, 173

Losartan Intervention for Endpoint Reduction in Hypertension (LIFE) study, 188
Lower extremity amputation
  above-knee amputation, 174
  amputation level determination
    below-knee amputations, 169
    limb length preservation, 169
    mobility capability, 169
    optical tomographic imaging, 170
    physical examination, 169
    segmental pressures, 169–170
    tissue viability, 169
    transcutaneous oxygen measurement, 170
    visual assessment, 169
  below-knee amputation, 172–174
  Chopart's amputation, 171–173
  complications, 176–177
  current trends, 168–169
  hip disarticulation, 175
  historical perspectives, 168
  knee disarticulation, 174
  Lisfranc amputation, 171, 173
  open amputations and guillotine amputations, 175–176
  rehabilitation, 178–179
  Syme's amputation, 172
  toe amputation, 170
  transmetatarsal amputations, 171
Lower extremity arterial disease
  diabetic foot ulceration, 63
  drug eluting stents (*see* Drug eluting stents (DES))open peripheral arterial reconstruction
    early lower extremity bypass graft failure, 150–152
    patent but failing lower extremity bypass graft, 152–153

M
Magnetic resonance angiography (MRA), 112–113, 115
Management of Atherothrombosis with Clopidogrel in High-risk patients (MATCH) study, 189
Matrix metalloproteinases (MMPs), 214–215
Medical nutrition therapy (MNT), 30
Metformin, 31–32
Methicillin-resistant *Staphylococcus aureus* (MRSA), 71
Metronidazole, 97
Motor neuropathy, 68
Moxy™ balloon, 232
Myocardial infarction (MI), 13

N
Nephrogenic systemic fibrosis (NSF), 112–113
Nephrotoxicity
  computed tomographic angiography, 111–112
  contrast arteriography, 114
Nerve–axon reflex, 58
Nerve–axon reflex vasodilation (NARV), 45
Nerve entrapment syndromes, 43
Neuropathic foot ulcers, 70

Neuropathy, 66–68. *See also* Diabetic neuropathy (DN)
Neurotrophic ulcers, 67
Noninvasive arterial studies (NIAS), 103
    Doppler waveform analysis
        biphasic velocity waveform, 105, 108
        low-resistance vascular beds, 105
        triphasic velocity waveform, 105, 108
        velocity frequency shifts, 105
    pressure measurements, 104
    pulse volume recordings
        bilateral PAOD, 107
        normal, 105, 106
        pressure cuffs, 104–105
    stress testing, 105
Normoglycemia in Intensive Care Evaluation-Survival using Glucose Algorithm Regulation (NICE-SUGAR), 34

O

Open peripheral arterial reconstruction
    autogenous graft failure
        intraoperative factors, 150
        long-term patency, 149
        thrombosis, 149
        vein graft failure, 149
    early lower extremity bypass graft failure
        early failure, 150
        early graft thrombosis, 150
        factors affecting, 150
        greater saphenous vein, 151
        heparin-bonded expanded polytetrafluoroethylene, 151
        intraoperative conduit manipulation, 150
        management algorithm, 152
        technical problems, 150–151
        unanticipated vein imperfections, 150
    graft infection and wound complications, 155
    late infrainguinal graft occlusions
        arm-vein grafts, 155
        thrombolytic therapy, 153–154
        veno-venostomy, 154–155
    patent but failing lower extremity bypass graft
        balloon angioplasty, 153
        Duplex criteria for, 152
        open surgical (OS) revision, 152–153
        percutaneous balloon angioplasty, 153
        vein mapping, 153
Optimal medical care (OMC), 201–202
OrbusNeich R Stent™ AR trial, 233
Orthostatic hypotension, 44
Osteomyelitis, 99–100
Oxidative stress, 48

P

PAD Awareness, Risk, and Treatment: New Resources for Survival (PARTNERS) study, 199
Peak systolic velocity (PSV), 109
Percutaneous transluminal angioplasty (PTA), 121–122

Peripheral arterial disease (PAD)
    clinical outcomes determinants
        chronic lower extremity ischemia, 129
        CLI prevalence, 129
        comorbidities and risk factors, 130
        disease location, 127–128
        factors affecting patency, 127, 128
        runoff vessels, 128
    diabetes mellitus
        diabetes control, 28–29
        diagnosis, 29–30
        lifestyle modification, 4–5
        medical management, 4–5
        morbidity and mortality, 28
        prediabetes, 29
        reduced revascularization, 28
        risk factors, 27
        T2DM treatment (*see* T2DM)drug eluting balloons (*see* Drug eluting balloons (DEB))drug eluting stents (*see* Drug eluting stents (DES))endovascular therapy (*see also* Peripheral endovascular intervention)angioplasty, 121–122
        arterial circulation assessment, 119–120
        atherectomy, 123
        bare metal stents, 122
        covered stents, 122–123
        crossing lesions, 120–121
        cryoplasty, 123
        diagnostic angiography, 120, 121
        drug-eluting technology, 124
        follow-up and surveillance, 125
        peri-procedural management, 124–125
    guidelines and clinical outcomes
        AHA recommendations, 125
        assisted and secondary patency, 126–127
        clinical success, 126
        hemodynamic success, 126
        limb salvage, 127
        primary patency, 126
        target lesion revascularization, 127
        TASC guidelines, 125
        technical success, 125–126
    prevalence of, 1, 119
Peripheral endovascular intervention
    arterial access complications, 156–157
        arteriovenous fistula, 158–159
        closure devices, 159–161
        diagnostic and therapeutic arteriography, 155, 156
        hematoma and pseudoaneurysm, 158–159
    lesion treatment complications, 160
    PTA/stent complications
        collateral blood flow loss, 162
        drug-eluting balloons and stents, 163
        duplex surveillance and pharmacologic adjuncts, 162
        stent maldeployment, 161–162
        stent restenosis, 162
Plasma osteoprotegerin (OPG), 201
Polytetrafluoroethylene (PTFE), 207

Index

Postocclusive reactive hyperemia (PRH), 56
Pramlintide, 33
Protein kinase C (PKC) pathway, 18, 59
Proximal asymmetric mononeuropathy, 43
Pulse volume recordings (PVR), 104–106

Q
Quiescent-interval single-shot (QISS) MRA, 200

R
RAndomized Study of Basal Bolus Insulin Therapy in the Inpatient Management of Patients with Type 2 Diabetes (RABBIT-2) trial, 34
Reactive oxygen species (ROS), 41
Receptor of advanced glycation end product (RAGEs), 58
Recombinant human NGF (rhNGF), 49
Regular insulin sliding scale (RISS), 34
Renal complications, foot ulceration, 71–72
Rifampin, 98
Rocker-bottom foot, 68, 69
Rosiglitazone, 33
Ruboxistaurin (RBX), 48–49

S
Segmental pressures, 104
Sensorimotor polyneuropathy, 67
SFA Treatment with Drug-Eluting Stents Study (STRIDES) Trial, 229
Sirolimus Coasted Cordis Self-expandable Stent (SIROCCO) trial, 227
Skinner–Gardner protocol, 105
Small fiber neuropathy, 42
Small vessel disease, 54
Staphylococcus aureus, 70-->
Stroke, 181
    dyslipidemia, 188–189
    hyperglycemia, 183–184
    hypertension, 184, 187–188
    ischemic strokes, 182
    lacunar strokes, 182
    management of, 191
Sudomotor dysfunction, 45
Sulfonylureas, 32

Superficial Femoral Artery Treatment with Drug-Eluting Stents (STRIDES) trial, 124
Supervised exercise (SE), 201–202
Surgical site infections (SSI), 155
Syme's amputation, 172
Symmetrical neuropathies
    distal sensory and sensory-motor neuropathy, 42
    large fiber neuropathy, 42–43
    small fiber neuropathy, 42

T
Target lesion revascularization (TLR), 127
Thiazolidinediones, 32
Tigecycline, 97
Time of flight (TOF) angiography, 112
Toe amputation, 170
Transmetatarsal amputations, 171
Treadmill function test, 200
Trimethoprim/sulfamethoxazole (T/S), 97–98
Truncal radiculopathy, 43
Type 2 diabetes mellitus
    atherosclerosis, 13
    treatment
        ADA recommendation, 30
        a-glucosidase inhibitors, 32
        DMSE, 30
        glucagon-like peptide-1, 33
        insulin, 32
        medical nutrition therapy, 30
        metformin, 31–32
        pramlintide, 33
        rosiglitazone, 33
        sulfonylureas, 32
        thiazolidinediones, 32

U
Ultravist™, 231
United Kingdom Prospective Diabetes Study (UKPDS), 184

V
Vascular endothelial growth factor (VEGF), 49, 59
Vascular permeability factor (VPF), 59

Printed by Printforce, the Netherlands